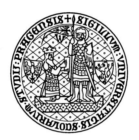

HEALTH AND DISEASE IN THE NEOLITHIC LENGYEL CULTURE

EDITED BY VÁCLAV SMRČKA
AND OLIVÉR GÁBOR

CHARLES UNIVERSITY
KAROLINUM PRESS 2021

With contributions by
František Bůzek, Alžběta Čerevková, Eva Čermáková, David Dick, Marta Dočkalová,
Vojtěch Erban, Martina Fojtová, Csilla Gáti, Zdeněk Hájek, Martin Hill, Ivana Jarošová,
Sylva Drtikolová Kaupová, Kitti Köhler, Vítězslav Kuželka, Martin Mihaljevič,
Zdenka Musilová, Ivo Němec, Lenka Půtová, Štefan Rástočný, Jakub Trubač,
Zdeněk Tvrdý, Ivan Zoc, Jarmila Zocová

The manuscript of the book was peer reviewed by T. Douglas Price (University
of Wisconsin–Madison) and Niels Lynnerup (University of Copenhagen)

KAROLINUM PRESS
Karolinum Press is a publishing department of the Charles University
www.karolinum.cz

Designed by Jan Šerých
Set in the Czech Republic by Karolinum Press
Printed in the Czech Republic by PRINCO International, s. r. o.

Cataloguing-in-Publication Data is available from the National Library
of the Czech Republic

ISBN 978-80-246-4514-8
ISBN 978-80-246-4521-6 (pdf)

CONTENTS

ACKNOWLEDGEMENTS

The expeditions to Pécs between 2017–2018 in order to explore the Zengő-várkony and other burial sites were financed by the university support scheme Progress number Q23 (History of university science and education). The authors appreciate the wide-ranging assistance received from Karel Černý, the Head of the Institute for History of Medicine and Foreign Languages at Charles University—the First Faculty of Medicine.

Chapters 8, 9, 10 and 11 in this book was accomplished with support from the project "Lifestyle as an unintentional identity in the Neolithic" (Project 19-16304S), financed by the Czech Science Foundation.

Chapter 10 was partially supported by the Czech Science Foundation (GAČR grant no. 206-26-1126).

The authors of chapters 6 and 12 are grateful to their external advisors, particularly to Jaroslav Jambor (Masaryk University, Brno).

The authors of chapter 8 are grateful to Jiří Kala from the Institute of Archaeological Heritage Care in Brno for providing information about the latest finds of skeletal remains of the people of the Lengyel Culture in Moravia.

Fig. 1 on the page 178 is used by courtesy of Julia I. Giblin (Quinnipiac University).

Much stimulating discussion and critical input were provided by our reviewers T. Douglas Price (University of Wisconsin-Madison) and Niels Lynnerup (University of Copenhagen).

1. INTRODUCTION

VÁCLAV SMRČKA

1.1 DEFINITION OF THE NEOLITHIC DEMOGRAPHIC TRANSITION

The discovery of a ceramic gradient from the Middle East to Europe was referred to as the "Neolithic Revolution" by Childe (1925). A significant change from the former lifestyle of foragers led to a substantial increase in human numbers. This was termed "transition" by demographers (Lazaridis et al. 2016; Price 2000a, b, c; Price and Feinman 2001; Bocquet-Appel and Bar-Yosef 2008; Ames 2010 ; Kristiansen et al. 2017; Furholt 2021) and was the basis of this phenomenon.

1.2 ADOPTION OF FARMING: INSECT PATTERNS, THE ORIGIN OF COMPLEX SOCIETY

In both insect and human populations, societies can only start to form after the incorporation of plants into their way of life i.e. after the emergence of agricultural practices (Smrčka and Žd'árek 2002; Smrčka et al. 2019; Hayden 2014). The most complex societies cannot develop until their network of social relations becomes sufficiently "dense" as a result of population growth. The development of agriculture and this incorporation of plants caused the growth of the human population and facilitated advances in communication between members of groups. This stage began when man started cultivating grasses for their seeds as nourishment. Similarly, the evolution of insect species that were able to form vast colonies with highly sophisticated, division of labour based on complex communication, was enabled by the development of special "agricultural" practices. This includes and is not limited to the employment of symbiotic bacteria, fungi and protozoa for the processing of cellulose as food (termites), and the cultivation of fungi (leaf-cutting ants) on plant material and faeces. The co-evolution with angiosperm plants and exploitation of flower products (nectar and pollen) facilitated the evolution of a complex societies in bees. An adoption of agricultural practices supposes a non-nomadic way of life. Members of social groups construct special dwellings: country-type common houses near fields in man, complex nests in bees, ants and termites. Dwellings have the biological function of protection, but also as an exchange places for obtaining other sources of food. The model of dwelling organisation can change from culture to culture, tribe to tribe, but it seems to remain fixed within a group. The location of a dwelling within the settlement reflects social relations among the families; those more closely related have closer contact between their dwellings while families of different clans are more separated. This organisation within settlement was such that higher-ranking groups were those that had inhabited the area first (Flannery and Marcus 2012). The distance between the dwellings of each culture seems to be standard (Gron 1997). After this amplification of agriculture, and establishment of a dependence on a vegetal diet, biological changes occurred in man, as well as in ants and termites. There is a significant decline in stature in Upper Palaeolithic populations through the Neolithic, and is best demonstrated in females (Meiklejohn et al. 1984). The shift from meat to vegetal food was demonstrated using analysis of trace elements (Zn, Fe) in human bones from the Neolithic to the early Middle Ages (Smrčka and Jambor 2000). This Neolithic gracilisation is directly linked with the concentration of Zn and other elements essential for growth (Cu, Fe) (Smrčka et al. 1989, 1998). Similarily, this difference in stature between the hunter and the farmer in the human population is seen in the hymenopteric world; the largest ant individuals can be found among the primitive predatory Ponerids, whose colonies are generally small, while ants that are primarily dependent on a vegetal diet (e.g. seed-eaters, leaf-cutters) form huge colonies of relatively small individuals with a strongly morphologically distinct worker casts. In humans, at least in the early stages, hierarchy was also based on aggression (Watts et al. 2016). Since the Neolithic Age, this societal stratification (Bentley et al. 2012) has meant those with the greatest individual power were also those that controlled the wealth (Gronenborn 2016; Heath 2017; Feinman 2016).

The history of the human species exhibits cyclical changes in its social network. Empires rise and fall. Therefore, it seems that history is repeated in the course of the development of states (Carmack 2015). Control over a certain territory by a group of aggressive individuals is the driving force behind the rise of the majority of founding states (Hrnčíř and Květina 2016). Aggression was the means by which order and social hierarchy, and subsequently the distribution of food, were maintained, before being replaced by rules, and finally formal laws (Smrčka and Žďárek 2002). Distribution of food in advanced eusocial insects is such that all sterile members of the society (the worker cast) receive an equal share of the colony wealth (social stomach) through mutual exchange of liquid food (trophalaxis). Only the reproductive females are preferentially fed, often with more nutritious food, in order to maximise the outcome of their reproductive potential. However, that is not the case in the human society; while the privileged social classes are also preferentially supplied, but their effect on overall reproduction within the population is negligible. Whitehouse et al. (2019) confirmed the association between moralizing gods and social complexity. Duration of eusocial insect communities may have seasonal or perennial character. Parallels between human and insect populations in factors surrounding population nutrition, which aided societal expansion, were observed. Such populations could form only after the process of the adoption of farming practices. This insect pattern shows that the Neolithic revolution was not a revolution, but a social phase of human evolution: the origin of complex society.

1.3 ARCHAEOLOGICAL EVIDENCE OF THE NEOLITHIC DIET

The earliest LBK agricultural crops included einkorn and emmer wheat, barley, millet, peas, lentil, and linseed (Kreuz 1990 in Jochim 2000). The wild ancestors of these plants are not native to Central Europe; therefore, their domesticated forms must have been introduced from elsewhere. Along with these, at least twelve different non-native weed species have been identified in the earliest LBK sites. Furthermore, domesticated animals at these sites include sheep, goats, cattle and pigs, with only the latter two have wild ancestors native to Central Europe. This impressive array of non-native foods suggests to many that they were imported as part of a functioning economy of immigrants, rather than as items of exchange (Jochim 2000). Settlements were located on gently sloping hillsides. These were often exposed to the east, and thus houses, mostly oriented NNW–SSE, were built parallel to the slope. Villages were built close to water courses (Gronenborn 1999). The focus on grain production gave rise to the manufacture of pottery (Schier 2015; Salisbury 2016), in which cereal meals and beverages could be prepared and stored. Close contact with animals is evidenced in small ceramic sculptures of animals.

1.4 BIOLOGICAL EVIDENCE OF THE NEOLITHIC DIET

Neolithic diets are remarkably uniform and based on terrestrial food sources. Neolithic burials from caves in Portugal generally show that Mesolithic diets had a strong marine component, and by the middle Neolithic there was a significant shift to mainly terrestrial foods. In the United Kingdom, the scarcity of Mesolithic human remains problematic, but a few studies do show the importance of marine foods in the diets of Late Mesolithic coastal peoples from the site of Oronsay (Richards and Mellars 1998). There is, however, a substantial amount of isotope data on Early and Middle Neolithic humans indicating a completely terrestrial diet (Richards et al. 2003). Samples from the Central European Neolithic period from the Vedrovice settlement (Buchvaldek et al. 2007), show collagen $\delta^{15}N$ values ranging from +8.8 to +12 per mil and $\delta^{13}C$, values of bone collagen fall between -20.5 and -21.9 per mil (Smrčka et al. 2008). In south-eastern and eastern European inland, there is stable isotope evidence of an aquatic-based diet (likely fresh-water fish) along the Danube (Bonsall et al. 1997) and the Dneiper (Lillie and Richards 2000) that continued to be important in Neolithic times.

1.4.1 TRACE ELEMENT ANALYSES

Concentrations of Zn in the skeletons of the first farmers of Central Europe (Linear Pottery Culture at Těšetice) are the lowest of all researched places (Smrčka and Jambor 2000). Meiklejohn et al. (1984) found that there is a significant stature decline from the Upper Palaeolithic through the Neolithic. The trend appears to manifest more strongly in the female sample than in the male. However, none of the subsamples show significant decrease from the Upper Palaeolithic to the Mesolithic. There is a significant decrease from the Mesolithic to the Neolithic in the female samples, and overall.

1.4.2 ISOTOPIC ANALYSES—DISTINGUISHING NEOLITHIC MIGRATORY POPULATIONS

Linear Pottery Culture (Linearbandkeramik—LBK) is traditionally used to describe the first farmers of Central Europe, named after the pottery they introduced approximately 7,500 years ago. Radiocarbon dating for LBK suggests it rapidly spread into Central Europe from its place of origin in the Hungarian Plain (Gronenborn 1999; Price et al. 2002). Bentley et al. (2002) identified Neolithic migrants who moved between geologic regions, the area uplands (^{87}Sr / ^{86}Sr > 0,715) and regional lowlands (^{87}Sr / ^{86}Sr < 0,710) near the Dillingen site. Strontium isotopic signatures make their way faithfully from local geologic materials and ultimately into the human skeleton. Comparing the isotope signature in adult teeth, which is incorporated into the teeth between four and twelve years of age, with that in bones, with characteristic turnover times varying between 6 and 20 years for different bones of the body. Ericson (1985) and Grupe et al. (1997) identified 11 out of 17 (65%) of the remains from Dillingen as nonclocal. Nonlocals in this LBK cemetery (and also in others—Flomborn and Schwetzingen) had social identities different from the locals. Nonlocal females were common. At Dillingen, all 5 (100%) females were above the local range compared with the 6/12 of the males being nonlocal (5 above the local range, 1 below). ^{87}Sr / ^{86}Sr may correlate with burial orientation. 80% of west-facing burials were immigrants at Floborn. At Schwetzingen, 30% (7/23 burials) with head directions ranging from north to east are nonlocals. Many nonlocals are buried without a shoe-last adze. At Dillingen, burials with shoe-last adzes are significantly more likely than those without. Among the 11 burials without a shoe-last adze at Dillingen, 9 (82%) are nonlocals, with tooth values above the local range. Of the 6 Dillingen burials with a shoe last adze, 2 (33%) are nonlocals and only 1 of whom was above the local range. The presence of nonlocal males without adzes confirms that the correlation is not merely between shoe-last adzes and males who happen to be locals. Nonlocal $^{87}Sr / ^{86}Sr$ values are mostly above the local range for their place of burial. Of the 27 immigrants from the three sites, 23 tooth values are above the local range for the site and only 4 below it. The last pattern is suggestive of the source of the nonlocal's diet in the younger part of their lives. The $^{87}Sr / ^{86}Sr$ values for the nonlocals are not high enough, however, to be "from" the granitic uplands, where water samples are generally above 0,720 The best interpretation at this point may be that the higher $^{87}Sr / ^{86}Sr$ values reflect a significant proportion of the diet from the regional uplands (Bentley et al. 2002).

1.5 AGRICULTURE, THE PROBABLE REASON FOR BONE PATHOLOGY

Throughout the entirety of the Neolithic period in Europe, gathering continued to be a supplementary part of the economy. Gathering and agriculture were not mutually exclusive, but they supplemented each other according to local natural conditions (Bickle and Whittle 2013). The change in diet, based on grains, triggered a population explosion which resulted in the formation of new socials contacts. However, from a biological point of view, humans were unable to adapt completely to these new conditions even though there are hints of partial genetic adaptation e.g. lactose tolerance in adults (Allentoft et al. 2015). In the period of agricultural development, the proportion of vegetal foods in the diet increased and meat consumption decreased. However, at the same time, the population became more slender and shorter. Angel (1984) and Schoeninger (1981) compared the average size of individuals in populations of Palaeolithic hunters and Neolithic agriculturalists. They concluded that the European *Homo sapiens sapiens*, who consumed animal albumin to the maximum extent in the Late Palaeolithic 30,000 years ago was 30 cm taller than his successor in the period of agricultural development. A meat diet contains zinc, which is necessary for both the development of the foetus and for the pregnant female. This element, as well as many other essential elements, can get caught up in the intestine on the fibrous material of grain husks, and can cause premature osteoporosis. This was identified in the populations which intensified their agriculture and consumed unleavened bread (Smrčka et al. 1998). Gluten from wheat flour or, more exactly, prola-min gliadin, can have a toxic effect and give rise to coeliac disease as demonstrated by Dicke and his colleagues (1953) in the Netherlands. The Greek doctor Aretaeus described this disease in the 2nd century A.D. (Adams 1856 in Simoons 1981). However, it was Gee (1888 in Simoons 1981) who presented the first clinical description: "A kind of chronic ingestion that can appear at any age, but more commonly in children 1–5 years old. Diarrhoea, vomiting, loss of appetite and weight loss, or failure to gain weight, are the symptoms." Gee concluded that the condition is brought about by errors in diet and that "if the patient can be cured at all it must be by means of diet." Gee noted that "death is common" and the disease, which had a 15% overall mortality rate in the 544 celiac patients included in articles published in Europe and the United States from 1909 to 1939. Moreover, those early patients who recovered tended to have stunted growth (Hardwick 1939). Falchuk et al. (1972) found a highly significant correlation between the disease and the HLA-B8 antigen: 88% of adult celiac patients in the United States and the United Kingdom had the HLA-B8 antigen, compared with 22–30% of the controls. Concentrations of Zn in the skeletons of the first farmers at Těšetice (Smrčka and Jambor 2000), in the Central-European territory (Linear Ceramics), are the lowest of any researched location. It was not until the arrival of Corded Ware and Bell Beaker cultures, with different diet types, that gracilization of the skeleton "stopped" in Europe. We suppose that "the Neolithic gracilization, which is the background of the wealth of agricultural populations and the increase of population," is directly linked with the concentration of Zn and various other elements of growth (Smrčka et al. 1998). In developing countries, where the chief nutrients are cereal grains and where the diet lacks animal protein, there is a prevalent nutritional Zn deficiency. Zinc deficiency interferes with the mechanisms necessary for mediating long-term memory (Wauben and Wainwright 1999). Those most vulnerable to zinc deficiency include (1) infants, (2) adolescents during rapid growth phases, and (3) women during pregnancy and lactation. A study of food samples from Iranian villages and from Nubia (Smrčka et al. 1998) indicated that zinc concentrations in the diet were suboptimal.

1.5.1 MANIFESTATION OF SHORTAGE AND DISEASE

In the Neolithic, periods of famine were probably repeated in cycles. This, including associated diseases with vitamin C deficiency (*scurvy*) and mineral deficiencies were indicated by interrupted enamel growth, *enamel hypoplasy*, or discontinued bone growth, *Harris lines* and *porotic hyperostosis* (Arnott 2005). In this context, parasitic infestations should not be omitted as it was one of the causes of *anaemias*.

1.6 AGRICULTURE AND ZOONOSES

Bone pathology was not only affected by the transition to a cereal grain-based diet, but also by the domestication and breeding of animals. Close contact with animals and milk utilization since the 7th millennium B.C. (Evershed et al. 2008) lead to a rise in diseases transmissible to humans—zoonoses. Due to transmission from cattle, *tuberculosis* occurred in various regions of the Neolithic world (Kohler 2012, 2013, 2014), and at the same time, due to the goat population exchange, sporadic *brucellosis* infections would occur.

1.7 THE AIM OF THIS PUBLICATION

The aim of this publication is to clarify the hitherto unknown or little explained facts regarding the daily life of individuals of the Lengyel Culture (LgC), Neolithic farmers who emerged from the Balkans to replaced the original early agricultural population of Central Europe of Linear Pottery Culture (LBK or LPC) and the successive Stroked Pottery Culture (SPC). This Neolithic culture lived in village communities with grain cultivation and in close contact with domesticated animal. The settlement organization, with its hierarchy and emerging individual specialisation (Řídký et al. 2018), was exposed to plant and animal lives in the agricultural cycle. The Lengyel culture differed from early Neolithic cultures by the introduction of metal, copper, its regional distribution, the distribution of volcanic glass and an increase in hunting proven by archaeozoologic research (Dufek et al. 2016).

This culture was presented to the world by the pastor of Szecvárd, Mór Wosinsky and the notary in the Moravian town of Znojmo, Jaroslav Palliardi, at the turn of the 20th century.

The eponymous type site was at Lengyel in Tolna County, Hungary, even though later settlements of this culture were also discovered in Vojvodina, Serbia, and in Croatia. This Neolithic culture migrated beyond Moravia, further west to parts of today's Austria and Poland.

The first amateur archaeologists, just like the succeeding professionals, were enthralled by the beautiful painted pottery, statuettes of animals and humans, as well as everyday objects.

An idea about the everyday life of the people in this population of the Middle and Late Neolithic started to form. Since the 1950s, following the discovery and analysis of rondels, the spiritual life and the religious ideas of these humans have started to emerge (Řídký et al. 2018).

In the first third of the 21st century, it might seem that all archaeological questions had been answered, yet more questions arise (Kristiansen and

Earle 2015; Řídký et al. 2015; Renfrew 2018). How was this population affected by the introduction of metal? Why was the need for hunting increased? What was the health and morbidity of the Lengyel Culture population before its migration from today's Hungary to the Moravian region of the Czech Republic, where it flourished unprecedently? Which diseases mostly troubled the inhabitants of Lengyel settlements? In what ways was the lifestyle during the expansion of this Neolithic culture different from those of the preceding Linear and Stroked Pottery Cultures? These questions will be addressed in the following chapters.

1.8 SUMMARY OF INDIVIDUAL CHAPTERS

CHAPTER 2
In this chapter, the rudimentary features of the Lengyel Culture in Hungary with special attention given to the Baranya and Tolna regions, where the eponymous site is located, are presented. It is conceived from the archaeological point of view with a brief overview of the analysed burials at the, now already classic, burial sites of Zenkövárkóny and Villánykővesd.

CHAPTER 3
In this chapter, the paleopathologic analyses of the sites Zenkövárkóny, Villánykővesd, Belvárgyula, Borjád and Alsónyék-Bátaszék are interpreted. An archaeological gender study of the Zenkövárkóny burial site introduced new findings about textile, hide, and metal processing at the site. These were also verified through bone material analysis. Pathological changes, exceptional from the medical aspect, were examined from the point of view of several scientific disciplines.

CHAPTER 4
In this chapter the dietary trends from the Zenkövárkóny and Villánykővesd burial sites are examined using stable nitrogen and carbon isotopes.

CHAPTER 5
Migration analysis using stable strontium isotopes conducted at the Zenkövárkóny, Villánykővesd, Belvárgyula and Borjád sites.

CHAPTER 6
In this chapter, the health of the Neolithic population members of the Zenkövárkóny, Villánykővesd and Belvárgyula sites is addressed through the use of multi-element analysis of trace elements in bones and tooth enamel.

CHAPTER 7

The archaeological characteristics of the Lengyel Culture (Moravian Painted Ware Culture) in Moravia are presented in this chapter, including the history of research.

CHAPTER 8

The population of the Moravian Painted Ware Culture (LgC) is compared with the preceding Linear Pottery Culture (LPC) and the Stroked Pottery Culture (SPC) from an anthropological viewpoint.

CHAPTER 9

In this chapter, the Neolithic cultures of Moravia (LPC, SPC, LgC and Moravian Painted Ware Culture) are compared from the perspective of paleopathological analysis of bone diseases.

CHAPTER 10

Dietary trends in Neolithic cultures of Moravia (LPC, SPC, LgC and Moravian Painted Ware Cultures) are compared based on stable nitrogen and carbon isotope analysis.

CHAPTER 11

The Neolithic cultures of Moravia (LPC, SPC, LgC and Moravian Painted Ware Cultures) are compared from the aspect of the population's mobility using stable strontium isotope analysis.

CHAPTER 12

Bone health in individual periods of the Neolithic cultures of Moravia (LPC, SPC, LgC and Moravian Painted Ware Cultures) is examined through multi-element analysis of trace elements.

CHAPTER 13

Conclusion on the health and morbidity of the Lengyel Culture populations including their paleopathological profile and reference to the importance of scientific examination of Neolithic bone material.

2. THE LENGYEL CULTURE IN HUNGARY

OLIVÉR GÁBOR

2.1 TIME AND TERRITORIAL BOUNDARIES

In Europe, the change from the hunter gathering lifestyle to the settled lifestyle took place during the 7-6 Millenium B.C. (Childe 1925; Lüning 1988; Andel and Runnels 1995; Fernández-Domínguez and Reynolds 2017). The most important innovations were settling in one place for a long time, deliberate food production, making polished stone tools, and the birth of pottery craft. A permanent settlement established near the cultivated area, and the larger area unit was covered by a settlement network. At that time was evolved the well known Dumbar's number (a measurement of the cognitive limit to the number of individuals with whom any one person can maintain stable relationships—Dunbar 2010). Neolith revolution: producing farming (agriculture, animal housbandry), an active attitude towards the environment (both creative and devastating) (Childe 1936; Bíró 2003a, 99; Barker 2009). At the beginning the stone tools used as chock and axe spread while the areas under newly cultivated land were cleansed (Bíró 2003a, 99). Constant shaped containers made of clay (inorganic material). The larger clay pots were used to store the crop more safely, the smaller ones mimicked the shape of bowls made of pumkins. The first artifical material in the history was the burnished clay. The farming population grew due to the food production, and caused the spread of the new population and its lifestyle to the detriment of the mesolithic people. The enrichment caused by the food production, created social differenties, which are reflected in the excavated graves.

The Lengyel culture was born in the late Neolithic age (around B.C. 4800) in Hungary (Bíró 2003b, 103), as a genetic offspring of the earlier Linear Pottery Culture (Zalai 2003, 110), but not directly. The last time limit of this culture was the early copper age (till B.C. 4000), because it saw the appeerence of the first copper beads. This period was the beginning of the Secondary Products Revolution during the copper age (Greenfield 2010; Szeverényi 2013, 58): milk, dairy products, wool use, inventing alcoholic products beverages (Gábor 2008, 77; Gábor 2009, 188).

In the Neolithic era was the late Neolithic the flower. This is also the richest period in archaeological finds: sophisticated craft products, long distance obsidian trade and large central sites. According to the highest density of contemporary settlements, the center of the late Neolithic Lengyel culture was in Southwest-Hungary.

2.1.1 AREA

The Lengyel culture was a part of a greater late Neolithic Central-European cultural-unity, which includes territories of West-Hungary, Austria, West-Slovakia, South-Moravia and South-Poland (Bíró 2003b, 102). But this unity was determined only in modern age (20th century), based on the similarity of archaeological finds—mainly the painted ceramics. That is why we do not know if this material similarity in that era also meant real ethnical and cultural unity or not. However we can figure an inner boundary, by help of Neolithic balkanian traditions, which reached to Hungary but not further north.

2.1.2 ORIGIN, SPREAD, DATING AND PERIODS OF THE CULTURE

In the territory of Slovenia and Croatia a new late Neolithic culture was born, which is called Sopot culture (Dimitrijević 1968; Kramberger 2014). The settlements of the 2nd phase of this culture appeared in South West Hungary, and later in North West Hungary (Regenye 2002). The material culture also changed, and cultural unification began. The base of the new Lengyel culture came from the remains of the middle Neolithic population. This late Neolithic culture was probably built on local foundations with the help of powerful South East European influence (Simon 2003, 102; Bíró 2003b, 102–103).

The time periods and phases of Lengyel culture were calculated using synchronology (e.g. ceramic typology and absolute chronology (Lichardus and Vladár 2003; Barna 2011, 243–246). The Lengyel culture was born about 4800 B.C. (Barna 2011). The tradition of ceramic painting was inherited from the previous Sopot culture (Kalicz and Makkay 1972) and not directly from the Linear Pottery Culture. The dishes were the finest in the most colourful (red, white, black and yellow) in the first period. Later fewer colours were used. In the latest period the colours were replaced by plastic ornaments (cams). The extent of the Lengyel culture was the South West Hungarian group (Baranya county and Tolna county), the North Hungarian, and the South Slowakian Aszód-Csabdi-Svodín group from the late period.

- 1st phase: lots of painted ceramics (mainly red), scrached ornaments, small knobs with horizontal opening, pedestaled bowls, mushroom vessels.
- 2nd phase: continousity of the earlier vessel-forms, red-white painted ceramics, schrached meander.
- 3rd phase: the surveillance of the culture reached to copper age, but only in West-Hungary (copper beads). The life of the settlements and usage of

circular ditch systems was unbroken. White coloured ceramics and big knobs (Raczky 1974).

- The existence of phase 4 is questionable (Pavúk 2004).

2.2 SITES

For a long time, the sites of South West Hungary were the most known. Today more than 300 sites of the Lengyel culture are known in Hungary. The best-known sites were: the eponymous site Lengyel-Sánc, excavated by Wosinsky Mór (Wosinsky 1885), and the settlement and cemetery of Zengővárkony, excavated by János Dombay in the 1930's and 1940's (Dombay 1960a). The Aszód site, excavated later by Nándor Kalicz (Kalicz 1985), showed the northernmost part of the culture in Hungary. The most important obsidian mines were in Tokaj, out of Lengyel cultres' territory. There were close connections to the east Hungarian late Neolithic groups. The tell of Tiszapolgár-Csőszhalom lies in the corridor between the Lengyel and the Tisza-Herpály cultures, as a common point (Raczky 2002).

2.2.1 SETTLEMENTS

After Werner Buttler (excavated the Neolithic settlement of Köln-Lindenthal: Buttler and Habarey 1936, tabs. 22–26) János Dombay believed, that the clay pits were the sites of the homes (Dombay 1960a, 181–192). Today we know that the rows of postholes show the location of the long late Neolithic Houses (Lüning 1979; Sherratt 1982; Mausch and Ziessow 1985). These large family houses continued the Central European Neolithic traditions. In the early period of the culture, people sometimes were buried in the settlements, but most of the cemeteries became an area entirely separate from the settlements. At that early time the type of cemeteries with great numbers of graves were formed. The great settlements played significant role in the long-distance trade of copper, sea shells and obsidian. The polished stone axes and bone tools were local products. (Bíró 2003b, 102–103) Firstly they were farmers, secondly craftsmen (craft settlements: Zengővárkony, Aszód), and miners expanding to the mountainous regions (Kalicz 1985). They lived in large family houses with pile structures (it was a Central-European Neolithic tradition). In Zengővárkony was a central settlement with farming, polished stonetool-making local mine (Szamárhegy et al. 2000, 9), and it was obsidian distance trading center. Here were found the earliest copper beads of Hungary.

2.2.2 CEMETERIES

The number of cemeteries is remarkably small compared to the great number of settlements (Zalai 2003, 110). The richest cemeteries were in Southwest-Hungary: Zengővárkony (368 graves in 24 grave groups), Lengyel-Sánc (2 grave groups), Mórágy-Tűzkődomb (109 graves Zalai-Gaál 2001, 2002; Zoffmann 2004), Alsónyék-Bátaszék (2400 graves!), Villánykővesd (28 graves), Pécsvárad-Aranyhegy (8? graves), Szekszárd-Ágoston-puszta (20 graves).

The cemeteries are mostly known in parts close to the Danube. Most of the known cemeteries were found in the abandoned parts of the settlements, because it was exactly the time period of history, when the settlement and the cemetery were separated from each other. The graves were usually sorted into rows (30-35 graves belonged to a group), but there were lots of graves outside the cemetery (eg. in the pits and ditches of the settlements).

Placing the corpses in flexed positions was a regular habit (Zalai 2003, 110). The most common grave goods were ceramics (with food and drink for the dead) interred by the mourners. The other type of grave findings were the personal objects owned earlier by the dead such as clothing items or tools. Typical grave findings found in the graves of men were wild boar tusks and pig jaws.

Orientation of the graves (Zoffmann 1965): The most common custom was: East-West and West-East, lying on the right or left side. The South-North orientation was rare (eg. Eastern cemetery group in Lengyel).

Special burial rites were cremation[1], burying little children in vessels (Mórágy), skull grave, grave without skulls[2], trepaned skull in a grave (Lengyel: Zalai 2003, 110), limb mutilation[3], graves containing several bodies[4], cenotaph with grave goods[5].

2.2.3 ZENGŐVÁRKONY (SETTLEMENT AND BURIAL SITE)

The Lengyel culture was named after the eponymous type site, the enclosed settlement of Lengyel in Hungary, right of the Danube. To the South of Lengyel, the site of Zengővárkony was discovered in 1933. The history

---

[1]   The cremation was a middle Neolithic local tradition. Györe: 9 cremations of 16 graves in a separated group (Zalai 2003, 110, 112).

[2]   Zengővárkony: 15 graves layed next to each other without skulls. Hard slaughtering of cadaver occured mainly in graves of male or boys. At the same time these were sometimes rich graves (Bándi, Petres, and Maráz 1979, 25).

[3]   Limb mutilation after death? It occured continously during the prehistoric age, as the sign of reburial or the fear from the dead (Zalai 2003, 110).

[4]   It is rare, mainly mother with her child—Zalai 2003, 110.

[5]   The cenopahs were relatively common. Bothros in the cemetery (eg. Mórágy): it is not known, if it was a cenotaph or bothros.

of archaeological research at the settlement and burial site was described by János Dombay in the introduction to his book, *Settlement and burial site Zengővárkony* (Dombay 1960a): "Most of the finds came from the minor excavations in 1936 and 1937, which had to be protected as they were endangered by agricultural activities. The observations showed that Zengővárkony was an important settlement. The clues were the traces of settlements near to burial sites as well as groups of graves rather far from other groups. In one such group of graves, as it seemed, blood relatives may have been buried, or families living together. One conspicuous feature was the quantity of artefacts in the settlement. This was proved not only by rich funerary equipment but also by the great quantity of untreated silex fragments, flint tools produced by the chipping technique, polished instruments of various kinds of stone and tools of bone, fragments of pottery and a large quantity of animal bones. This suggested that there was a centre of production of silex tools and painted pottery.

In the summer and autumn of 1938, 147 graves were excavated at various sites within the settlement, and another 77 in the autumn of 1939. We had to be satisfied with saving the endangered graves, situated on small hillocks. In such places, the graves are endangered even nowadays by soil washed away after heavy rains or by agricultural activities. We first attempted exploration of the settlements in 1941. In 1944 we found another 15 graves while exploring the settlement. The excavations and explorations fully confirmed our previous observations. We estimated the number of as of yet unearthed graves at about 1,500 and that of the as of yet unexplored groups of graves at 50-60. We supposed it would be possible to find more homes of square ground plan which had been built above the ground level and perhaps that some remnants of buildings would be discovered that served economical purposes.

In 1947 we performed the first major research at the settlement. At that time, we had the first chance to observe the phenomena of the everyday life that cannot be judged by the material from graves and we widened the scope of research to the type of the settlement, economic and social life to such an extent that we might arrive at a complete picture. The goal of the systematic unearthing of the whole settlement was explanation of the most important issues of the type of economic life, the connection between the settlement and the graves, the structure of the family and social relations as much as needed to prove that the complexes of pits were remnants of earth-houses and associated farm buildings. We could only try to collect enough material to show the everyday life of the inhabitants and provide the best reconstruction of life in those times.

We tried to achieve these goals through the excavations in 1948. As, considering the experience of 1947, the partial and particular excavations did not prove the anticipated result, we started to explore whole respective areas in order to see a larger complex of pits and, at the same time, study the details in their interconnections."

The burial site of Zengővárkony originally included 368 graves arranged in 14 grave groups, but only 64 graves, i.e. barely 18%, have been excavated.

2.3 POTTERY

The pottery of the Lengyel culture is exceedingly rich and varied (Kalicz 1998; Barna 2011, 168–181). Its description is important, as it suggests, at least vaguely, the food the people consumed. The typical ceramic forms of the Lengyel culture (figs. 1, 2, 3) are the follows: thin-walled cups, with a small bottom; small double-cone shaped vessels; big round flat dishes; indented deep dishes; high dishes on a stem, with a shallow dish part and a stem which is narrow at the top but with a funnel-shaped widening downwards; and big jugs with a high neck. On comparison of the decorations of the pottery of

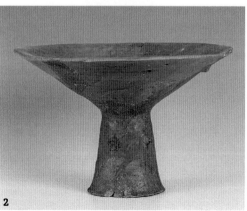

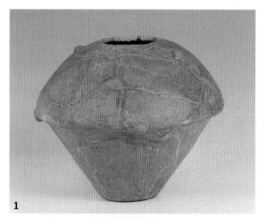

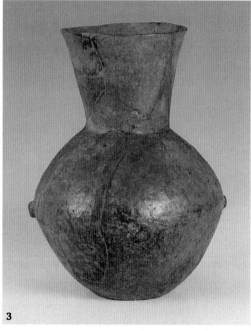

Fig. 1. Zengővárkony, grave no. 14.
Photo: Sinkó Anikó.

Fig. 2. Zengővárkony, grave no. 176.
Photo: Sinkó Anikó.

Fig. 3. Zengővárkony, N11–55. Photo: Sinkó Anikó.

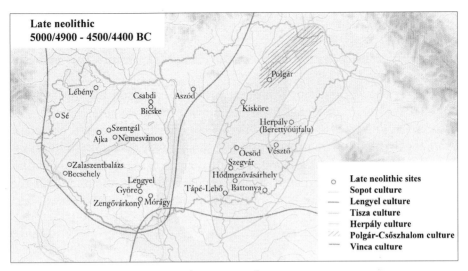

Fig. 4. Late Neolithic age in Hungary (Visy 2003, 98).

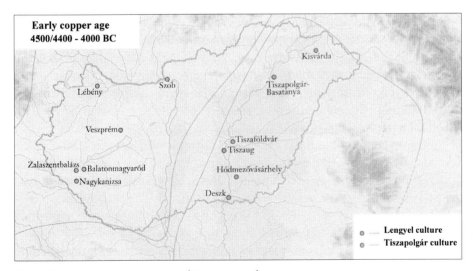

Fig. 5. Early copper age in Hungary (Visy 2003, 124).

the Tisza culture and of the Lengyel culture, it is obvious that in the Tisza culture the spiral pattern on the vessels is not as important as in the Lengyel culture. In case of the meander pattern, it is the other way round. In artefacts of the Tisza culture, combinations of spirals and meanders, so conspicuous in the Lengyel culture and in Zengővárkony in particular, do not occur (figs. 4, 5).

2.4 METALLURGY

In the areas of the Lengyel culture and the Tiszapolgár culture, copper jewelleries were found.

The earliest worked copper pieces appeared already during the late copper age. They were collected from the surface the malachite, azurite, and natural ore, and were used for jewellery beads, needles, rings and bracelets. From the first half of 5th millennium B.C. the number of copper findings increases in sites. Besides working/shaping objects using hammers, the first signs of copper extrusion appeared in Zengővárkony, in the middle of the 5th millennium B.C. Prosperous South Eastern European metalwork was created (Virág 2003, 129–130).

2.5 EVERYDAY LIFE UTENSILS AND CRAFTSMENS' TOOLS

Axes were found in men's graves. Only in exceptional cases do the cutting edges show signs of use. The edges were mostly sharpened only from below, on one side, and with a bulge just above the edge, which interfered with the use of the instruments as an axe. Also, rather narrow specimens with a rounded neck exist, but these are rare. Their shape is different, and so is the stone material they were made of. They were obtained through barter.

Knives for skinning were first roughly shaped, then ground to the required shape on a grindstone and eventually the cutting edge was sharpened. Often they were re-sharpened.

Tools resembling the *chisel* (like that used by sculptors) are smaller, narrow and rather long, like incisor teeth, but they also resemble the edges of a shoemaker's last. They are polished. The arch-shaped cutting edge was ground and sharpened from below but sometimes from the above as well.

The *club head* was cylindrical. It was polished into the round shape after the hole for the handle was drilled.

The number of grindstones and grinding boards testifies that most stone tools were manufactured on the spot, in the settlement. *Small grindstones* were 8–10 cm long. Their bottom sides are smooth and robust. The back sides are arched. They are light and convenient, easy to hold on one hand. They were moved during sharpening rather than being ground against passively. Beyond doubt, their primary use was working wood. The heavy *grindstones* could have been used as a plane, as the grip part was held in the right hand while the left hand was holding the narrow back of the grindstone. *Smooth stone plates* were used to rub pigments into powder with grindstones. Ferric red ochre was first milled and then the chips were ground to fine powder.

In *lumps* of clay from the huts, impressions of wooden parts, square in shape, were found. This suggests that construction timber was squared off first. For this purpose, heavy grindstones, 55 cm in length, may have been used. Their bottom side is 12 cm wide, smooth and worn, the top side is narrow. The back part is narrow and ends with a grip part, facing the left.

2.6 ARCHAEOZOOLOGICAL EVIDENCE OF CHANGES IN ABUNDANCE OF ANIMALS IN LATE NEOLITHIC AND ENEOLITHIC (CHALCOLITHIC) PERIOD

Animal farming in migrating populations that came to the Carpathian Basin from the South-East became part of the Tiszapolgár culture in the early Chalcolithic period, in the northern part of the region between the Danube and Tisza, as well as in the Lengyel culture in the Transdanubian region. The Neolithic type of animal farming and hunting survived to the Eneolithic period but acquired some new forms.

Considering the proofs of composition of the fauna, the first part of the Chalcolithic period in these cultures was different. In the Lengyel culture the animal farming and hunting survived and stayed similar to that of the Neolithic period.

Domestic animals did not include the horse. Cattle were the most frequent animal, followed in number by pigs, sheep, goats and dogs. The composition of the domestic fauna was very similar to that of the Tisza and Herpály cultures.

The population of wild animals was not typically Neolithic. Aurochs and red deer occurred approximately in the same quantities, which suggested some recession of Neolithic hunting activities. The occurrence of auroch bones, however, was still high—at the same level as in the Tisza culture. A high number of transient forms between aurochs and cattle occurred, but not as many as in the Herpály culture.

At all Lengyel culture settlements, the composition of the fauna was very similar, although the distances between them were big. Between the two settlements with the richest specimens of fauna, Zengővárkony and Aszód, the distance was 200 kilometres. In Aszód, the hilly countryside of the northern Hungary, finds of the boar were the most common in game animal remnants (Bökönyi 1974, 21–33).

2.7 BELIEFS AND CIRCULAR DITCH SYSTEMS

The clay idols (usually women) were present throughout the Stone Age in Hungary. Almost all of them were found in settlements. A cult corner can be deduced in the dwelling houses (Bánffy and Goldmann 2003, 112–113), that is, that part of faith was a family matter, in accordance with the Neolithic Balkan traditions. The number of idols declined in Late Neolithic.

The circular ditch systems were of Central-European origin, located mainly in Western-Hungary. They were created outside the settlements and composed of "V" shaped concentric ditches, which were not made for defense purposes, rather as sacred community facilities. The circular ditch systems had some entrances (oriented to the cardinal points), but there were no setlements within. Little archaeological material was found in them, among which the idols indicate a sacral function (Szeverényi 2013, 51).

2.8 SOCIETY, ETHNICITY

The grave goods of cremated graves are similar to the inhumated graves. There may be two separated ethnical groups represented (Zalai 2003, 112)? Likewise, different types of grave orientations can also show differences in origins of the groups. At the same time, the decapitation in a separate cemetery group can also show a cultural togetherness (Bándi, Petres, and Maráz 1979, 25, 27). Copper beads, which occur as grave goods only in certain groups (but not necessarily as a sign of wealth) may be as a sign of cultural differences (Bándi, Petres, and Maráz 1979, 27).

The richest graves belong to men. The finds from the graves were: polished stone axes, chipped stone tools, a couple of pendants made of wild boar tusks, and bone pricker. The dog skeleton or antler axe in a grave also show the high rank of the burried man. Based on the rich child-graves, social rank was inheritable. The poorest graves did not have any grave goods (about one-third of all graves).

2.9 ANALYZED GRAVES

2.9.1 ZENGŐVÁRKONY

Grave no. 5: Male, flexed on right side, E–W. Pedestaled bowl, 11 shell beads (Dombay 1939, 7) (fig. 6).

Grave no. 7: Male, flexed on right side, E–W. Polished stone axe, 2 vessels, pedestaled bowl, mushroom vessel (Dombay 1939, 8, JPM Fotótár: 231) (fig. 7).

Grave no. 13: Male, flexed on left side, E–W. Polished stone axe, chipped jaspis scraper, animal dent, pedetaled bowl, bone tool, mushroom vessel, 8 chipped stone blades, 2 obsidian fragments (Dombay 1939, 11–12) (figs. 8–9).

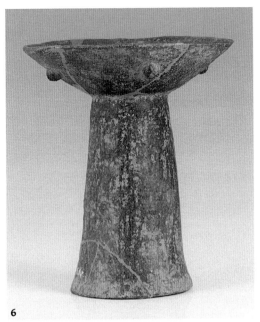

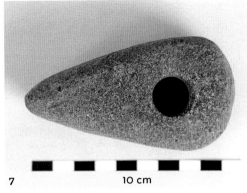

Fig. 6. Zengővárkony, grave no. 5.
Photo: Sinkó Anikó.

Fig. 7. Zengővárkony, grave no. 7.
Photo: Sinkó Anikó.

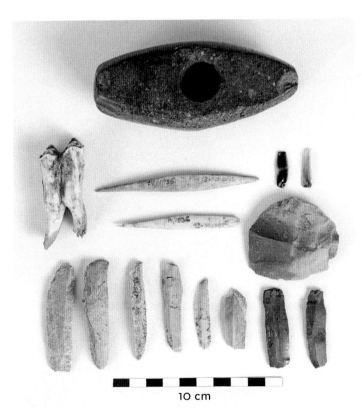

Fig. 8. Zengővárkony,
grave no. 13.
Photo: Sinkó Anikó.

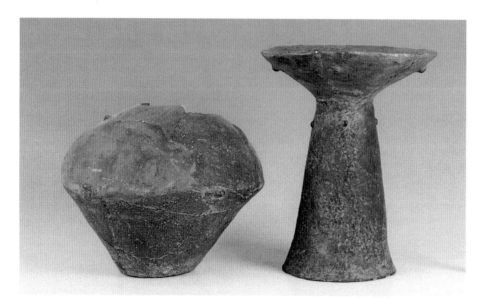

Fig. 9. Zengővárkony, grave no. 13. Photo: Sinkó Anikó.

Grave no. 14: ?, flexed on right side, E–W. Bowl, pedestaled bowl, 2 vessels, mushroom vessel. (Dombay 1939, 12, VI/3) (figs. 10–13).

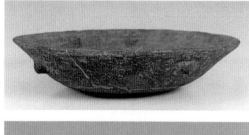

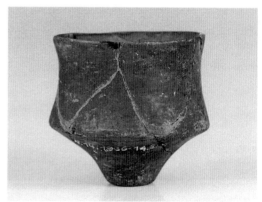

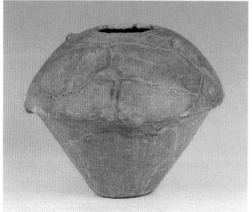

Fig. 10–12. Zengővárkony, grave no. 14. Photo: Sinkó Anikó.

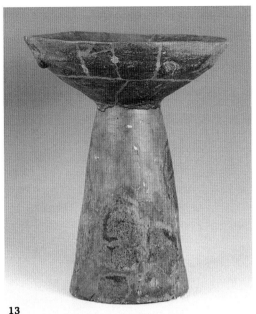

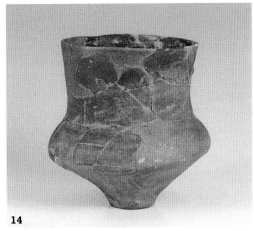

14

13

Fig. 13. Zengővárkony, grave no. 14.
Photo: Sinkó Anikó.

Fig. 14: Zengővárkony, grave no. 34.
Photo: Sinkó Anikó.

Grave no. 34: Male, flexed on back, SW–NE. 2 bowls, 2 vessels (Dombay 1939, 16–17, X/1) (fig. 14).

Grave no. 43: ?, flexed on left side, W–E. Vessel (Dombay 1939, 19).

Grave no. 84: Male, flexed on left side, O–W. Pedestaled bowl, 2 bowls, mug, stone axe. (Dombay 1960a, 75–76, XXXV/11) (figs. 15–16).

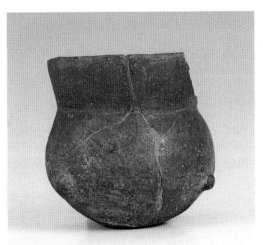

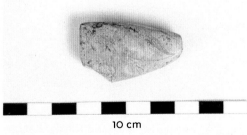

10 cm

Fig. 15–16. Zengővárkony, grave no. 84.
Photo: Sinkó Anikó.

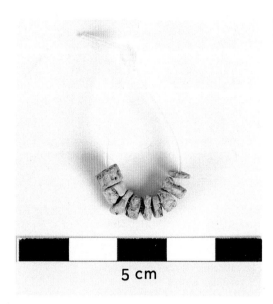

Fig. 17. Zengővárkony, grave no. 87.
Photo: Sinkó Anikó.

Grave no. 87: Female flexed on left side, O–W. 2 pedestaled bowls, 2 bowls, copper beads. (Dombay 1960a, 77) (fig. 17).

Grave no. 88a: Female, flexes on left side, NE–SW. 3 pedestaled bowls, 2 bowls, bone pricker. (Dombay 1960a, 77, XXXVI/5—JPM Fotótár: 237) (figs. 18–21).

Grave no. 88b: Baby? (Dombay 1960a, 77).

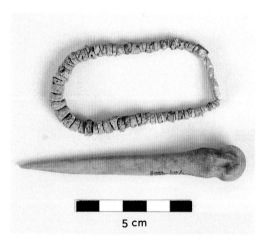

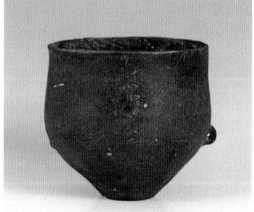

Fig. 18–19. Zengővárkony, Grave no. 88. Photo: Sinkó Anikó.

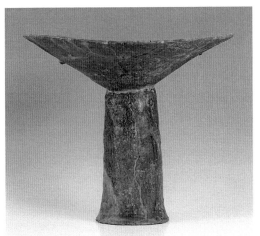
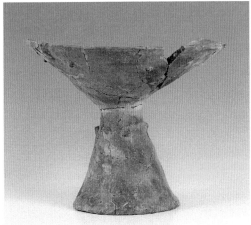

Fig. 20–21. Zengővárkony, Grave no. 88. Photo: Sinkó Anikó.

Grave no. 90: Male, flexed on left side, E–W. Pedestaled bowl, vessel, bowls, silex knife. (Dombay 1960a, 78, XXXVI/8a—JPM Fotótár: 238) (figs. 22–23).

Grave no. 91: Female, flexed on left side, E–W. Bowls, bone needle, copper beads, animal bones, shell (Dombay 1960a, 78, XXXVI/8b—JPM Fotótár: 238) (figs. 24–26).

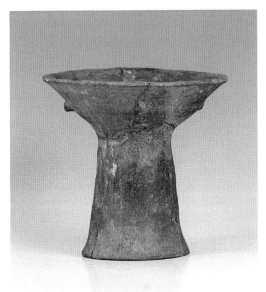
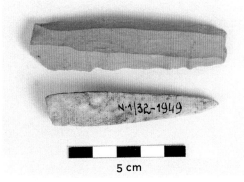

Fig. 22–23. Zengővárkony, grave no. 90. Photo: Sinkó Anikó.

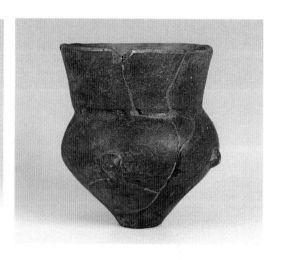

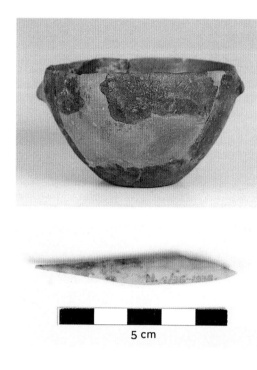

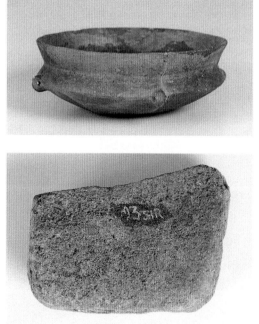

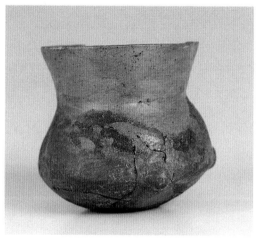

Fig. 24–26. Zengővárkony, grave no. 91.
Photo: Sinkó Anikó.

Fig. 27–29. Zengővárkony, grave no. 93.
Photo: Sinkó Anikó.

Grave no. 93: Male flexed on left side NE-SW. 4 bowls, pedestaled bowl, vessel, 2 stones, stone axe (Dombay 1960a, 79, XXXVI/12—JPM Fotótár: 200) (figs. 27-29).

Grave no. 99: Male, flexed on left side E-W. 3 pedestaled bowls, 3 bowls, vessel, animal bones, nucleus stone (Dombay 1960a, 80-81) (figs. 30-31).

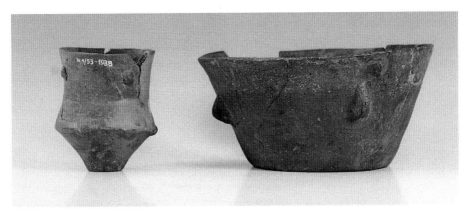

Fig. 30. Zengővárkony, grave no. 99. Photo: Sinkó Anikó.

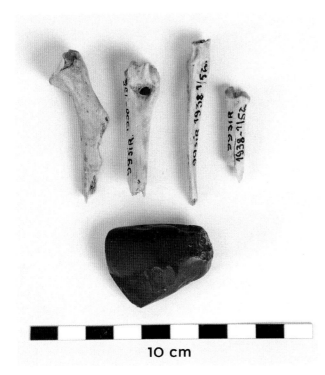

10 cm

Fig. 31. Zengővárkony, grave no. 99. Photo: Sinkó Anikó.

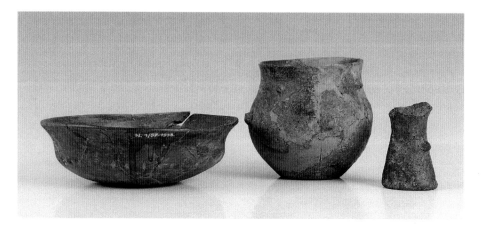

Fig. 32. Zengővárkony, grave no. 101. Photo: Sinkó Anikó.

Grave no. 101: Female (and child) flexed on left side NE–SW. Pedestaled bow, bowls, vessel, cup (Dombay 1960a, 81—JPM Fotótár: 202) (fig. 32).

Grave no. 102: Male, flexed on left side E–W. 2 pedestaled bowls, 2 polished stone axes, chipped stone blade, clay cone (Dombay 1960a, 81–82) (fig. 33).

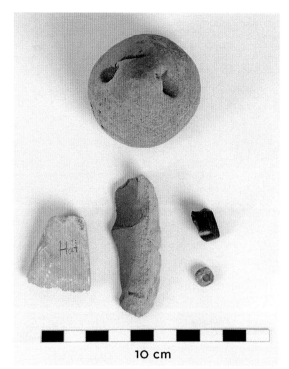

10 cm

Fig. 33. Zengővárkony, grave no. 102. Photo: Sinkó Anikó.

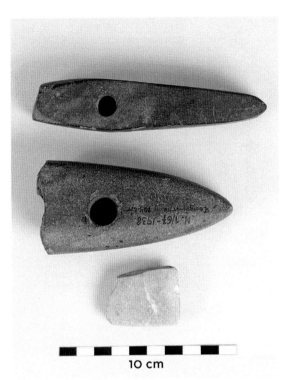

Fig. 34. Zengővárkony,
grave no. 104. Photo: Sinkó Anikó.

10 cm

Grave no. 104: Male, flexed on left side E–W. 2 bowls, 2 polished stone axes, 2 pedestaled bowls, vessel (Dombay 1960a, 82, XXXVIII/1—JPM Fotótár: 204) (figs. 34–35).

Grave no. 125: Male, flexed on left side E–W. Obsidian blade, stone knife, flat axe, pedestaled bowl, 5 silex chipped stone tools (Dombay 1960a, 90–91—JPM Fotótár: 213) (fig. 36).

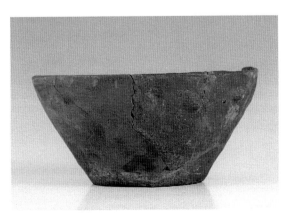

Fig. 35. Zengővárkony,
grave no. 104. Photo: Sinkó Anikó.

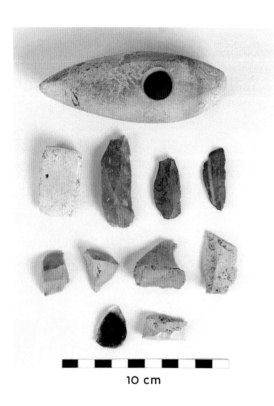

Fig. 36. Zengővárkony,
grave no. 125. Photo: Sinkó Anikó.

10 cm

Grave no. 135: Female, flexed on left side E–W. 3 bowls, vessel, pedestaled bowl (Dombay 1960a, 94) (fig. 37).

Grave no. 137: Male, flexed on left side NE–SW. 8 bowls, pedestaled bowl, animal bones, wild boar tusk, polished stone axes, chipped jaspis knife (Dombay 1960a, 94–95, XLIII/4) (figs. 38–39).

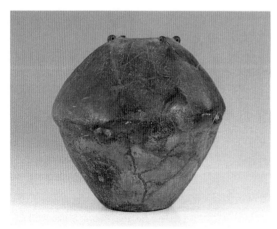

Fig. 37. Zengővárkony,
grave no. 135. Photo: Sinkó Anikó.

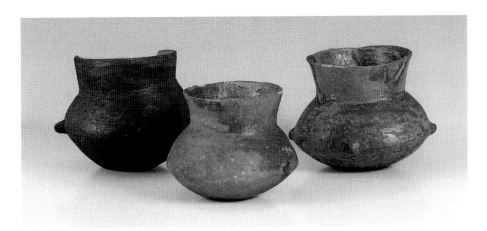

Fig. 38. Zengővárkony, grave no. 137. Photo: Sinkó Anikó.

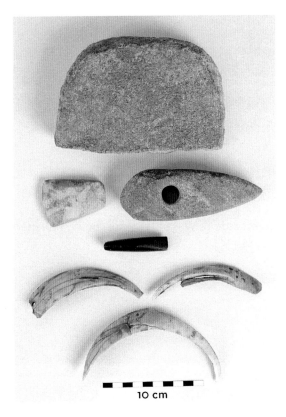

Fig. 39. Zengővárkony, grave no. 137. Photo: Sinkó Anikó.

10 cm

Grave no. 238: Male, flexed on left side, E–W. Jaspis knife, polished axes, 2 pedestaled bowls, 2 bowls, 2 vessels, stone (Dombay 1960a, 125–126) (figs. 40–41).

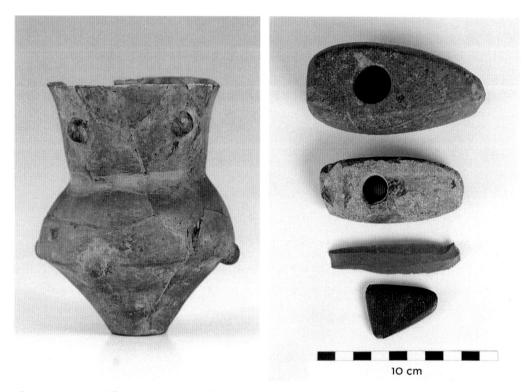

10 cm

Fig. 40–41. Zengővárkony, grave no. 238. Photo: Sinkó Anikó.

Grave no. 272: Male, flexed on left side, E–W. Pedestaled bowl, bowl, 2 vessels, 2 polished stone axes, 4 chipped stone tools (Dombay 1960a, 133) (figs. 42–43).

Grave no. 281: Female, flexed on left side E–W + child skull. Bowl, polished stone axe (Dombay 1960a, 135) (fig. 44).

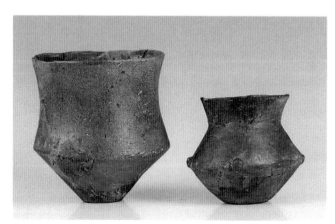

Fig. 42. Zengővárkony, grave no. 272. Photo: Sinkó Anikó.

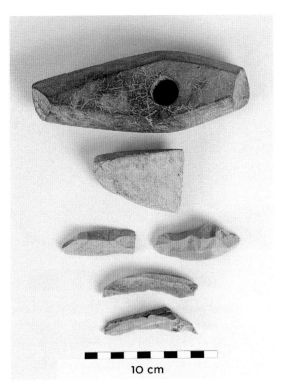

Fig. 43. Zengővárkony,
grave no. 272. Photo: Sinkó Anikó.

10 cm

Grave no. 286: Female flexed on left side, SW–NE. Copper bracelet, copper ring, copper beads, pedestaled bowl (Dombay 1960a, 136, LXXII/3) (figs. 45–46).

Grave no. 299: ?, flexed on left side, NE–SW. Vessels (Dombay 1960a, 138).

Grave no. 301: ?, flexed on right side, SW–NE (Dombay 1960a, 139).

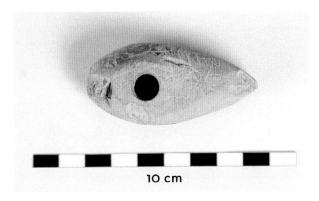

10 cm

Fig. 44. Zengővárkony,
grave no. 281.
Photo: Sinkó Anikó.

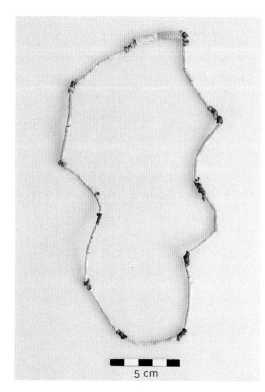

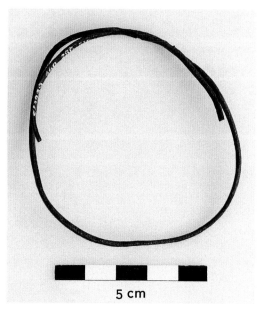

Fig. 45–46. Zengővárkony, grave no. 286.
Photo: Sinkó Anikó.

Grave no. 313: Female, flexed on left side, NE–SW. 4 bowls, pedestaled bowl, shell beads, dentalium beads, shell bracelet, bone awl (Dombay 1960a, 140–141, LXXV/18) (fig. 47).

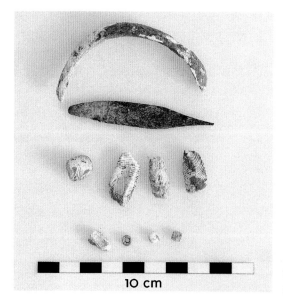

Fig. 47. Zengővárkony, grave no. 313. Photo: Sinkó Anikó.

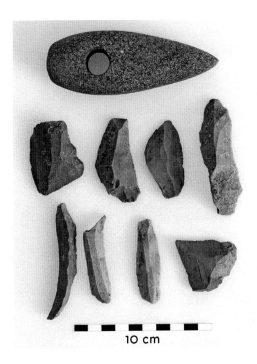

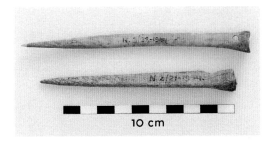

Fig. 48–49. Zengővárkony, grave no. 314.
Photo: Sinkó Anikó.

Grave no. 314: Male flexed on left side, E–W. 2 polished stone axes, bone needl, bone awl, 2 silex blades, 2 pedestaled bowls, 2 bowls, grindstone, vessel (Dombay 1960a, 141, LXXV/17) (figs. 48–51).

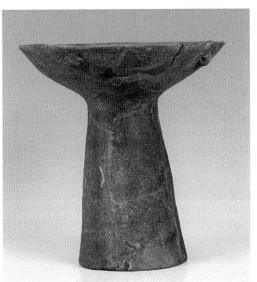

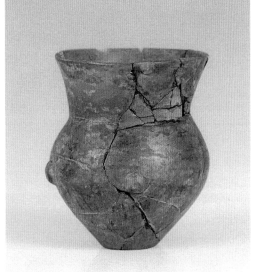

Fig. 50–51. Zengővárkony, grave no. 314. Photo: Sinkó Anikó.

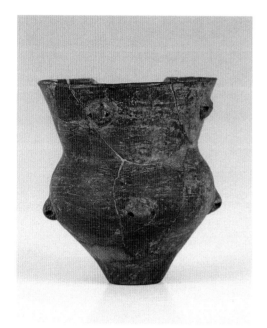

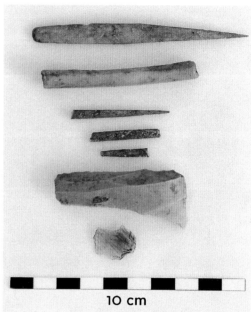

Fig. 52. Zengővárkony, grave no. 316. Photo: Sinkó Anikó.

Fig. 53. Zengővárkony, grave no. 319. Photo: Sinkó Anikó.

Grave no. 316: Child flexed on left side, NE–SW. 4 bowls, pedestaled bowl, vessel, bone bracelet (Dombay 1960, 142) (fig. 52).

Grave no. 317: ?, flexed on left side, NE–SW. 2 vessels, 2 pedestaled bowls, animal bones, bowl (Dombay 1960a, 142–143).

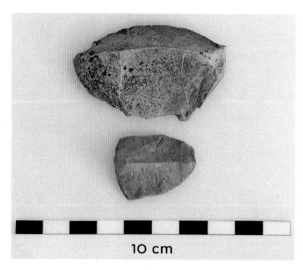

Fig. 54. Zengővárkony, grave no. 323. Photo: Sinkó Anikó.

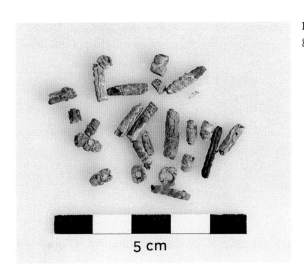

Fig. 55. Zengővárkony,
grave no. 323. Photo: Sinkó Anikó.

Grave no. 319: Female, flexed on left side, NE–SW. Vessels (Dombay 1960a, 143) (fig. 53).

Grave no. 320: Female, flexed on left side, E–W. 2 pedestaled bowls, 2 bowls (Dombay 1960a, 143–144).

Grave no. 323: Female, flexed on left side, E–W. Pedestaled bowl, copper beads, silex tools (Dombay 1960a, 144) (figs. 54–55).

Grave no. 325: Male, flexed on left side, E–W. Pedestaled bowl, 2 stone axes, wild boar tusk, jaspis scratch (Dombay 1960a, 144–145) (fig. 56).

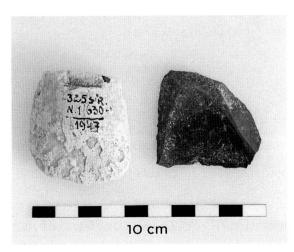

Fig. 56. Zengővárkony,
grave no. 325. Photo: Sinkó Anikó.

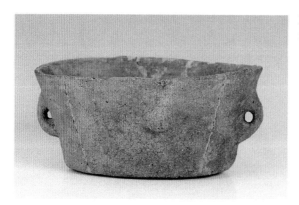

Fig. 57. Zengővárkony, grave no. 326. Photo: Sinkó Anikó.

Grave no. 326: Male, flexed on left side, E–W. Bowl, stone axe, pedestaled bowl, stone drill tap (Dombay 1960a, 145) (fig. 57).

Grave no. 327: ?, ?, NE–SW. Vessels (Dombay 1960a, 145).

Grave no. 329: ?, flexed on left side, NE–SW. Ceramic fragments (Dombay 1960a, 145).

Grave no. 331: Baby, flexed on left side, E–W. Bowl (Dombay 1960a, 145).

Grave no. 336: ?, flexed on left side, NE–SW. Bowl, vessel (Dombay 1960a, 147).

Grave no. 337: ?, flexed on left side, NE–SW. Bowl, vessels (Dombay 1960a, 147).

Grave no. 338: ?, ceramic fragments (Dombay 1960a, 147).

Grave no. 340: ?, ceramic fragments (Dombay 1960a, 147).

Grave no. 341: ?, ceramic fragments, polishd stone axe, silex tool (Dombay 1960a, 147) (fig. 58).

Grave no. 342: ?, flexed on left side, NE–SW. Ceramic fragments (Dombay 1960a, 147–148).

Grave no. 345: ?, pedestaled bowls, ceramic fragments (Dombay 1960a, 148) (fig. 59).

Grave no. 347: Adult, flexed on left side, NE–SW. 4 vessels, 2 pedestaled bowls (Dombay 1960a, 148–149).

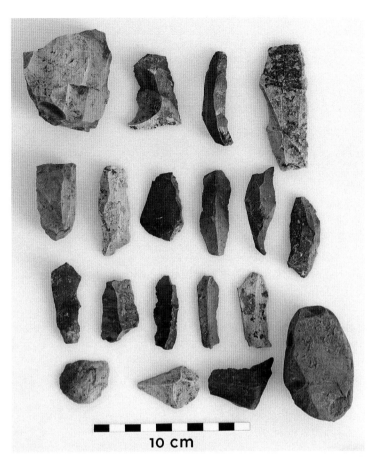

Fig. 58.
Zengővárkony,
grave no. 341.
Photo:
Sinkó Anikó.

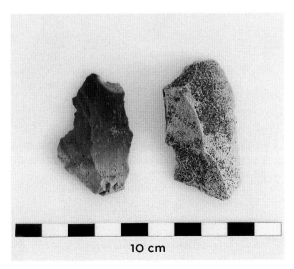

Fig. 59. Zengővárkony,
grave no. 345. Photo: Sinkó Anikó.

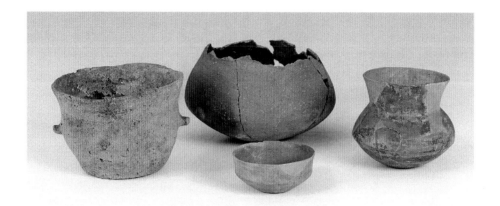

Fig. 60. Zengővárkony, grave no. 355. Photo: Sinkó Anikó.

Grave no. 355: ?, flexed on left side, NE–SW. 2 bowls, animal bone, pedestaled bowl, 2 jugs, vessels (Dombay 1960a, 151) (figs. 60–61).

Grave no. 365: ?, flexed on left side, NE–SW. Bowl, pedestaled bowl, vessel (Dombay 1960a, 155) (fig. 62).

Grave no. 366: ?, ?, E–W. 2 vessels, jaspis blade (Dombay 1960a, 155) (fig. 63).

Grave no. 368: ?, flexed on left side, NE–SW. Jug. (Dombay 1960a, 155).

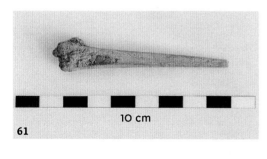

10 cm

61

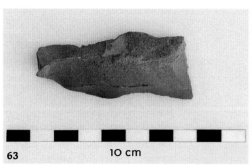

63   10 cm

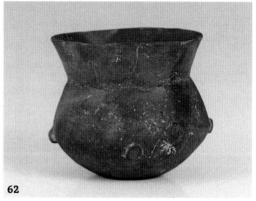

62

Fig. 61. Zengővárkony, grave no. 355. Photo: Sinkó Anikó.

Fig. 62. Zengővárkony, grave no. 365. Photo: Sinkó Anikó.

Fig. 63. Zengővárkony, grave no. 366. Photo: Sinkó Anikó.

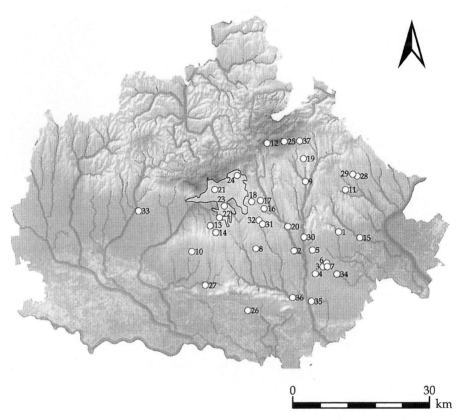

Fig. 64. Map of the Late Neolithic Lengyel Culture Sites around Pécs (SW-Hungary) (Szeverényi 2003, 48). 1. Babarc-Babarcpuszla, 2. Belvárdgyula-Szarka-hegy, 3. Borjád, M6/58, 4. Borjád-Kenderföld, 5. Bóly-Békás, 6. Bóly-Sziebert-puszta, 7. Bóly-Téglagyár, 8. Egerág-Hoszcú-földek, Kelet, 9. Erzsébet, 10. Görcsöny, 11. Himesháza-Rigó-dúló, 12. Hosszúhelény, 13. Keszü-Gyöngyösi csárda, 14. Kökény, 15. Lánycsók-Égettmalom, 16. Magyarsarlós-Kerekes-dúló, 17. Nagykozár, 18. Nagykozár-Zámájur-dúló. 19. Nagypall, 20. Olasz, 21. Pécs-Makárhegy, 22. Pécs-Málom, 23. Pécs-Megyeri réi, 24. Pécs-Szabolcs-Kedves u., 25. Pécsvárad-Aranyhegy, 26. Siklós-Kórház, 27. Szava, 28. Szebény-Farkaslik-dúló, 29. Szebény-Sajtos, 30. Szederkény, 31. Szemely-Hegyes, 32. Szemely-Bregova, 33. Szentlórinc, 34. Töttös-Téglagyár, 35. Villány-Virágos, 36. Villánykövesd, 37. Zengövárkony.

2.9.2 VILLÁNYKŐVESD

Grave no. 1: ?, flexed on right side, NW–SE. Bone awl, silex chisel (Dombay 1959, 61; fig. 65).

Grave no. 2: Female, flexed on left side, NE–SW. Pedestaled bowl, vessel, red paint piece, beads (made of shell, dent and copper) (Dombay 1959, 61; fig. 66).

Grave no. 3: Child, flexed on left side, NE–SW (Dombay 1959, 61).

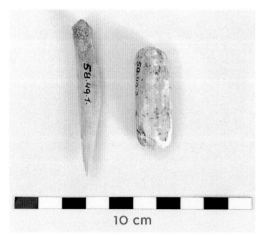

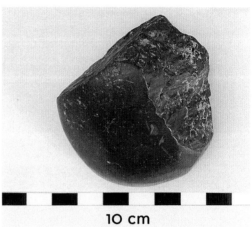

Fig. 65. Villánykővesd, grave no. 1. Photo: Sinkó Anikó.

Fig. 66. Villánykővesd, grave no. 2. Photo: Sinkó Anikó.

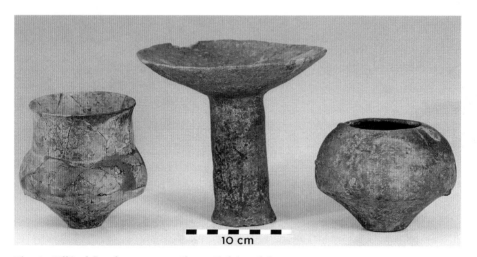

Fig. 67. Villánykővesd, grave no. 4. Photo: Sinkó Anikó.

Grave no. 5: Male, flexed on left side, NE–SW. Polished stone axe (Dombay 1959, 62).

Grave no. 7: Male, flexed on left side, NE–SW. Polished stone axe, stone chisel, chipped stone messer (Dombay 1959, 62; fig. 69).

Grave no. 8: Male, flexed on left side, NE–SW. Polished stone axe, chipped silex messer, vessel (Dombay 1959, 62; fig. 70).

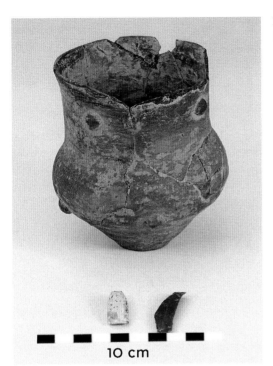

Fig. 68. Villánykövesd, grave no. 6.
Photo: Sinkó Anikó.

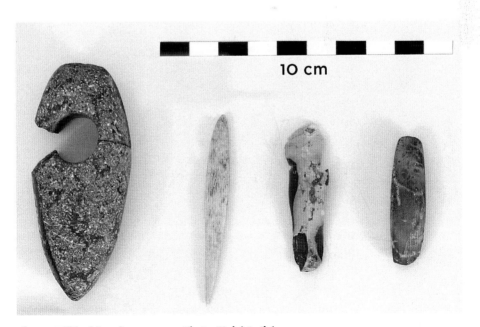

Fig. 69. Villánykővesd, grave no. 7. Photo: Sinkó Anikó.

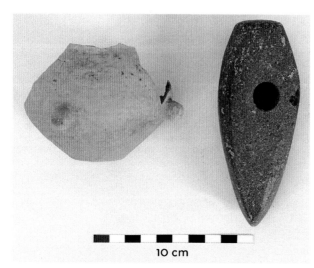

Fig. 70. Villánykővesd, grave no. 8. Photo: Sinkó Anikó.

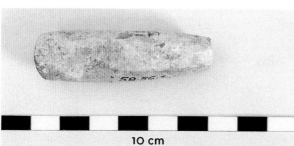

Fig. 71. Villánykővesd, grave no. 9. Photo: Sinkó Anikó.

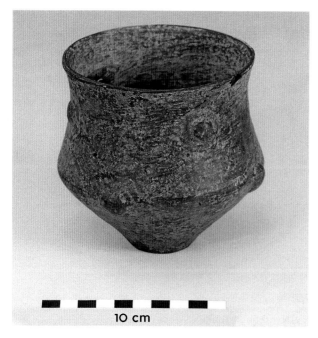

Fig. 72. Villánykővesd, grave no. 10. Photo: Sinkó Anikó.

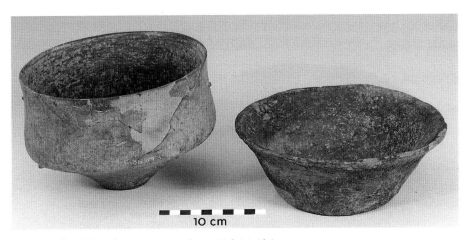

Fig. 73. Villánykővesd, grave no. 12. Photo: Sinkó Anikó.

Grave no. 9: ?, flexed on left side, NE–SW. Silex chisel, yellow clay (Dombay 1959, 62–63; fig. 71).

Grave no. 10: Female + baby, flexed left side, SE–NW. 3 vessels, bone needle, pedestaled bowl (Dombay 1959, 63; fig. 72).

Grave no. 12: ?, flexed on left side, NE–SW. 2 bowls, pedestaled bowl, vessel, dental beads, copper beads (Dombay 1959, 64; fig. 73).

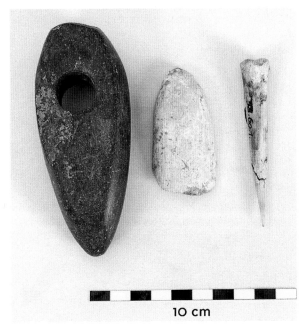

Fig. 74. Villánykővesd, grave no. 13. Photo: Sinkó Anikó.

Grave no. 13: Male, flexed on left side, NE–SW. Polished stone axe, polished stone messer, bone awl (Dombay 1959, 64; fig. 74).

Grave no. 14: Child, flexed on left side, NE–SW (Dombay 1959, 64).

Grave no. 16: Child, flexed on left side, E–W. Pedestaled bowl, 2 vessels, bone needle, polished stone axe (Dombay 1959, 64–65; fig. 75).

Grave no. 17: ?, flexed on right side, W–E (Dombay 1959, 65).

Grave no. 18: Child, flexed on left side, SE–NW. Vessel, shell bead (Dombay 1959, 65).

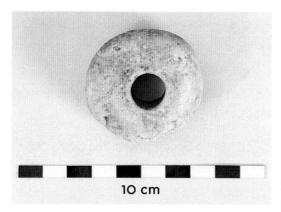

10 cm

Fig. 75. Villánykővesd, grave no. 16. Photo: Sinkó Anikó.

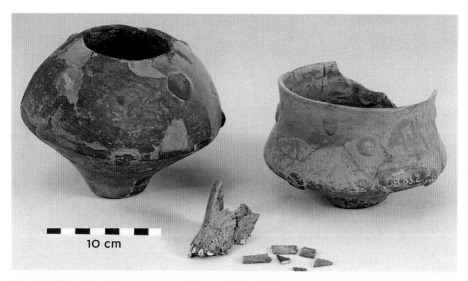

10 cm

Fig. 76. Villánykővesd, grave no. 20. Photo: Sinkó Anikó.

Grave no. 19: Child, flexed on right side, SW–NE (Dombay 1959, 65).

Grave no. 20: ?, flexed on left side, E–W. 2 vessels, bone needle, pig bone (Dombay 1959, 65; fig. 76).

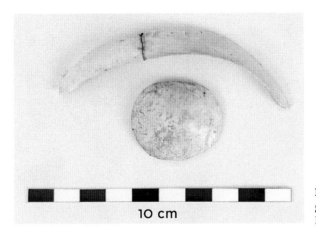

Fig. 77. Villánykővesd, grave no. 22.
Photo: Sinkó Anikó.

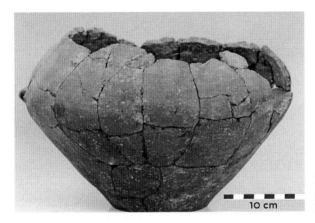

Fig. 78. Villánykővesd, grave no. 23.
Photo: Sinkó Anikó.

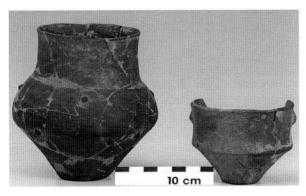

Fig. 79. Villánykővesd, grave no. 23.
Photo: Sinkó Anikó.

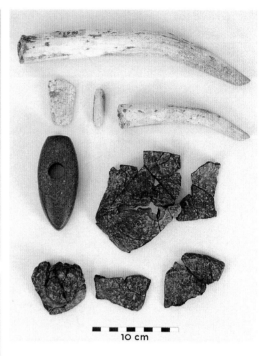

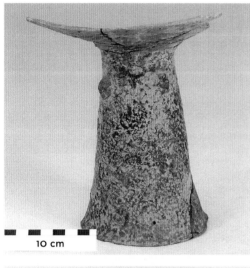

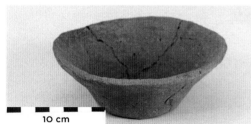

Fig. 80-82. Villánykővesd, grave no. 27.
Photo: Sinkó Anikó.

Grave no. 21: ?, Pedestaled bowl (Dombay 1959, 65).

Grave no. 22: ?, flexed on left side, E–W. Wild boar tusk, stone diadem, shell bead, vessel (Dombay 1959, 66; fig. 77).

Grave no. 23: ?, flexed on right side, SW–NE. 5 vessels (Dombay 1959, 65-66; fig. 78, 79).

Grave no. 24: Male. flexed on left side, E–W. Pedestaled bowl, vessel, polished stone axe, 2 chipped silex knife, chipped silex chisel, antler (Dombay 1959, 66).

Grave no. 25: Child, flexed on left side, SE–NW (Dombay 1959, 66).

Grave no. 26: Child, flexed on left side, SE–NW (Dombay 1959, 66-67).

Grave no. 27: Female, flexed on left side, NE–SW. Vessel, bowl, animal bone (Dombay 1959, 67; fig. 80-82).

3. LENGYEL CULTURE SITES IN BARANYA AND TOLNA COUNTY: PALEOPATHOLOGICAL, ANTHROPOLOGICAL AND ARCHAEOLOGICAL DESCRIPTION

3.1 ZENGŐVÁRKONY

3.1.1 PALAEOPATHOLOGICAL ANALYSIS
VÁCLAV SMRČKA, ZDENKA MUSILOVÁ, VÍTĚZSLAV KUŽELKA

The Lengyel Culture (LgC) includes the population migrating to Central Europe from South-East at the end of the Neolithic and the turn of Eneolithic (Chalcolithic) period. The Lengyel Culture was named after the eponymous type site, the enclosed settlement of Lengyel in Hungary, right of the Danube. To the South of this site, the burial site Zengővárkony was discovered by Dombay (1939, 1960) (fig. 1).

The burial site Zengővárkony originally comprised 368 graves in 14 grave groups, but only 64 were unearthed, i.e. slightly less than 18%.

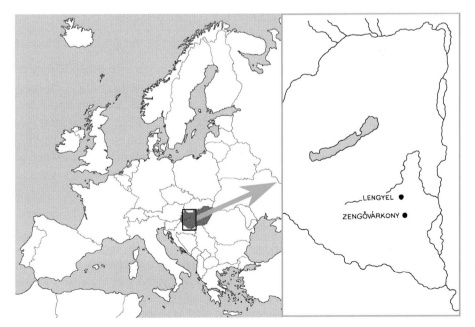

Fig. 1. Relation of the burial site at Zengővárkony to the eponymous site, the fenced settlement of Lengyel. Map: Jan Kacinský.

Our objective was to establish, using the skeletal material, a set of signs of diseases that would characterize the Lengyel population in Hungary and could serve as a tool of comparison to Moravian Painted Ware culture in Moravia, the successor of the LgC in Moravia (Smrčka, Tvrdý 2009).

During the exploratory research and literature search we found that the research done at Zengővárkony was a repeated palaeopathological research. The first palaeopathological description of the skeletons there was done by Gy. Regöly-Merei and another by L. Bartucz in 1966, and the resulting opinions of the two researchers differed. Thus it was necessary to revise and specify the diagnoses and perform a new classification according to the diseases. From the skeletons available (N = 59), we chose 31 skeletons where both the skull and postcranial skeleton were preserved. These were analysed in the spring of 2017 and preliminary results were published (Smrčka et al. 2018) The other incomplete burials that only contained the skull or postcranial skeleton alone (N28) were analysed at the second stage of the research, including their detailed statistic processing, in the autumn of 2017 and spring 2018.

The treated set of 59 skeletons at the Zengővárkony burial site included the remains of 25 men, 30 women, 3 children and one unidentified individual. Each skeleton was matched to the basic anthropologic data (age, sex and body height) taken from the publication by Zsuzsanna K. Zoffmann (1969), who had done the anthropologic research of the burial site.

PALAEOPATHOLOGICAL CHARACTERISTICS OF THE ANALYSED COHORT (N = 59)

The Lengyel burial site at Zengővárkony was processed at the depository of Janus Pannonius Muzeum in Pécs. The skeletons were examined macroskopically. The detected pathologic lesions were recorded in charts and documented in photographs. Together with description of the pathologies, we assessed the state of preservation of bones in the skeleton where the finding was established. This enabled us to calculate the prevalence of incidence of disease entities.

EXCESSIVE WORK STRAIN
BONE RIMS ON PHALANGES OF FINGERS

In 7 women, phalanges of fingers of the right hand were examined, and in four out of the total, bone rims on proximal phalanges were found (57% prevalence). In four women, phalanges of the left hand were examined, and in one of them the bone rims were found as well (25% prevalence).

The bone rims were due to excessive strain of short muscles of the hand, interosseous muscles and lumbricals of the hand, probably on weaving. At the same time, they testify to the working dominance of right hands in the women.

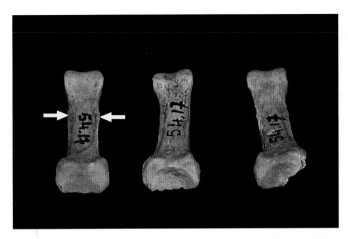

Fig. 2. Fringe 2 mm *bone rims* on *proximal phalanges* of the fingers in a woman in grave number 99. Photo: Zdenka Musilová.

In one man, bone rims on proximal phalanges of the right hand were found too.

Fringe 2-mm rims (fig. 2) occurred on the proximal phalanges of the fingers in graves number 90, 99, 88a and 336.

CONGENITAL ANOMALIES
AXIAL SKELETON (SKULL, VERTEBRAL COLUMN)
The total 41 skulls at the burial site (18 male, 22 female and 1 child's) were examined.

In the group of 20 skulls with well-preserved parietal bones at the burial site (8 male, 11 female and 1 child's), we found congenital anomalies with defects of fusion at the sutures.

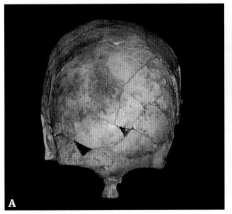
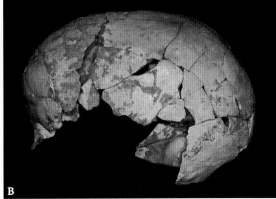

Fig. 3a–b. *Scaphocephaly*—A: front view in the 23-year-old woman from grave number 7. B: view from the left. Photo: Zdenka Musilová.

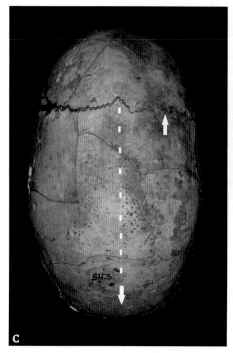

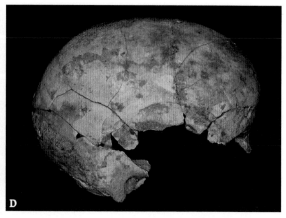

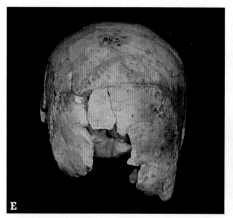

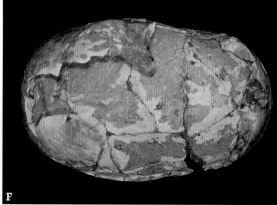

Fig. 3c–d. C: *Scaphocephaly* with agenesis of the sagittal suture in the 23-year-old woman from grave number 7. The arrows indicate the preserved sutures (coronal and lambdoidal), which direct the growth in longitudinal direction. D: view from the right. Photo: Zdenka Musilová.

Fig. 3e–f. *Scaphocephaly*—E: view of the occipital region with the preserved lambdoid suture. F: view of the inner surface of the calvaria with the blood vessel imprints. Photo: Zdenka Musilová.

These included craniosynostosis, *scaphocephaly* (5.6% prevalence) with premature fusion of the sagittal suture (figs. 3a, 3b, 3c, 3d, 3e, 3f). The skull, thanks to the preserved coronal and lambdoid sutures, continued growing lengthwise (fig. 3c).

In one case, a man aged 40-80 years (grave number 125), *oxycephaly* was found (with 5.6% prevalence).

In a man aged 29-33 years (grave 104) and another man aged 52-55 years (grave 338), *batrocephaly* was identified (with 11.1% prevalence).

In a woman aged 30-59 years (grave 281), *metopism* was found (with 4.5%prevalence). In a man aged 40-80 years (in grave number 238), an interstitial *Inca bone* was found (with 5.6% prevalence). So was one in a woman, aged 40-80 years, in grave number 6 (with prevalence 4, 5%).

In another woman, aged 16-17 years (in grave number 62), the cervical vertebrae were covered with calcareous crust, however, *Klippel-Feil syndrome* with fusion of cervical vertebrae cannot be excluded.

The lower jaw bones examined were 22 in number (8 in men, 11 in women and 3 in children). Congenital deformity asymmetry of the head of the right jaw articulation was described in a man, aged 30-59 years (grave 355). The head of the right jaw articulation is of an altered oval shape (12.5% prevalence).

VERTEBRAL COLUMN

In a man, aged 38-48 years (grave 325), a congenitally *cleft sacral bone* was found.

EXTREMITIES

The bones of the forearm, the radius and ulna, were examined bilaterally in men (right in 11, left in 13 individuals) as well as in women (16 on the left and

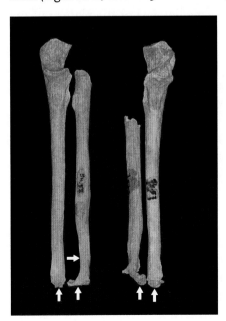

Fig. 4a. *Bilateral amputation* of bones of the forearm in a man, aged 30-59 years, in grave number 345. Photo: Zdenka Musilová.

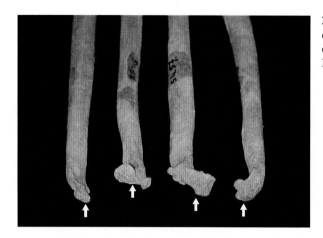

Fig. 4b. Narrowing and dish-like deformity of distal ends of the bones of the forearm. Photo: Zdenka Musilová.

16 on the right) and in one child, left. In one man of the cohort, aged 39–59 years (grave 345), *amputation of both forearms*, probably congenital, was found (with 9.1% prevalence on the right and 7.7% on the left forearm) (figs. 4a, 4b).

DEFORMITIES DUE TO ARTHROSIS

TEMPOROMANDIBULAR JOINT

Development of the changes due to arthrosis in the area of the socket of the temporomandibular joint (in the man, aged 30–50 years, from the grave number 355) was caused by the asymmetry of the socket of the temporomandibular joint. In the same skeleton, *alabaster gloss* was observed on the medial condyle of the right femur (fig. 5) and the medial part of the plateau of the right tibia, with 3 mm osteophytes in its surroundings.

VERTEBRAL OSTEOPHYTES

Cervical vertebrae were examined in 14 individuals (6 men, 7 women and 1 child). Out of them, 2 mm osteophytes were found in 3 men (with 50% prevalence), but in one child as well.

The lumbar part of the vertebral column was examined in 16 individuals (6 men, 9 women and one child). Osteophytes sized 2 mm affected one man (16.7% prevalence) and 4–10 mm osteophytes were found in six women (with 66.7% prevalence).

In the part cervical of the vertebral column we found 3–5 mm osteophytes in two men.

Spondylosis with 2 mm osteophytes occurred on thoracic vertebrae in a man aged 52–55 years (in grave number 338). Osteophytes sized 3 mm were present on the vertebrae of the lower part of the lumbar portion of the spine in a woman aged 50–56 years (in grave number 337), and larger than 5 mm on the caudal five lumbar vertebrae of another woman, aged 62–75 years (in

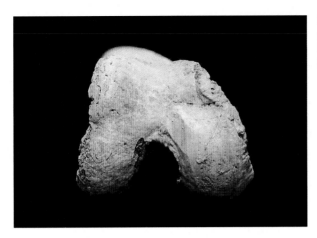

Fig. 5. *Arthrotic alabaster gloss* on the right femur in grave number 355. Photo: Zdenka Musilová.

grave number 341). In the same woman we found *rhizoarthrosis* of a phalanx of the thumb.

The most pronounced changes due to *spondylosis* (vertebral osteophytosis) with 3–5 mm osteophytes were found in the man, aged 48–58 years (grave number 5).

ARTHROSIS OF THE FEMUR

The total number of 81 femurs were examined, 37 in men (19 right, 18 left), 41 in women (23 right and 18 left) and 3 in children (1 right and 2 left).

In the right femur of a man, aged 30–59 years (grave 355) (fig. 5), there is *alabaster gloss* due to grinding (with 5.3% prevalence), and in the right femur of a woman aged 62–75 years (grave 341), a 4 mm arthrotic rim is present (4–3% prevalence).

ARTHROSIS OF THE TIBIA

The total number of 72 tibias were examined, 35 tibias in men (18 right and 17 left), 34 tibias in women (17 right and 17 left), 3 tibias in children (1 right and 2 left).

On medial part of the right tibia (man, aged 30–59 years, grave 355) alabaster gloss was seen with 5.6% prevalence.

ARTHROSIS OF THE FIBULA

The total number of 28 fibulas were examined, 15 fibulas in men (8 right, 7 left), 13 fibulas in women (7 right and 6 left).

In fibulas we did not find any lesions due to arthrosis.

On other part of the skeleton, arthrosis occurred on the right patella, rhizoarthrosis in a woman on the 1st metacarpal of the right thumb, and on the pelvic bone in another woman.

TRAUMA

At the said burial site, 53 parietal bones of skulls were examined, including 20 male (10 right and 10 left), 30 female (15 right and 15 left) and 3 children's (2 right and 1 left).

In the left parietal region of a man, aged 30–42 years (grave 314), an artificial orifice was found, probably caused by a *trauma* (with 10% prevalence), sized 25 × 12 mm (fig. 6a).

On the inside of the skull around the opening, there are well-visible splinters that are characteristic of a hit (fig. 6b). Location of the wound in the left parietal region suggests a right-handed attacker. A photo of the edge of the orifice taken in a slanting angle clearly shows the one-millimetre reparation rim on the edge of the bone (fig. 6c), which suggests survival for at least *3 months*. The injury was probably inflicted with a slender axe-hammer of the Lengyel type.

Another traumatic lesion was found in a woman, aged between 40 and 80 years (obj. 54–59). On the skull, there are two traumatic lesions. One is an *impression fracture* in the right temporoparietal region (25 × 15 mm) with the

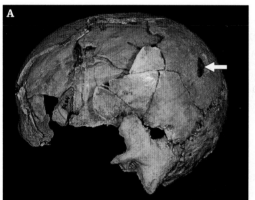

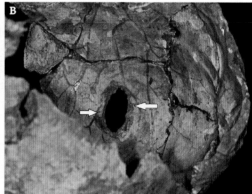

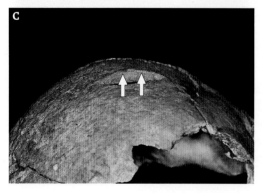

Fig. 6a–c. A: *Injury in the left parietal region* in a man, aged 36–42 years, in grave number 314. B: Injury in grave number 314—chipping on the internal surface of the cranial wall. C: Injury in grave number 314—the milimetre rim at the edge of the orifice suggests survival for at least 3 months. Photo: Zdenka Musilová.

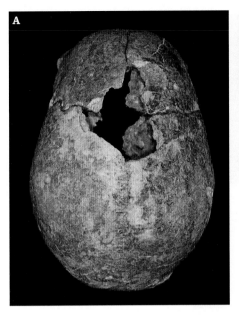

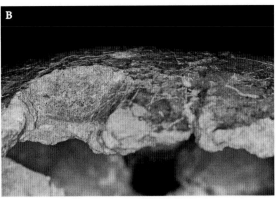

Fig. 7a–b. A: *Impressive fracture* in a woman, aged 40–80 years (object 54–59). B: Separation of a 60 × 20 mm fragment with a fracture in a woman, aged 40–80 years (54–59). Photo: Zdenka Musilová.

pressed into the cranial cavity as deep as 8 mm (fig. 7a). In the other case, a fragment sized 60 × 20 mm is broken off right to the foramen magnum along the lambdoid suture, with a fracture into the right parietal region (fig. 7b) (with 13.3% prevalence).

On examination of 81 femurs, including 37 male ones (19 right and 18 left), in a man aged 30–39 years (in grave number 84) we found an *unhealed fracture* of the middle and upper portion of the right thigh bone (fig. 8).

INFLAMMATIONS
PERIOSTITIS OF THE CALCANEUS
In women, we examined 13 left and 12 right calcaneus bones, without detecting any periostitis. In men, 6 right and 8 left calcaneus bones were examined,

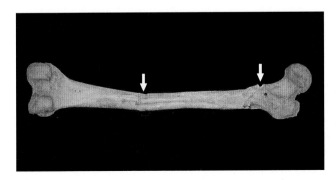

Fig. 8. *Unhealed fracture* of the middle and upper portion of the thigh bone in a man, aged 30–39 years (grave number 84). Photo: Zdenka Musilová.

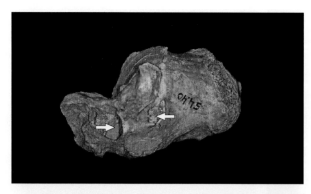

Fig. 9. *Specific inflammation, probably of TB origin,* affecting the heel bone of a man, aged 38–48 years, in grave number 325. Photo: Zdenka Musilová.

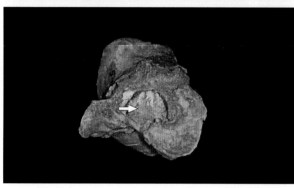

Fig. 10. Tuberculosis in grave number 325—short and straight fistulas with TB lesion to the tarsal bone, type *"spina ventosa."* Photo: Zdenka Musilová.

and periostitis was only found on one left calcaneus, in a man aged 38–48 years (grave 325). This is probably a *specific inflammation due to tuberculosis* (fig. 9), with 12.5%prevalence.

In the same individual, also the tarsal bone showed a lesion of the type of *"spina ventosa"* with a short straight fistula (fig. 10).

PERIOSTITIS OF THE RIBS
Ribs were examined in 4 men, 11 women and 2 children. Periostitis was only found in one child (grave 316, age 7–8 years) at the outer part of the rib, with 50% prevalence.

PERITOSTIS OF THE TIBIA
In men, 19 right tibias were examined to find one case of periostitis (with 5.2% prevalence), and also examined were 20 left tibias with one periostitis (5% prevalence).

In women, 18 right tibias were examined, none of which were affected by periostitis, and left tibias examined were 18 in number as well, with one periostitis on the upper part of the left tibia, sized 80 × 35 mm, in a 46-to-55-year-old womanin grave number 13 (5.6% prevalence).

In total, 37 right tibias were examined, with on case of periostitis found (2.7% prevalence) and 38 left tibias with 2 cases of periostitis, with 5.3% prevalence.

PERIOSTITIS OF THE FIBULA

In men, 10 right and 8 left fibulas were examined, and no periostitis was found.

In women, 9 right fibulas were examined with no periostitis and 7 left fibulas with one case of periostitis, with 14.3% prevalence.

In total, 19 right fibulas without periostitis and 15 left ones with one case of periostitis (6.7% prevalence) were examined.

TUMOURS

In a woman, aged 62-75 years (grave number 341), the blood vessel imprints and large pacchionian granulations are marked intracranially in the occipital region (fig. 11). In our opinion, it is *meningioma*.

CRIBRA ORBITALIA

In Zengővárkony we examined 3 right and 3 left children's orbits. *Cribra orbitalia* were not found in these children.

In women, five right orbits were examined (with one case of cribrification of the *2nd type* and one of the *3rd type*; with 40% prevalence) and six left orbits (with two cases of cribrification of the *2nd type* and one of the *3rd type*; with 50% prevalence) (fig. 12).

In men, six right orbits (with one case of cribrification of the *1st type* and two of the *2nd type*; with 50% prevalence) and six left orbits (with one case of cribrification of the *1st type* and two of the *2nd type*; with 50% prevalence) were examined.

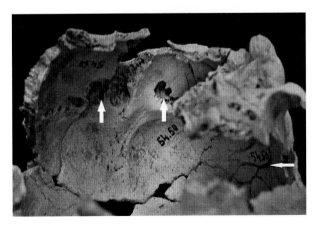

Fig. 11. *Meningioma* in the occipital region in a woman, aged 62-75 years, in grave number 341. Photo: Zdenka Musilová.

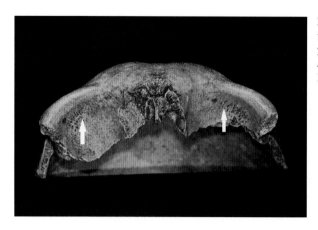

Fig. 12. *"Cribra orbitalia" type 2* in the woman, aged 39–45 years, in a woman, aged 40–80, in grave number 34. Photo: Zdenka Musilová.

Out of the total 14 right orbits, five were affected by cribrification 5 (35% prevalence), and in 15 left orbits, six skulls were affected (40% prevalence), and only women reached the *typu 3* cribrification.

DENTAL ABRASION

Dental abrasion allows estimation of the age (Dobisíková 1999; Lovejoy 1985). In our case, however, the abrasion did not correspond to the age. We classified the degree of dental abrasion in three types. Type 1 includes the degrees 0, 1, 2 of the classical six-point scale, type 2 the degrees 3 and 4, and type 3 degrees 5 and 6 on the six-point scale.

Therefore, type 1 included the cases with no abrasion (degree 0), abrasion within the enamel (degree 1), and exposure of the dentine at the top of the cusps (degree 2).

Type 2 means exposure of dentine on the whole occlusion surface (degree 3) or abrasion progressing into the pulp cavity of the crown (degree 4).

Type 3 is abrasion also affecting the area of the neck of the tooth (degree 5), or even the pulp cavity of the root (degree 6).

In 30 individuals at the burial site, the teeth of the upper and lower jaws were examined (in 11 men, 17 women and 2 children).

MEN

In four men out of the 11 examined, *type 2* abrasion was found in three cases and *type 3* in one case (with 36.4% prevalence).

Type 2 abrasion was found in men in the following graves: in grave 368 a man aged 30–59 years; in grave 355 another aged 30–59 years too; and in grave 135 the man's age was 40–80 years.

Type 3 abrasion was found in a man aged 40–80 years (in grave 120). Another man aged 40–80 years (in grave 125) showed excessive alveolar resorption and multiple dental abscesses.

It is obvious that *type 2 abrasion* occurs in men of the LgC after the age of 30 years, and *type 3 abrasion* after the age of 40.

WOMEN

In four cases out of the 17 women examined, *type 1 abrasion* was found in one woman, *type 2 abrasion* in one woman as well, and *type 3* in two women (with 23.5% prevalence).

Type 1 abrasion was found in a woman in grave 88a (age 53-57 years) (fig. 13a).

Type 2 abrasion occurred in a woman in grave 87 (age 51-57 years) (fig. 13b).

Type 3 abrasion was found in two women, one in grave 341, age 62-75 years (fig. 13c), and the other in grave 6, age 40-80 years. In one woman, aged

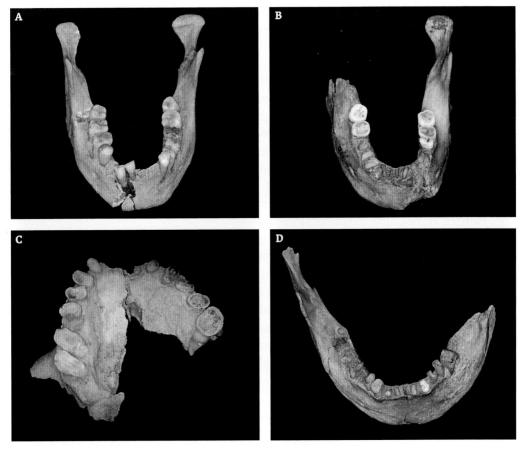

Fig. 13a–d. A: *Type 1 dental abrasion* in a woman, aged 53-57 years, in grave number 88a. B: *Type 2 dental abrasion* in a woman, aged 51-57 years, in grave number 87. C: *Type 3 dental abrasion* in a woman, aged 62-75 years, in grave number 341. D: *Type 3 dental abrasion* in woman 62-75, in grave number 341 (mandible). Photo: Zdenka Musilová.

50–56 years (grave 337), a narrow-vaulted palate occurred (with 5.9% prevalence).

Type 1 and type 2 abrasion occurred in women after 50, but *type 3* only in a woman after 40 years of age as well as after the age of 60 years. The most serious *type 3 abrasion* did not depend on the age.

DISCUSSION

In terms of body height, the Lengyel population was one of the shortest Neolithic populations in Europe. Using the measurement according to Manouvrier, K.-Zs. Zoffmann (1969–1970) measured the average height 164 cm in 14 male skeletons, and 151 cm in 16 female skeletons, but women who were only 145 cm tall were no exception.

In the skeletons, the bones of extremities were well-preserved but the skulls and especially their facial parts were much worse preserved.

EXCESSIVE WORK STRAIN
BURIAL RITES WITH INTERMENT OF SKULLS
For palaeopathological examination we only chose complete skeletons, 31 in number. In other more than twenty graves, either skulls alone or headless skeletons were buried. This corresponds to our knowledge of the Moravian Painted Ware Culture in Moravia, where ancestors' skulls were exhibited in homes and then probably buried separately. This custom probably survived in the whole migrating population of the Lengyel culture, both in the area of present-time Hungary and in the successor population of the Moravian Painted Ware Culture (Podborský 1993).

BONE RIMS ON PHALANGES OF THE FINGERS
Bone *rims on the base phalanges* are caused by excessive strain of interosseous muscles (mm. interossei) and lumbricals, which flex the proximal phalanges but at the same time extend the medial and distal ones.

2-mm rims on the borders of the bone (fig. 2) occurred on proximal phalanges of the fingers in the graves number 90, 99, 88a and 336.

In 7 women, phalanges of the right hand were examined, and four of them showed bone rims on the proximal phalanges (57% prevalence). In four women, phalanges of the left hand were examined, and one of them showed the bone rims as well (with 25% prevalence).

The movement pattern that with excessive strain on the short interosseous muscles and lumbricals of the hand caused the development of bone rims on proximal phalanges of the fingers would suggest making the clothes—weaving and sewing. At the same time, it is an indicator of the right hand dominance at work in Lengyel women.

Bone rims on proximal phalanges of the right hand were observed in on man as well.

Bone rims on medial phalanges—"phalanx flexor hypertrophy"—caused by extensive strain of the superficial flexor of the hand (m. flexor digitorum superficialis), which flexes the medial phalanges of the 2nd to 5th finger, were not observed in the Lengyel population.

WEAVING OF FABRICS, SEWING

Weaving of fabrics must have been a female activity, considering the pronounced bone rims at the edges of the palmar side of the proximal phalanges.

In the LPC population from the burial site at Vedrovice, the percentage of adult individuals with bone rims on the phalanges of finger even exceeded 80% (Dočkalová 2008). It is likely that production of textile employed a good part of the population in the Linear Pottery Culture, probably women and children, and the fibres that were processed were probably obtained from nettles.

In the LgC at Zengővárkony, a 25% prevalence of bone rims on the proximal phalanges of fingers. This biological evidence of weaving, proving extra strain of interosseous muscles on the phalanges of fingers, also corresponds to archaeological evidence of this activity from the finds at Zengővárkony, where Čermáková (2007) found a number of graves with funerary gifts of needles and awls.

These artefacts, connected with textile production, were most typical of female graves, and so were the bone rims on phalanges of the fingers. By and large, male graves with needles and awls were less common, nevertheless in grave number 314 even a set of two pieces was discovered.

The Lengyel population (LgC) had to dress as much as the Linear Pottery (LPC) population. Then, how to explain the fact that weaving of fabrics in the LgC was by nearly four times reduced as compared to the LPC?

One explanation may be the increased use of fur and leather for clothes in the LgC, which is indicated by the increased incidence of dental abrasion at Zengővárkony.

DENTAL ABRASION

In 30 individuals at the burial site, the teeth of the upper as well as lower jaws were examined (in men 11, in women 17 and in children 2). Under our assessment of abrasion using the above three types it is obvious that *type 2 abrasion* occurs in men of the LgC after the thirtieth year of age, and *type 3 abrasion* after the age of 40 years.

In women, *type 1 and type 2 abrasion* occurred after the age of 50 years, but *type 3* was found in a woman over 40 as well as in another over 60 years.

DENTAL ABRASION AND PROCESSING OF LEATHER

At the burial site of Zengővárkony, the highest degrees of dental abrasion were found, above all, in old women, the most in one at the age between 62 and 75 years (fig. 11).

An anonymous reviewer reminded us (Smrčka et al. 2018) that the excessive dental abrasion may have been due to processing of leather. This is also suggested by the fact that it mainly occurred in elderly women, it was roof-shaped and parallel in upper and lower teeth, with a higher lingual and lower buccal position, and the teeth with abrasion showed dark pigmentation.

This biological finding and evidence of the process of leather production in the Lengyel population, however, had to be supported by archaeological evidence as well. On detailed research into funeral equipment from the LgC burial site at Zengővárkony it was revealed that the number of scraping tools found in female graves (N = 3; 6.82%) and children's graves (N = 2; 4.35%) was much higher than in male graves (N = 1; 1.56%). According to the author (Čermáková 2007), this probably testifies to the fact of domiciliary production of leather, in which particularly the two said groups participated.

If both biological and archaeological evidence seems to confirm the fact of processing of leather, then the following question arises naturally: How was the process performed and what was the tanned and processed leather used for?

The first part of the question can only be answered through ethnographic comparison with the populations that processed skins. Nansen (1891, 80) described the use of the teeth by Eskimo women on production of leather:

> On the whole, the Greenland women make great use of their teeth, now to stretch the skins, now to hold them while they are being scraped, and again for the actual scraping. It is rather startling to us Europeans to see them take up a skin out of the tub of fetid liquor in which it has been steeping, and straightaway fix their teeth in it and begin to dress it. The mouth, in fact, is a third hand to them, and therefore the front teeth of old Eskimo women are often worn away to the merest stumps.

Nansen (1891, 78) also described the process of chewing on preparation of skins and the men's role in this work:

> The operator takes the dry skin, almost dripping with fat, and chews away at one spot until all the fat is sucked out and the skin is soft and white; then the chewing area is slowly widened, the skin gradually retreating further and further into the mouth, until it often disappears entirely, to be spat out again at last with every particle of fat chewed away. This industry is for the most part carried on by the women and children, and is very highly relished by reason of the quantity of fat it enables them to absorb. In times of scarcity, the men are often glad enough to be allowed to do their share.

If the sealskins are to be used for kamiks (shoes), the blubber and the inner layer of the skin itself are scraped away with a crooked knife (ulo) upon a board made for the purpose out of a whale's shoulder blade. When the skin has been scraped thin it is steeped for a day or so in stale urine until the hairs can be plucked off with a knife. This done, the skin is stretched, by means of small bone pegs, upon the earth or the snow, and dried. Then it is rubbed until it is soft, and the process is complete. As this sort of skin has its outer membrane intact, it is of a dark colour.

White kamik-skins are prepared up to a certain point like the foregoing, but when the hairs have been removed they are dipped in warm water (not too warm) until the black membrane is loosened, and then steeped in sea water, as cold as possible. If all the membrane is not removed, the skin is again dipped alternately in warm water and sea water until it comes away. Then the skin is pegged out and dried like the black skin.

The white skins, not being as strong and watertight as the black, are used almost entirely by women, who either keep them white or dye them in different ways.

Sole leather for the kamiks is prepared in the same way as the black kaiak-skin, but is pegged out while drying.

Kaiak-skins are dressed either black or white.

The black skin (erisak) is obtained by scraping the blubber from the under side of the skin while it is fresh, and then steeping it in for a day or two in stale urine, until the hairs can be plucked out with a knife. These being removed, the skin is rinsed in sea water, and in summer it is then dried, but not in the sun. in winter, it is not dried, but if possible preserved by being buried in snow. Whether in summer or winter, however, it is best if, immediately after being washed, it can be stretched on the kaiak so as to dry upon the framework. These skins are dark because the grain or outer membrane of the skin of the seal is either black or dark brown.

White kaiak-skins (únek) are prepared in this way: While they are quite fresh, and after the blubber has been roughly removed, they are rolled up and in a tolerably warm place either of of doors or in. There they lie until the hairs and the outer membrane can easily be scraped away with a mussel-shell. For this purpose, however, the Greenland beauties generally prefer to use their teeth, since they can thus suck out a certain amount of blubber, which they consider delicious. Then, in summer, the skins are hung up to dry—not in the sun—upon a wooden rail, and are often turned in order that they may dry evenly. In winter they are preserved. Like the black skins, in the snow. The dark membrane being scraped away, these skins are quite light-coloured or white when they are finished.

Using Nansen's observations, we could speculate about similar use of large dark skins for roofs of houses or shelters and smaller skins for foot ware and articles of clothing.

CONGENITAL DEFECTS

CONGENITAL AMPUTATION OF THE FOREARM

In the above mentioned man (30–59 years, in grave number 345), atrophied and badly deformed distal end of the bones of the forearm in both arms (fig. 4a). In the first anthropological description of the skeleton of 1960 (Dombay) there is no mention of metacarpals and small bones of the hands in the material preserved.

It follows from the above that it was a case of amputation of both hands at the wrist. Another question is whether the amputation was congenital or traumatic.

In our view, hypoplasia of both bones of the forearm and their dish-like bend (figure 4b) suggest *bilateral congenital amputation of the forearm, transversal defect in the distal part of the forearm* (classification Swanson 1976, Ogino 2000, Oberg et al. 2010).

This type of congenital amputation, once called meromelia (Barnes 2012), occurs rarely. More often are amputations found in the proximal and medial thirds of the forearm, and the bone ends are sometimes fused (Gladykowska-Rzeczycka and Mazurek 2009).

The social environment in this Neolithic culture allowed the individual with bilateral amputation of hands to survive to adulthood.

However, amputation as a form of punishment or other incident in early childhood cannot be completely excluded either, with distal deformities shaped within the period of growth acceleration.

TRAUMAS

PENETRATING SKULL TRAUMA

On the skull of a man, aged 36–42 years (grave number 314), an orifice, sized 25 × 12 mm can be found in the left parietal region, which in 1960 was ascribed by Regöly-Merei to post-mortem trephining. L. Bártucz, on the next examination in 1966, found "chippings" on the internal lamina and concluded that the injury was caused before the death, probably by a stone axe (fig. 6b).

On the internal surface of the skull around the orifice, distinct bone chips can be found which characterize a hit (fig. 6b). Location of the wound orifice in the left parietal region suggests a right-handed attacker. A photo of the edge of the orifice taken in a slanting angle clearly shows the one-millimetre reparation rim on the edge of the bone (fig. 6c), which suggests survival for at least 3 months. The injury was probably inflicted with a slender axe-hammer of the Lengyel type.

FRACTURE OF THE THIGH BONE

Apart from the injury to the skull in the 30 to 39-year-old man (in grave number 84), an unhealed fracture of the upper part of the right femur was found (fig. 8).

NON-SPECIFIC INFLAMMATION

Periostitis measuring 100 × 60 mm was discovered in the left part of the occipital pit of a woman, aged 27–34 in grave no. 45 (54.7) and would have manifested as *meningitis*.

Periodontitis with multiple abscesses in the upper jaw was found in a male, aged 40–80, in grave 125 (54.23). The skull of this individual was keel shaped, which is indicative of congenital *oxycephaly*.

Otitis media was described in a woman, aged 39–45, in grave no. 34 (54.8).

Periostitis of rib was discovered in grave no. 316 (54.35) in a child, aged 7–8. Tuberculosis and brucellosis are possible aetiologies of this periostitis.

Tibial periostitis was found in a woman, aged 46–55, in grave no. 13 (54.4) and in a man, aged 36–46, in grave no. 108 (54.21). This was found to be an example of the *striated type of periostitis*, measuring 130 × 30 mm in the left tibia and 150 × 30 mm in the right.

Fibular periostitis was discovered in a woman, aged 35–55, in grave no. 342 (54.54).

TUBERCULOSIS INFLAMMATION

Obvious is the relation between inflammatory changes and *periostitis* on the skeleton (Gladykowska-Rzeczycka and Mazurek 2009). In the calcaneous and tarsal bones of a man, aged 38–48 years (from grave number 325), Regöly-Merei in 1960 presumed arthritic changes. When we compared this finding to a similar case in our atlas (Smrčka, Kuželka, and Povýšil 2009), it was clear it was a specific tuberculosis inflammation (figs. 9 and 10) with short fistulas, without complicated pockets (Hoppe and Polívka 1968, 108) and with changes of the type of "spina ventosa" (Smrčka et al. 2018).

MENINGIOMA

The changes in a woman, aged 62–75 years (grave number 341), were described as a tumour by Regöly-Merei in 1960. Considering our finding of medieval trephining with the same type of meningioma in the calvaria of Sedlčany (Smrčka et al. 2003), here we also presume development of meningioma in elderly age. Another example of this type of tumour was discovered in a woman, aged 40–80, in grave no. 6 (54.2); this was a left sided meningioma displaying the same features as the calva of Sedlčany, occurring alongside multiple arachnoid granulations in the area of the sagittal sinus. Meningioma in a younger age produces hyperostosis on the skull.

WOMEN'S METALLIC ORNAMENTS

Women wore ear-rings and neck collars or other ornaments on the neck. On nipple-like projections of skulls, we identified several instances of copper corrosion (graves number 88a, 88b and 87). On the first three thoracic vertebrae, where a metallic neck collar was probably worn, we found copper corrosion in grave number 88.

Beads of copper were confirmed archaeologically by Čermáková (2007) in 10 graves at Zengővárkony (25%). She states that if the dead person had more jewels, then one of them were nearly always beads, and copper ornaments were related to women endowed with rich funeral gifts.

CONCLUSION

In the survey of pathological findings on 59 skeletons from the burial site of the Neolithic Lengyel culture at the location of Zengővárkony, there were found congenital defects, arthrotic deformities, traumas, inflammations, tumours, manifestations of anaemia and changes due to excessive work strain.

Of congenital defects, inborn amputation of both hands in the area of the forearm was found (right with 9.1% prevalence, left with 7.7% prevalence) and craniosynostosis of the type of scaphocephaly (5.6% prevalence), oxycephaly (5.6% prevalence) and batrocephaly (with 11.1% prevalence).

Arthrotic deformities occurred in the area of the temporomandibular joint and knee joint.

Spondylotic changes in the form of vertebral osteophytosis mainly affected the thoracic and lumbar spine (with 2 mm osteophytes in a man, with 16.7% prevalence, and 4–10 mm osteophytes in 6 women, with 66.7% prevalence), when the size of the osteophytes in the thoracic portion reached 2 mm, and in lumbar portion 3–5 mm.

Of the traumas, one special group was injuries to the head, both penetrating (with 10% prevalence) and non-penetrating (with 13.3% prevalence) and an unhealed fracture of the upper part of the thigh bone.

Of inflammations, specific tuberculosis inflammation of the tarsals of the type "spina ventosa" (with 12.5% prevalence) occurred, as well as periostosis on a rib and shin bone (prevalence 2.7% on the right and 5.3% on the left).

Of tumours, meningioma in the occipital region was detected. Out of the signs of anaemia, "cribra orbitalia" occurred bilaterally in the vault of the orbit (with 35% prevalence in the left orbit and 40% in the right), of which one case was type I and two type 2, but type 3 was only found in women.

Excessive strain on short muscles of the hand—interosseals and lumbricals—caused the occurrence of fringe 2 mm bone rims on proximal phalanges of the fingers, mainly on the dominant right hand in Lengyel women, which testifies to weaving of fabrics for clothes or making fisher nets.

Increased dental abrasion, which does not correlate with the age but rather with the archaeological findings of gifts, is probably connected with leather industry in the population of the Lengyel culture.

3.1.2 GENDER ROLES OF THE MAKERS OF THE LENGYEL CULTURE IN TERMS OF THE ZENGŐVÁRKONY GRAVE FINDS
EVA ČERMÁKOVÁ

INTRODUCTION

The possibilities of gender role reconstruction of the makers of the Lengyel cultural complex based on grave finds, especially from the Hungarian Zengővárkony burial site, are examined in this paper. The text is based on a more detailed study on gender roles of the Upper Neolithic in general, and the origins and development of gender archaeology (Čermáková 2007, 207–255).

METHOD

The study of gender roles based on analysis of burial complexes places specific demands on the selection of sources. Only a limited number of individuals is suitable for further processing. The bodies need to be well preserved and their sex, and potentially age, anthropologically determined. Only a restricted number of such individuals exists within the Lengyel complex. At the outset, I decided to assess a larger grave collection, in which the closest possible time-space connection can be presumed, thus allowing for a representation of the society at a given stage of development. This demand is best met by burial sites. The original idea of combined assessment of sources distant in both space and time (yet within the Lengyel complex) would have probably led to a distorted idea of the society of the era, particularly, considering the regional differentiation of the culture. Findings acquired through the analysis of one burial site, no matter how specific in terms of time and space, allow for a "case study" of the Neolithic society. The Zengővárkony burial site was chosen for my analysis as it contains a relatively large number of individuals allowing for a suitable database to be created. My results are compared by analogy with other Lengyel or Neolithic sites and burials. However, these other sites are primarily mentioned for illustration as sufficiently detailed or linguistically accessible publications are lacking.

LENGYEL GRAVES AS OBJECTS OF GENDER STUDIES

Throughout the Neolithic, a phenomenon referred to by Hodder as the "invisibility of death" (Hodder 1990, 72) is encountered to great extent. Considering the density of Lengyel settlements, the corresponding amounts of burials, especially in its Western part, are lacking. In the case of Eastern settlements, death becomes slightly more visible. Slovak (Svodín) and especially Hungarian (Zengővárkony, Aszód, Morágy-Tüzködomb) locations with Lengyel burial sites provide valuable sources for learning about the society of the era. Nevertheless, even here caution is necessary. Apparently, even in these areas only a fraction of the population was inhumed. Unfortunately, the incentives for inhuming one individual and cremating another, or (and that is probably the case of majority) treating the corpse in a different manner without leaving any traces, are unknown to us.

It is therefore necessary to admit that it is not known whether inhumation was a privilege or fate of a specific part of the population. In any case, inhumations provide such valuable information about Neolithic individuals that they cannot be disregarded by pointing out their limited representativeness of the living population.

GRAVE UNITS DATA ASSESSMENT

The Zengővárkony site is found in the southern part of Hungarian Transdanubia. J. Dombay's research from the 1930's and 40's uncovered a large settlement intertwined with groups of graves. Zengővárkony has become one of the most famous Lengyel burial sites ever, both for its indisputable importance, but also for the high quality and linguistic accessibility of presentation (Dombay 1960).

Out of the total of 367 inhumed, 64 males, 44 females and 46 children could be identified. That is a total of 154 individuals suitable for more detailed analysis. In the remaining cases, information about sex or age could not be determined usually due to the bad condition of the skeleton. From the cases of multiple burials, triple burial no. 88, containing the remains of two women and one child, three double burials (no. 101, 119 and 275) containing the remains of two females and a child, one double burial of a male and child (no. 114), one double burial with a male and a female (no. 113) and one double burial containing a child and an unidentified individual (no. 115), were considered.

Position, orientation and possible evidence of skull manipulation were observed in the interred individuals together with the number, distribution and character of grave goods. Results of statistical analysis are presented below. The significance of grave goods is elaborated in a special subchapter.

Tab. 1. Position on the right / left side—Zengővárkony.

	Left side	Right side	?
men	60 (93.35%)	3 (4.69%)	1 (1.56%)
women	42 (95.45%)	1 (2.27%)	1 (2.27%)
children	38 (82.60%)	6 (13.04%)	2 (4.35%)

BURIAL RITE

The deceased at the examined location rest in crouched position and a clear majority of burials is furnished with grave goods.

POSITION OF THE DECEASED

At the Zengővárkony burial site, inhumation in the crouched position on the left side prevailed. Out of the 154 examined individuals, 140 were interred in this manner. The number of individuals positioned on the right side is considerably lower—a total of ten individuals. In four cases, the position was different or impossible to reconstruct. In tab. 1 below, the distribution of positions according to gender is shown.

While the preference of position in terms of right/left side during burials is almost identical for both males and females, there is greater variability in the case of children. This can also be observed in the Lower Neolithic period (Čermáková 2002, 14). The choice of a particular position in child burials can be presumed in cases when the individual had undergone a form of initiation or reached a specific (biological, cultural?) stage.

ORIENTATION OF THE DECEASED

The orientation of the deceased in graves is shown in tab. 2.

Tab. 2. Orientation of the graves.

	E–W	NE–SW	W–E	Other
men	42 (65.63%)	17 (26.56%)	2 (3.13%)	3 (4.69%)
women	28 (63.64%)	13 (29.55%)	0 (0.00%)	3 (6.82%)
children	25 (54.35%)	15 (32.61%)	3 (6.52%)	3 (6.52%)

Most of the inhumed were placed so as "to face" the Sun throughout the day; i.e., typically on the left side, with the head towards the East and feet towards the West. The E–W orientation was clearly preferred. Out of the 154 individuals, 95 were positioned in this way. Head towards the North-East and feet towards the South-West was the second most common orientation (45 occurrences). Other orientations were quite rare. Nevertheless, the unusual West-East orientation is worth mentioning: it occurred in five cases and in all of them the individuals were resting on the right side so the condition of facing the sun even in these, for some reason, anomalous burials was preserved. The orientation in the cardinal directions of the buried males and females is practically identical. Again, differentiation adult—child rather than male—female can be observed and is seen in the greater variability in orientation of the children. The same was observed at the burial site of the Linear Pottery Culture (hereinafter referred to as LPC) in Vedrovice: "In contrast to children, men and women have similar "rules" for the orientation of skeletons" (Rajchl 2002, 281). The author links children's burials with winter solstice, as the renewal of life, based on astronomical analysis (ibid.). As though the children were being called back to life. Archaeoastronomical analysis of the Zengővárkony burial site has not been conducted yet, however, an analogical link between the orientation of Lengyel child burials and astronomical phenomena cannot be excluded.

SKULL MANIPULATION AS A SIGN OF RESPECT?
A distinct phenomenon observed not only at the examined site but also in the broader Neolithic context is the frequent manipulation with the heads (skulls?) of both humans and animals.

In Zengővárkony, 14 of the inhumed individuals whose sex was determined had undergone such treatment. An overwhelming majority of these were males, particularly those with the most abundant grave goods (11 cases in total: graves no. 92, 93, 114, 128, 137, 155, 179, 180, 205, 206, 261), two cases were child burials (graves no. 126 and 335) and one female grave (no. 119a).

Two types of manipulation with the skulls are recognized: either the whole skull is absent (which is less common) or the mandible remains in the grave in its natural anatomic position. It seems that the presence or absence of the mandible is of special significance. While both above mentioned child skeletons lacked the skull completely, i.e. including the mandible, men's "headless" skeletons lacked the mandible only on three occasions, and the female skeleton also had the mandible preserved. Such manipulation with skulls had already appeared in Jericho, in Pre-Pottery Neolithic B (Parker-Pearson 2003, 159) and it probably implies a very important and strong tradition. According to M. Parker-Pearson it proves ancestor worship of prominent adult individuals. The Jericho skulls were carefully modelled and stayed on with the family throughout its everyday life. It is worth noting, that these modelled skulls do not depict mouths; not even in cases where the mandible remained on the skulls (ibid. 159).

Key to understanding this phenomenon may lie in the function of the mandible—besides chewing it is also related to speaking, and therefore also incantations. If the mouth is not indicated, or when the mandible is removed from the skull, then the dead is simply "kept from talking." Perhaps it is a sign of a certain complex and ambivalent attitude towards the dead—the heads of deceased ancestors were perhaps displayed in Lengyel homes (see e.g. Ruttkay 1985), but on the other hand caution was taken so they could not cast a spell on or enchant the bereaved.

Such fears could also be related to the find of a singular human mandible from pit 1/55 in Cezavy u Blučiny (Ondráček and Podborský 1954, 774). Analogous treatment of the dead is documented from Romano-Celtic Britain.

Occasionally, the heads of old females were cut off prior to the funeral and from these, mandibles were removed. M. J. Green explains this procedure as possible prevention from witches' incantations (Green 1998, 103–104).

Besides the presumed display of "ancestors' heads" in homes, there were other forms of manipulation. In Blučina, four human skulls belonging to individuals between 2 and 17 years of age were kept on a hearth. Incisions on one of the mandibles even indicate cannibalism (Ondráček and Podborský 1954; Tihelka 1956). A similar find exists from Poigen, Lower Austria. In a settlement pit a total of five human skulls with cut marks was discovered (3 female, 1 child, 1 male; Berg 1956). An inhumed infant skull was found in the Hungarian site of Mórágy-Tüzködomb (Zalai-Gaál 1984, 335). A unique case is known from Rajhrad. In a multiple (family?) grave a male was buried together with a female and three children. His skull was separated from the body but it lay in the grave by his side (Wankel 1873). These might be cases of some magic rites in which the human head could have played a role. An interesting parallel with the Celtic world can be found: in Welsh myths, there were magic heads that could foretell the future (Green 1998, 14). A similar occurrence is described K. J. Erben's adaptation of a Slavic myth in which a girl tries to call back her missing beloved by boiling a corpse's head, which then calls the boy (Erben 1988, 152).

This magical treatment of skulls could be taken into consideration in the case of children, as those were not counted among ancestors (Parker-Pearson 2003, 163). Both headless child skeletons of Zengővárkony also lack the mandibula, which could imply that fear of incantation did not apply to them, and that their heads, even with the mandibles, did not invoke fear (and were therefore used for magical purposes). A more complex case is known from Moravia, storage pit no. 159, in Těšetice. At the site, a ritually interred child was found. Its separate skull was discovered near the skeleton, however, the mandible was missing (Podborský 1988, 109–110). That is a very unusual occurrence and could possibly document a sacrifice to vegetative powers, which the child should have invoked through its youth without endangering it by incantation.

It follows from the above, that the separation of skulls from the bodies always affected individuals respected by the society, who were counted among ancestors (and who probably invoked some fear) or who were important for the society in some way. I suppose that two different habits can be attributed to manipulation with skulls. Firstly, it could be the preservation of heads of significant ancestors, which is prevalently the case of the "beheaded men with mandibles." The second tradition, represented by "skull nests" from Poigen and Blučina, is probably connected to the magical function of the head regardless of the "donor." In my opinion, it should be noted that in this category skulls of juvenile individuals prevail. Children, as mentioned above, do not count among ancestors and so their skulls could have been used for certain rites.

It is also possible, that some animals were also viewed in this way as finds of a "buried" bear skull in Těšetice, a bull in Branč (Vladár 1969) as well as beheaded pig and hare skeletons in a Lengyel grave in Brno-Královo Pole imply (Král 1956).

GENDER IN THE LIGHT OF GRAVE GOODS

A unique source for learning about ancient gender roles are artefacts and objects accompanying the dead and symbolically or factually illustrating the world of women, men and children of the Upper Neolithic. They can provide evidence of specific work activities as well as traces of actual ideas related to the roles of women, men and children. Objects found in graves often show individuals splayed between earthly material existence and metaphysical spheres. The number of recovered grave goods alone is noteworthy. In contrast to the previous categories of body positions and orientation, there is apparent differentiation based on the gender of the deceased. The situation at the Zengővárkony burial site is illustrated in tab. 3. The figures represent the average amount of grave goods for each of the categories. For clarity, the male category was divided between regular burials and burials without skulls.

This pattern can be considered quite typical for the Upper Neolithic. An analogous situation can be observed at the late Lengyel (Ludanice group) burial site in Jelšovce, Slovakia (see tab. 4)—adapted from: Pavúk and Bátora 1995, proceeding from the 23 determined individuals, 12 females, 6 children, 5 males.

Tab. 3. Average amount of grave goods (Zengővárkony).

	Grave goods
children	3.3
women	4.0
men	5.9
men without skull	11.2

Tab. 4. Average amount of grave goods (Jelšovce).

	Grave goods
children	1.5
women	3.1
men	5.2

I presume that the proportion of grave goods for the given categories (male—female—child) and particularly the richness of the elite male graves is representative of the whole Lengyel era. For comparison, let us consider the situation in the Lower Neolithic at the LPC burial site in Vedrovice—Široké u lesa. At this site, the average number of grave goods in male graves was 8.08 while in child graves only 1.95 and in female graves a mere 1.65 (Podborský et al. 2002, 311–312, 315). In Vedrovice, just like in Zengővárkony, a special group of rich male burials stands out, perhaps "patriarchs" or "exchange organisers" (Podborský et al. 2002, 315). It is striking that in female burials such social stratification is encountered to a much lower extent. In order to learn more about the social status of these males and other members of the society, it is necessary to examine the character of the grave goods that accompanied them more closely.

POTTERY

The most common grave goods were pottery. This category includes all preserved vessels, shards and weights. In the examined graves in Zengővárkony there was a total of 488 ceramic artefacts. Their distribution in graves and the corresponding averages are illustrated in tab. 5 below.

Tab. 5. Pottery grave goods (Zengővárkony).

	Amount of pottery grave goods in total	Average per person
men	253	3.95
women	124	2.81
children	111	2.41

When examining the individual pottery types, it is noted that some are more universal in terms of gender and some are more gender specific. In tables 6–9 below, the variability of values within the different categories is shown: beakers and beaker-like vessels, footed bowls, other bowl-shaped pottery, and pots.[6]

Tab. 6. Distribution of beakers in graves (Zengővárkony).

Beakers (168 pcs)	In total	Number of graves with beaker/s	Average per person
men	83	40 (62.50%)	2.01
women	42	27 (61.36%)	1.56
children	43	28 (60.87%)	1.55

---

6   Besides the aforementioned ceramics categories, other and non-reconstructable shapes should be mentioned. 32 of these were found in the graves, however, they are not suited for further processing. Similarly, the isolated occurrences of ceramic weights (four items) originating from one male grave, one female grave and one child grave (two pieces), are not being considered.

Tab. 7. Distribution of footed bowls in graves (Zengővárkony).

Footed bowls (141 pcs)	In total	Number of graves with bowl/s	Average per person
men	76	52 (81.25%)	1.46
women	40	30 (68.18%)	1.33
children	25	22 (47.83%)	1.14

Tab. 8. Distribution of other bowl-shaped pottery in graves (Zengővárkony).

Other bowl-shaped pottery (79 pcs)	In total	Number of graves with other bowl-shaped pottery	Average per person
men	42	26 (40.63%)	1.62
women	20	14 (31.82%)	1.43
children	17	14 (30.43%)	1.21

Tab. 9. Distribution of pots in graves (Zengővárkony).

Pots (64 pcs)	In total	Number of graves with pot/s	Average per person
men	35	31 (48.44%)	1.62
women	18	17 (38.65%)	1.06
children	11	9 (19.13%)	1.22

The aforesaid data clearly indicate the special status of beakers in several aspects. Firstly, they are the most frequent type of pottery grave goods. 34.4% of all ceramic grave goods are beakers and, in most cases, more than one piece is present in a grave. The even representation of beakers in graves is also remarkable. Their presence was documented to some extent in 61% of all graves almost independently of gender. What is not so "fair" is the number of beakers in individual graves. The largest collections of beakers were recovered from male graves, especially those of males buried without heads (skulls). The largest numbers of beakers, six, were found in two instances (grave no. 137 and no. 114). For the sake of completeness, it should be noted that grave no. 114 contained the greatest amount of grave goods overall: 26 in total. Grave no. 137 contained "mere" 16 items of grave goods. Three beakers were also present in the "headless" female grave no. 119a and the "headless" child grave no. 335. The female grave no. 119a and the male grave no. 114 correspond in one more aspect—in both, besides the adult skeleton a child's skeleton was present.

It is not easy to interpret the aforesaid results. Based on the collections of beakers in male graves, the introduction of "drinking parties" analogous to those of the Hallstatt period seems a tempting interpretation, yet that would probably be an incongruous anachronism. So far, it can be presumed that a beaker as such is not a gender specific grave offering. When present in larger collections, beakers can indicate an important person, usually male. A different situation is observed within the remaining categories: bowl-shaped vessels, pots and footed bowls, which are more frequently found in male graves. Footed bowls can be considered an imaginary counterpoint to beakers. These pottery shapes show relatively greatest gender affinity, namely for male graves, nevertheless, they cannot be simply viewed as gender specific either. These shapes scarcely appear in larger numbers (although in the aforesaid male grave no. 114 there were 5 of them). In Svodín, bowls appeared in large numbers in the funerary context but were quite rare in the settlement (Němejcová-Pavúková 1986, 153). Nevertheless, if pottery shapes were to be organised according to their gender sensitivity, the order would be following: footed bowls, other bowl-shaped goods and pots, beakers. The results may indicate some correlation between the gender of the deceased and the individual pottery types. Yet, this correlation needs to be viewed as quite a loose one and most probably varied in the different areas of the Lengyel culture. For instance, in Svodín, the frequent presence of mushroom-shaped vessels in male graves is striking (Němejcová-Pavúková 1986, 145), however, cannot be confirmed in the case of Zengővárkony, where this category was relatively rare and not limited to a particular gender category of burials.

Ceramic vessels, at least from the morphological point of view, are not the most readable medium for gender recognition, however, detailed analysis of painting and decoration of the vessels could greatly contribute to it. In Zengővárkony, painting appeared most distinctly on the vessels in "headless" male graves (Dombay 1960, 200). This fact seems to testify to the existence of a connection between the social status of the buried and the embellishment of the pottery grave goods. I believe that in the case of Zengővárkony we may, in all probability, surmise information "encoded" in the decorative elements on pottery as suggested by I. Pavlů (Pavlů 1997, 106) and as proved to some extent in Vedrovice (Květina 2004, 385). Unfortunately, without the possibility of close examination of the originals or at least high-quality image documentation, it is impossible to state anything particular about these correlations.

It is worth noting that there are some pottery shapes which may have an affinity with children. They are vessels with a teat and anthropomorphic vessels. The former category is represented by two pieces from the Mórágy—Tüzködomb burial site where they were found in graves of infants and for this reason were identified as feeding vessels for youngest children (Zalai-Gaál 1984, 337). Anthropomorphic vessels are known mostly from Slovak Lengyel child burials (Němejcová-Pavúková 1986, 143). I believe that these pottery shapes present a unique source for learning about the perception of women in the given period. A clay vessel in the shape of a woman may signify an inner affinity: earth—clay—woman—mother. Certain hints may also be derived from etymology. Compare the Latin word *terra*, which indicates both earth and pottery. Terra (Tellus) or *Terra Mater* is the Roman goddess of the earth and its prolific power. Analogously, Gaia in ancient Greek stands for either Earth Goddess or earth alone. It is probable, that Neolithic humans perceived earth, pottery and Mother goddess as various aspects of the same entity. A "profession" of this view of woman-mother-goddess in the earth (or the earth in woman-mother-goddess) could be done through two types of artefacts: clay statues of women or anthropomorphic vessels. However, this poses the question as to why the production was not limited to statues of women and "common" vessels. I believe that representing the woman as a vessel accentuates one particularity. In essence, the main difference between a vessel and a statue is its hollowness, that is, being empty inside allowing it to become a carrier for something. This connection is strikingly apparent, for instance, in Hebrew; the word for woman or female is "nkėvâ," which is derived from the word "nikkėv" = "to make or be hollow, that is waiting to be filled" (Weinreb 1995, 94).

Analogously, a woman, is physiologically "hollower" than a man so that a child can be conceived and created within her. The cyclic rhythm of farmers (compare, e.g. with myths about Demeter), indicates belief in the cycle of life and death, that is, the dying and rebirth of the soul. A woman-mother can therefore serve as a mediator (medium) between the world of immaterial souls and the material world. In accord with the viewpoint about the "broader" Neolithic thinking, I believe that physical fertility (of women) could be understood by the Neolithic people as "mediumship on the material level," that is, only one (yet highly important) aspect of female "mediumship." Perhaps this might be the reason for the frequent occurrence of anthropomorphic vessels in child graves in Svodín (Němejcová-Pavúková 1986, 143; 1981, 188). In this way, children are symbolically given the opportunity to return to their mothers who are ready to accept them and give birth to them again. An analogy could probably be seen in the later burials of children in *pithoi*.

An interesting phenomenon, probably related to the previously described perception of women, is seen in the famous Maltese temples. Their ground plan conspicuously resembles the silhouettes of the figures of seated women found in this area (Bouzek 1979, 87). Duerr mentions the Maltese cult of the Mother Goddess, "who periodically absorbed life back into her womb to give birth to it again" (Duerr 1997, 181). He goes on to point out the fact that Christian temples were, in some contexts, perceived as the "Holy Virgin's body" or the "Mother's body" (ibid. 184).

Here, the highest, sacred level of mediumship is reached; when the woman (priestess, "sybil") is filled up by the highest Reality (obviously named var-

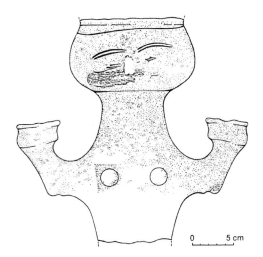

Fig. 1. Anthropomorphic (gynomorphic) vessel from Těšetice, borrowed from Kazdová (2002).

iously in accordance with the cultural-religious context) that prophesies or otherwise acts through the woman. Even though there is also evidence of men performing this sacred role, it can be said that mostly this was the domain of women. Men engaged in this field would quite often wear women's clothes and speak about themselves in feminine gender (more in Bouzek, 1996).

Rendering a woman as a vessel may therefore accentuate this mediating aspect of the female who is able to grasp that which is difficult to grasp and subsequently pass it on. For this reason, I believe that the interpretation of the Svodín type vessels as a rendition of women carrying vessels with offerings, as it is sometimes stated (e.g. Pavúk 1981, 42), is not quite correct. The woman does not hold the vessel—she becomes the vessel, and often she has a vessel in place of her head and even in place of hands (most clearly seen in the Těšetice specimen, fig. 1). This symbolism is also encountered in the Christian world, namely in legends of the Holy Grail, a vessel often associated with femininity and physicality (more in Neubauer 2002, 11–41).

STONE ARTEFACTS

While ceramic grave goods usually do not present types characteristic for a specific gender (with a few exceptions), chipped and polished stone artefacts are quite the opposite. In terms of chipped tools at the Zengővárkony burial site, blades, blade tools and scrapers prevail. In total, 75 items of chipped stone tools were found in the graves. Data for the various categories of burials are presented in the tables 10–13 below.

Values indicating the representation of the different types of chipped industry in graves according to gender are highly varied. The three most distinct types of artefacts are shown in the following tables:

Tab. 10. Distribution of chipped industry in graves (Zengővárkony).

	Chipped industry—in total	Average per person
men	44	0.69
women	16	0.36
children	15	0.33

Tab. 11. Distribution of blades in graves (Zengővárkony).

Blades (38 pcs)	In total	Number of graves with blades
men	23	19 (29.69%)
women	9	7 (15.91%)
children	6	5 (10.87%)

Tab. 12. Distribution of blade tools in graves (Zengővárkony).

Blade tool ("knife"); (15 pcs)	In total	Number of graves with "knife"
men	11	11 (17.19%)
women	0	0 (0.00%)
children	4	4 (8.70%)

Tab. 13. Distribution of scrapers in graves (Zengővárkony).

Scrapers (6 pcs)	In total	Number of graves with scraper
men	1	1 (1.56%)
women	3	3 (6.82%)
children	2	2 (4.35%)

Apart from the described types of stone tools, other shapes (cores, flakes and unspecified artefacts), 15 in total, were discovered in the graves. Nevertheless, a sufficient source basis for statistical assessment was not found. Chipped industry seems to be prevalently associated with the male population. An exception to this is the category of scrapers mostly encountered in female and child burials. It may be evidence of home hide working, which seems to have been women's domain. This assumption is also supported by the osteological analysis conducted on the skeletons of Zengővárkony and which documented teeth abrasion characteristic for hide working in two females and one male (Smrčka et al. 2018, 60–61).

Remarkable information can also be obtained from the material composition of chipped industry from this burial site. The majority of tools was made of silex followed by jasper. Relatively rarer were tools made of obsidian and there was one occurrence of flint. All four types of material were documented in female graves, male graves contained artefacts from all aforementioned materials but flint, and child graves only contained tools from the two most frequent materials: silex and jasper. If we work on the assumption that grave artefacts were produced by the buried, then an explanation could lie in the rareness of imported material which was to be worked by experienced individuals while children could "practice" on more common materials. However, it is not possible to determine who the makers of the tools were from the obtained data. The find of a core, which could imply the burial of a maker of chipped industry comes from a male grave, but it is a unique find.

Polished stone tools (hereinafter PST) form another distinct group of grave goods in terms of gender. Three categories of these artefacts were examined: axes, whetstones, other polished industry. Their presence in the graves is shown in the following tables 14–15.

Tab. 14. Distribution of axes in graves (Zengővárkony).

Axes (90 pcs)	In total	Number of graves with axe/s
men	81	55 (85.94%)
women	3	2 (4.55%)
children	8	7 (15.22%)

Tab. 15. Distribution of whetstones in graves (Zengővárkony).

Whetstones (15 pcs)	In total	Number of graves with whetstone/s
men	9	8 (12.50%)
women	2	2 (4.55%)
children	4	4 (8.70%)

Other PST such as shoe-last adzes, drilling cores and other undefined artefacts appeared in four instances in four male graves.

The connection of men and axes is one of the most distinct traits of (not only) the Neolithic burial rite but also of the whole Neolithic era. Hodder (1990, 111) considers this fact to be not only evidence of warfare and felling trees but also of "controlling that which is wild." An axe is therefore one of the artefacts with very strong symbolical meaning (in more detail e.g. Květina 2015, 527–537). In Zengővárkony, only nine of the 64 male graves did not contain any axes. These artefacts can truly be regarded as "manly attributes" indicating power as well as work outside the home.

The occurrence of whetstones in male graves is also noteworthy. Out of the nine items, seven come from the richest, "headless" male graves. Even in child graves, these artefacts are concentrated in the largest collections of grave goods (e.g. grave 79). In all likelihood, these can be seen as indicators of important individuals within the society or perhaps of a specific occupation. The special significance of whetstones at the Zengővárkony site is indisputable, however surprising it may seem. Yet, it is not quite clear what special fact is symbolized by these items in the funerary context.

ORGANIC GRAVE GOODS
The category of organic grave goods was divided into two thematic subchapters for better clarity. The first one is dedicated to bone adjuncts, bones, teeth and antler artefacts, the second mostly to shells and items made thereof. Other grave offerings are mentioned when there is a connection with one of the groups.

BONES, TEETH, ANTLERS AND ARTEFACTS MADE THEREOF
Wild boar teeth and jaws were a popular grave offering at the Zengővárkony burial site. Their distribution in graves is shown in tab. 16 below.

Tab. 16. Distribution of teeth and/or jaws of wild boar in graves (Zengővárkony).

Teeth and/or jaws of wild boar (16 pcs)	In total	Number of graves with teeth and/or jaws
men	11	11 (17.19%)
women	3	3 (6.82%)
children	3	3 (6.52%)

The most typical adornment of men was a pendant made out of two boar teeth worn around the neck. In five instances a whole boar mandible was found in the grave (two in male graves, two in child graves and one in a female grave). A wild boar mandible was found in the double grave no. 119 of a woman and child. The female was buried without her skull but with her mandible. An identical situation was observed in the double grave of a man and child, no. 114. The male was also buried without the head, but with the mandible and the wild boar jaw.

The occurrence of jaws and pendants made of boar tusks is quite common throughout the Lengyel area. V. Němejcová-Pavúková considers boar jaws and tusks part of the typical male equipment (together with axes, chipped tools, spondylus shells and red pigment); (Němejcová-Pavúková 1980, 146). For some reason, these animals held an important role in the Lengyel world. From later periods, we know wild boar as a symbol of warlike strength and power for the Celts, but also as a sacred animal associated with the Germanic fertility gods Freyr and Freyja (Becker 2002, 113). The connection of boars and fertility may lie in their habit of digging into the soil in search of food. For many indigenous peoples every such encroachment on the "body" of Mother Earth is seen as a very sensitive issue. The Baiga peoples of India do not plough the earth and only sow into the ashes of burnt jungle not to scratch the breast of their Mother (Eliade 2004, 249). Certain restrictions in manipulation with the land were also observed in the case of the Zuni tribe of North America. Only women were allowed to excavate clay for making pottery, for men, this activity was taboo (Mills 1994, 6). It is highly probable that in the Lengyel culture interventions into the earth were viewed in a similar manner and therefore animals that got in such close contact with soil drew attention.

M. Gimbutas mentioned finds of face masks representing boar heads from Vinča and Karanovo cultures. According to the author, pigs were consecrated to the Great Mother and she points out the frequent sacrifices of these animals to Demeter and Persephone (Gimbutas 1989, 146–147). Frazer even speaks about the original identification of Demeter (Persephone) with a boar which was regarded a godly creature. However, when the goddesses were given anthropomorphic forms, the animals were no longer killed in the role of gods but as field pests, that is, enemies of vegetation and the goddess (Frazer 1994, 408). It is not easy to determine whether wild and domesticated animals were interchangeable (in symbolism). Due to the contrast between "domesticated—wild" in which Neolithic populations lived, I believe that not quite. Artistic rendering of boars (zoomorphic vessels, sculptures, applications on pottery) is hardly ever encountered, which is quite surprising considering the abundant occurrence of boar teeth as pendants. It seems that in the Lengyel era boars were hunted mostly for land and field protection. A trophy of the killed animal could be symbolic of a partial victory over "wilderness."

Other gender specific organic grave goods were bone needles, and, eventually, awls. Their distribution in graves is illustrated in tab. 17.

Tab. 17. Distribution of needles and/or awl/s in graves (Zengővárkony).

Needles, awls (16 pcs)	In total	Number of graves with needle/s, awl/s
men	5	4 (6.25%)
women	9	8 (18.18%)
children	2	2 (4.35%)

These artefacts associated with textile manufacturing are most typical of female graves. Male graves with needles and awls are generally rarer, nevertheless, there was one with a set of two such items (grave no. 314).

Predominantly in the richer graves, animal bones are found, probably as remains of meaty grave goods. The situation is presented in the following table. (Only the presence of bones was considered regardless of their exact amount.)

Tab. 18. Distribution of animal bones in graves (Zengővárkony).

Animal bones (13 ×)	Number of graves with animal bones
men	8 (12.50%)
women	3 (6.82%)
children	2 (4.35%)

Of the eight aforementioned male graves, four were "headless," and one child skeleton was also without a skull. A meaty grave goods is typical for rich graves. It is not a mere supply of food for the dead on their journey to the world beyond (just the fact that the skeletons often lack skulls seems to imply the symbolical meaning of the good, which probably was not meant as food for the deceased). It cannot be excluded that they are evidence of farewell ceremonies for important members of the community. Meat placed in the grave was perhaps meant to testify to the dead about the funeral feast held in their honour.

A special case is the adjunct of a whole animal. In Zengővárkony one such case is documented. In grave no. 128, along with a male interred without the skull but with the mandible, a dog was inhumed. The man's skeleton is not quite complete, and the placement as described by J. Dombay (1960, 91) indicates secondary burial, which would suggest a longer period of displaying the body and the evident manipulation with the skull. It seems that in grave no. 128 the remains of a truly important person were interred. In addition to the dog skeleton, the grave contained other animal bones and bovine horns (further on bull symbolism Čermáková 2007, 244–246). The dog probably accompanied its powerful master during his life and added to his prestige.

A dog could be used for hunting, as a companion but also as a weapon. The great popularity of dogs in the Lengyel culture is manifested by frequent finds including contexts indicating special, even magical, significance of these animals. In Hluboké Mašůvky a dog sacrifice is assumed in the ditch enclosing the settlement (Stuchlík 2004). A burial of a man with a dog is also known from Friebritz, Austria (Lenneis, Neugebauer-Maresch, and Ruttkay 1995, 94) and Svodín, Slovakia (Němejcová-Pavúková 1986, 148). In the latter occurrence, the dog was covered by a bowl, which Němejcová-Pavúková considers to be the most beautiful exemplar found in Svodín (ibid.) that may really testify the respect shown to these animals. I. Zalai-Gaál states that in both, Tiszapolgár and Lengyel cultures, dog skeletons are often present in rich graves and quotes I. Bognár-Kutzián who associates the finds of dogs with "men—hunters" (Zalai-Gaál 1994, 54).

Antler artefacts at the Zengővárkony burial site were discovered in two anthropologically identified burials: in male grave no. 229 and child grave no. 273. In the former case it was a bar-shaped antler artefact. Based on the depiction (Dombay 1960, lxiv:5) I would favour the interpretation of this object as a soft percussor used in chipped industry production. A flat bone stick of unclear purpose and a jasper blade were also recovered from the grave. It is possible that these grave goods indicate the burial of a maker of chipped tools.

In the latter case, the grave offering contained an antler hammer-axe placed in the grave of a 5–6-year-old child. Other adjuncts were not discovered. Possibly, it might suggest, just as in the cases of stone axes, a symbolical grave offering indicating the special status of the child's family.

MOLLUSC SHELLS, SHELL PRODUCTS AND THEIR SUBSTITUTES

Other organic grave goods encountered since the Lower Neolithic are shells and artefacts made of shells. As expected, these grave goods are mostly discovered in female graves. At the examined site, the most commonly processed shells are of the Ostrea Fossilis species found naturally in the surroundings of Zengővárkony (Dombay 1960, 229). The most common artefacts are necklaces, which, in addition to the above-mentioned shells also contain dentalia and copper beads.

Tab. 19. Distribution of shell beads in graves (Zengővárkony).

Shell beads (10 ×)	Number of graves with beads
men	2 (3.13%)
women	6 (13.64%)
children	2 (4.35%)

A remarkable discovery was that of one bead in the "headless" male grave no. 180. Single mollusc shell finds are quite rare in Zengővárkony; one in a female grave and one in a child grave (no. 79 and 91), both of which belong among the richer burials. A bracelet of shell was discovered in the richer female grave no. 313. At other Lengyel sites we also encounter sea mollusc shells both in raw and processed state. Spondylus shells, the material characteristic for Neolithic jewellery is mentioned by N. Kalicz as a typical item of women's grave goods in the form of beads and bracelets in Aszód. Even multiple rows of spondylus beads are found on various parts of bodies: around the neck or hips (Kalicz 1985, 100). Similar spondylus bands are known from Svodín, from rich female graves (e.g. 113/80, see tab. ii:1) and one of the richest child burials (no. 112/80); (Němejcová-Pavúková 1986, 145, 146). In comparison with the Lower Neolithic periods, spondylus jewellery becomes rarer and various imitations, for instance of white marble, can be encountered especially in the more Northern areas (Podborský 2002, 236). This fact is probably illustrated in the graves of Jelšovce, belonging to the Ludanice, i.e. final, phase of the Lengyel culture. The two richest female graves (no. 189 and 252; both of category maturus) contained among other grave goods also bands of marble beads placed at the waist (Pavúk and Bátora 1995). Spondylus shells could be substituted by shells of other molluscs. At the Mórágy-Tüzködomb burial site a 36-45-year-old female was interred with a band of 78 dentalia (Zalai-Gaál 1984, 335). Considering the conspicuous connection of these bands to females of the maturus category (with the exception of the child grave from Svodín) and the richness of grave goods I believe that these bands could be an attribute of the "clan mother." Bands of shells or marble beads around the hips were perhaps meant to symbolize the abundance of offspring that these women brought into the world during their lifetime. Shells are frequently associated with fertility (Becker 2002, 182). In connection with women who were, in most cases, probably past their reproductive optimum, these could be a gesture of respect towards their fulfilled maternal role. In the case of a child (girl?); (infans III according to J. Jakab, Němejcová-Pavúková 1986, 146) from Svodín, such status was probably expected and that might have been the reason for adding a anthropomorphic vessel into her (?) grave. I suppose these bands were only part of the funeral (eventually ritual) attire, for their implied symbolism and for their probably significant weight (especially in the case of marble beads) and their overall impractical character (more also in: Čermáková 2008).

An interesting piece of jewellery, typical for the child population of Aszód, is described by N. Kalicz. They are pendants from small shells, which were, at this site, limited only to child graves (Kalicz 1985, 100). Unfortunately, pictorial documentation was unavailable.

Ornaments from shells seem to be typical of female and child (girl?) burials within the Lengyel complex. There are fewer occurrences in male burials and those are mainly associated with the richer graves—as is the case at Zengővárkony and Svodín (Němejcová-Pavúková 1986, 145), however it seems that the model of older periods—when spondylus shells were scarcely present in male graves, but if they were, they occurred in great amounts and in ostentatious form—does not apply, see e.g. Vedrovice (Podborský 2002, 238, table 1).

COPPER

The Lengyel Culture is the first time period in which copper products are encountered in Central Europe. One of the first indirect pieces of evidence of the knowledge of copper is a pendant painted onto the chest of a female sculpture from the Austrian Falkenstein-Schanzboden site (Podborský 1993,

145). Symbolically, copper appears on a "Venus" figurine. Both in astrology and alchemy, copper is associated with the planet Venus and both are symbolized by the sign of female gender: ♀. Cuprum, the Latin name for this metal, is derived from the name of the island Cyprus, which is an important source of this material. According to myth, at the coast of this island, Aphrodite—Venus, was born out of sea foam (Neubauer and Hlaváček 2003, 111). No matter how these associations are viewed, it is certain, that copper, at least in Central Europe, appeared during an era that enhanced feminine symbolism, and is most frequently discovered in female burials—see the following tab. 20.

Tab. 20. Distribution of copper artefacts in graves (Zengővárkony).

Copper artefacts in graves	Number of graves with copper artefacts
men	6 (9.38%)
women	11 (25.00%)
children	3 (6.52%)

More detailed overview of the individual categories of copper artefacts in graves is presented in the following tables 21-23.

Tab. 21. Distribution of copper beads in graves (Zengővárkony).

Beads (17 ×)	Number of graves with copper beads
men	6 (9.38%)
women	10 (22.73%)
children	1 (2.17%)

Tab. 22. Distribution of copper rings in graves (Zengővárkony).

Rings (6 pcs)	In total	Number of graves with ring/s
men	1	1 (1.56%)
women	4	3 (4.69%)
children	1	1 (2.17%)

Tab. 23. Distribution of copper bracelets in graves (Zengővárkony).

Bracelets (5 pcs)	In total	Number of graves with bracelets
men	1	1 (1.56%)
women	3	2 (4.55%)
children	1	1 (2.17%)

In two instances, only traces of patina were discovered (child grave no. 154 and male grave no. 218). The most common and often sole copper grave offering were beads. If the dead had several types of copper jewellery, then almost always, one of them consisted of beads. Rings and bracelets without beads were recovered on two occasions only (female grave no. 276 contained a sole ring, and child grave no. 115 contained a bracelet). Female grave no. 85 can be considered to be the richest. On the ring and middle fingers of her left hand she wore spiral rings (one on each finger), in the neck area there were copper beads. There were eleven other items of grave goods including a needle, a jasper scraper, a rare flint and even a fragment of a boar's tooth.

Very special symbolism of copper jewellery is presumed by J. Sofaer Derevenski. Based on the research of the Tiszapolgár-Basatanya burial site (Tiszapolgár culture) she proposed a system of categories (based on age and the side on which the dead was positioned) for which certain copper items of jewellery are characteristic. The author suggests, that these artefacts indicate a specific life phase. For instance, juvenile individuals would typically have spiral shapes (rings, bracelets) which "grow," i.e. can be stretched correspondingly with the growth of their owner. For adults, enclosed shapes should be typical as proof of the completion of a cycle (Sofaer Derevenski 2000). However, in Zengővárkony, all round jewellery was spiral—so it can only be stated that copper ornaments correlate with richly furnished female graves. Rich male ("headless") burials contain copper only in two instances.

SPATIAL GRAVE RELATIONS AND SOCIAL INTERPRETATION

The burial site in Zengővárkony did not form a homogenous unit. Larger or smaller groups of graves merge with the settlement and form fourteen relatively independent groups, not all of which have been fully examined (Dombay 1960, 193). Other Lengyel burial sites exhibited a similar structure (e.g. Aszód; Kalicz 1985).

As far as burial rules are concerned, J. Dombay mentions conspicuous concentrations of graves with common traits. The cumulations of rich male "headless" burials are distinct particularly in group VI, or more precisely VIc., and IX, where these men were often inhumed in immediate proximity (Dombay 1960, 199). Likewise, there are concentrations of markedly poor graves (groups III-V, X, XI and XIV), or these are found on the edges of the richer groups. An analogous situation seems to occur in Aszód; in the middle of the cluster, there is an inhumed couple, where the male burial was very richly furnished. Other graves surround this central pair. In instances similar to this one, they could be family arrangements as proven at the Mórágy-Tüzködomb site (Zalai-Gaál 1984, 338). Nevertheless, in the case of rich male graves, these might be areas dedicated to prominent members of the community regardless of bloodline.

Child burials also seem to form clusters, e.g. in Aszód (Kalicz 1985, 98) and even in Zengővárkony, albeit within larger groups, e.g. groups 6 and X. The last mentioned cumulation is all the more interesting as the children are prevalently positioned on their right side. Even adult individuals positioned on the right side are placed near each other (three males and one female from group XI). All the three burials were discovered at the edge of the group. The male graves no. 292 and 293 were extremely poor (1 and 2 grave goods items), while the male grave (no. 288) and female grave (no. 287) were relatively rich and both contained copper jewellery.

The significance of the right-side position is not quite clear from the context. Personally, I believe that they were individuals with a problematic affiliation with the community—that would be testified by the burials of children where this position was employed most frequently. It is known, that children were not automatically integrated into the society. In the case of adults, the interpretation that they were foreigners or guests deceased while travelling or visiting away from their home comes into consideration. Their graves are both poor and rich, they could have been hunters or merchants. The position on the outskirts of the group seems to imply the status of outsiders or foreigners. Out of the four thus positioned adults, three are male. Men were more "mobile" in Lengyel society (see next chapter) and so the probability of dying "abroad" was higher than in the case of women. In the instance of the aforementioned rich burials on the right side, considering the grave goods, they could have been merchants with copper artefacts.

Nevertheless, the proposed explanation would only be valid for the Zengővárkony site, because in later periods as well as in northern areas, the right-side position was common.

In any case, Lengyel burial sites show evident social stratification. Graves of important individuals formed the "cores" of the sub-graveyards. Sometimes, it was a couple, on other occasions they were important persons. Based on research of the Vedrovice burial site, P. Květina recognizes two instances from which the prominent status of certain individuals stems. For one thing, it is the origin, affiliation with a certain line of descent, and for another, special skills, so-called "big men" (Květina 2004, 387). This viewpoint is also plausible for the Lengyel complex.

Probably the most important social role was held by the "headless" men. Who were they, though? According to J. Dombay, they were leaders of larger family groups (Dombay 1960, 231). Based on anthropological research in Mórágy-Tüzködomb, matrilineal filiation and exogamy were proposed, at least for this site (Zalai-Gaál 1984, 338). These circumstances, in my opinion, prepare ideal conditions for the evolution of "big men." A man married into a relatively new environment will probably be more motivated to manifest his special skills (hunting, knowledge of deposits of precious materials etc.). I suppose that these most capable men would have reached the highest ranks in the social hierarchy. After their death, they would have been treated in the aforementioned special manner and their head could have become part of an "ancestors gallery."

In the case of women, I presume the most prominent status was held by those inhumed with shell or marble bead belts. It can be assumed that these women contributed to the multiplication of the family and for that they were duly respected. A very special role in the funeral context is given to children. Children's burial rites deserve a special chapter.

THE STATUS OF CHILDREN IN THE LIGHT OF THE SPECIFICS OF BURIAL RITE

It should be stated that for the purpose of this essay children are usually individuals referred to as such by authors of publications on which this work is based. Therefore, it is a biological aspect that defines children on the basis of physical immaturity. However, the viewpoint of the given culture could have been different and the transition to adulthood did not necessarily correspond with physical development. Nevertheless, at the given stage of knowledge it is still possible to trace some typical aspects in the attitude of the Lengyel society towards children. The effort to isolate burials of children aside or to the periphery of graveyards was mentioned already. This phenomenon can be understood as a trend enduring from the Lower Neolithic period (Čermáková 2002, 15) and persisting up to the historical era. A remarkable example is known from Ireland. Children were inhumed in special graveyards called "cillín" localized in the border areas of the community, often in derelict churches or old megalithic tombs (Finlay 2000). Irish fairy tales narrating of children swapped by supernatural beings illustrate this insecurity associated with their origin. Logically, after death, children were interred in places associated with these "other worlds" (ibid.). In the Neolithic, caves could be considered such "cillíns." I have already looked into this subject before, especially in the context of Lower Neolithic cultures (Čermáková 2002, 12). However, in the context of the Lengyel complex these locations did not go unnoticed either. In the Slovak Dúpna Diera cave, 26 prevalently children's skeletons positioned ritually in a crouched position on the right side with numerous grave goods were discovered. The find is dated into the Ludanice phase of Lengyel culture (Bárta 1983, 22). In contrast to a similar find from the German Lower Neolithic Jungfernhöhle site (Matoušek and Dufková 1998, 71), in Dúpna Diera no evidence of violence was detected on the skeletons. In fact, as J. Bárta states, it is the largest burial site of the Ludanice group in Slovakia (ibid.). Another child cave burial was found in Deravá Skala (Plavecký

Mikuláš, Slovakia). It is also dated into the Ludanice phase of the Lengyel culture (Bárta 1983, 31).

Child internment in caves is also known from the Neolithic in central Italy. Skeletal remains of a larger number of people were found for instance at the Grotta Continenza site. Children comprised almost half of the interred individuals (Skeates 1991, 126). Solely children's remains were discovered in caves S. Angelo and Grotta dei Piccioni. The latter site served as the place of last repose to children in two different time periods about one thousand years apart (ibid.). Nevertheless, occurrences of adults interred in such context are also known (e.g. the cave Čertova Pec u Radošiny contained three adult burials; ibid.). Still, the prevalence of children buried in this manner is conspicuous. In caves, the theme of isolation is combined with the specific characteristics of the environment. R. Skeates points to the "difference" of karst areas, their specific unchanging atmosphere reminiscent of other worlds and thus facilitating communication with them. According to the author, children could have been sacrificed to these other worlds so that the community would have won the favour of certain supernatural powers (Skeates 1991, 127). Such child burials could also be interpreted as returning children to the womb (earth) for them to be reborn (more in Čermáková 2002, 12). It cannot be excluded that both approaches were somehow interlinked. Nevertheless, the isolation of child and adult burials was not all that consistent. On the contrary, numerous multiple burials of children along with adults are known. Oftentimes, they are females with children: Moravský Krumlov, Krumlovský les VI (Oliva 2004); Zengővárkony (graves 88, 119, 275; Dombay 1960); a double burial of child and male is also known from Zengővárkony (grave 114). The last example is all the more interesting because the child was interred in a rich grave of a "headless" male.

The ambivalent attitude towards children is reflected in the existence of both poor and relatively rich burials. It can therefore be supposed that there existed some projection of the status of the closest relatives onto the child's personality which could have been demonstrated in very rich grave furnishing (see last chapter).

It seems that children and juvenile individuals played an indispensable role in some ritual and sacrificial practices. I have already mentioned the possible association of children with sacrifices and manipulations with heads. The significant connection of children and caves and the possible participation in particular rituals associated with these places was also pointed out. Another piece of evidence, this time of foundation sacrifice, is the discovery of a child's remains in the construction of a wall of a Lengyel house in Veszprém (Raczky 1974). Even though mass sacrifices of children were not common in the Lengyel culture, under certain conditions they were possible and apparently this would not have been an isolated occurrence. Out of all the community members, children would be chosen for such purposes perhaps due to their unequal standing in the society.

GRAVE GOODS INTERPRETATION SUMMARY

The aforementioned partial results clearly indicate that there are more gender specific grave goods categories and less gender specific ones. In the following tab. 24, grave goods that, according to my observations, show relatively strongest affinity with the individual genders are presented.

Tab. 24. Gender specific grave goods

Men	Women	Children
axes	needles	anthropomorphic vessels
whetstones	scrapers	mug with spout
blades, tools from blades	shell jewels	
teeth and jaw from boars	belts from beads	
animal bones, dog	copper jewels	

Data characteristic of children often fall between values illustrating the female and male populations. Children's graves, for instance, contain relatively more axes and whetstones than female graves but at the same time fewer than male burials. Similarly, scrapers and shell beads occur more frequently in connection with child graves than with male graves but less often than with female graves. This fact might indicate the gradual involvement of children in working processes corresponding to their sex, or, in the case of youngest children or non-work-related artefacts, a symbolical expression of their gender.

Several categories of grave goods appear less frequently in association with children in comparison to the adult population (regardless of gender). They are copper jewellery, animal bones, and bone needles and awls. The latter seem to be associated exclusively with female graves. The first two categories of grave goods (copper jewellery and animal bones) seem to be indicative of socially prominent women (copper artefacts) and men (animal bones) (argumentation above). Children therefore cannot be included in this group—generally, these graves are relatively the poorest (see figs. 7 and 8), often on the periphery of the burial grounds. However, that does not mean that rich child graves do not occur within the Lengyel complex. Several instances are known both from Zengővárkony (e.g. "headless" grave no. 126) and from other sites (Svodín grave no. 112/80, among other things containing a anthropomorphic vessel). Nevertheless, it is difficult to determine whether these children were important for some reason "per se" or if the rich grave goods implied their belonging to some important family line.

The distribution of grave goods allows for a reasonably reliable reconstruction of the division of labour into "house" and "field" work, that is, the connection with "domus" and "agrios" to use Hodder's terminology (Hodder 1990). Men seem to be closely connected to the field, the areas outside the home (axes, wild animal remains, dog). It is known that during the Lengyel culture period there was a great recovery of hunting and at many sites, especially in the Eastern part of the complex, hunted-down animals outnumbered the domesticated population (Ambroz 1986; Podborský 1993, 145). That is a remarkable difference compared to the Lower Neolithic periods. Hunting and exploitation of natural resources (wood, stone material) were, in my opinion, major activities of the male population. Participation in long distance exchange, especially of stone material, which was imported over hundreds of kilometres in the researched period (Mateiciucová 2001, 220; Mateiciucová and Trnka 2004, 91) can also be assumed. In association with these activities the origination of male roles such as exchange arranger, activity leader, and so on, can be expected.

"Agrios" was probably not exclusively limited to men. That can be implied by the rich female grave no. 85 from Zengővárkony. The buried woman had a boar tusk and a piece of flint with her, that is, two items associated with the out-of-home area. Alongside these two artefacts, the grave goods also contained a needle and a scraper, which are considered to be items of a very homely character, "balancing out" (perhaps intentionally?) the connection with "agrios." It cannot be excluded that females, before starting a family, could have been involved in the mentioned "manly" activities. A similar model is known in Scythian women, who would abandon the "manly" lifestyle only after marriage (Полосьмак 2001, 276). It is unclear, though, how long such a life period would have been in the case of Neolithic females or if it should be taken into consideration at all. The majority of feminine grave goods are definitely indicative of employment in the household, which could be considered the natural consequence of motherhood. The finds of feeding vessels in infant graves are very meaningful. If children were weaned on a more general basis, or if breastfeeding was cut back on, as is implied by these vessels, then an increase in natality can be expected. Women probably had to look after several younger children which obviously limited or even prevented various activities outside the home and its immediate surroundings. Needles and scrapers can be associated with making textiles and hide working. We do not have sufficient direct evidence for other house chores. Nevertheless, women are also claimed to have been the makers of pottery (e.g. Podborský 1993, 136) which would be consistent with this notion.

It is mentioned that the affiliation of women with the house, the hearth and pottery was emphasised by I. Hodder, who also attached great importance to it. The house, or "domus," was the place and symbol of the final transformation of the "wild" into the "domesticated," whether in terms of transforming food from raw to cooked, clay into fired pottery etc. (Hodder 1990, 64). This transformative role was played by women (ibid.). This model, in my opinion corresponds very well with the maternal role of women, in which the infant, who seems to be alive only in the biological sense, is transformed into a "cultured" being. The notion of "transformation" is, after all, closely linked to the population of children in general without any time or space circumstances. In most cultures the birth of a child is associated with several protective measures and the community usually accepts the new member only later, after passing some kind of initiation ritual. In this sense, presumably, the Lengyel society was not an exception.

The transformative role of women was probably perceived on many levels. From simple tasks such as food preparation (raw → cooked) or making a piece of pottery (natural material → culturally significant artefact) to "transforming" a child (natural being → cultural being). I think that ancient and perhaps even Neolithic sybils may be viewed analogously as they would enter extrasensory visions when soothsaying and then mediate them to the community (spiritual, ecstatic experience → their interpretation, prophecy, specific information for the community). I assume that the transformative role of Neolithic women is closely connected to "mediumship" as mentioned above.

On the one hand, the woman in the Lengyel context appears to be distinctly physically tied to a particular place, home. This fact is further intensified by the possible matrilocality of the Lengyel population (based on the Mórágy-Tüzködomb site; Zalai-Gaál 1984, 338). On the other hand, in the ideological-religious sphere it appears that women could "move" more easily in various different context and "parallel realities" and subsequently connect and combine some of their aspects. Men, contrarily, exhibited greater mobility in the physical world—the presumed matrilineality and exogamy are prerequisite for migration. Evidence of hunting and the presence of exotic materials at the settlements also testify movement of some kind. Men present themselves as those in closer contact with agrios and the rise in importance of hunting might be a gesture of conquering the wild rather than necessary means of subsistence.

In short, the organisation of "worldly matters" was most probably the domain of men, who probably also were the leaders of Neolithic communities. Women applied themselves in cult. They were the mediators between the physical and spiritual worlds and between the domesticated and non-domesticated realms.

CONCLUSION

The Lengyel civilisation presents a stratified society with apparent division of work between men and women and with specific status of both genders. The attachment to the house and house chores (especially textile processing) is characteristic of women. It might be enhanced by matrilocality and increased natality, which is related to the documented habit of complementary feeding of infants. Distinct feminine symbolism pervading the whole culture illustrates the important role of women in terms of cult. The existence of "sybils" who mediated between the physical and "metaphysical" worlds can be expected. "Mediumship" of women was probably metaphorically expressed by the anthropomorphic vessels. Women held a key role in the domestication process, that is, in the transformation of "wild" phenomena into "cultural" ones.

In comparison with women, Lengyel men exhibit greater mobility. Evidence of hunting, the presence of dogs in graves and plentiful imported materials point to "agrios" as their main domain. Men were probably active in "worldly matters" such as the coordination of exchange. As some rich burials indicate, especially those of men interred without heads, men were the leaders of communities and after death they received special treatment. An ambivalent attitude can be seen in relation to children. A common occurrence is the peripheral placement, or isolation, of their graves. Finds of child remains in caves are relatively common. It seems probable, that the community fully accepted children only after certain initiation rituals, which, however, remain unknown. In some instances, relatively rich child burials are found, which might reflect the importance of the child's bloodline. The Lengyel society knew and sometimes employed child sacrifices, which, again, testify the problematic affiliation of children with the community.

3.2 VILLÁNYKŐVESD: ARCHAEOLOGICAL AND ANTHROPOLOGICAL DESCRIPTION, PALEOPATHOLOGIC ANALYSIS
VÁCLAV SMRČKA, ZDENKA MUSILOVÁ

3.2.1 ARCHAEOLOGICAL AND ANTHROPOLOGICAL DESCRIPTION

Location: north of the village of Villánykővesd, in a wide, flat area west of the dirt track that leads to Jakabfalu (Villánykővesd geographic coordinates 601224 60804 (EOV, 04-211)).

Archaeological and Anthropological Description: J. Dombay, the director of the County Museum conducted a small-scale excavation near the village of Villánykővesd in 1957. His investigation showed that the site comprised of a settlement with scattered groups of graves covering an area as large as one square kilometre. Among the land-filled pitches, there were graves with crouched skeletons. Based on the burial rite and additional archaeological finds he attributed these graves to the Lengyel Culture (Dombay 1959).

29 graves were excavated, 23 of which contained anthropological material and 2 contained copper. During the excavation, the graves were uncovered in two separate areas of the site (graves 1–25 and 26–29).

Bone material was highly fragmental. It was deposited under inventory numbers 58.4–24 and 58.106–108 in the anthropological collection of the Archaeological Department of the Janus Pannonius Museum in Pécs.

There, it was analysed from the anthropological aspect by Z. K. Zoffmann (1968). She concluded that the fragmental material was unsuitable for demographic analysis. Osteological material in the Infans I age group comprised of 6 individuals and in the Infans II age group of 4 individuals, which meant that 44% comprised of juvenile individuals.

In the Adultus age group there were 4 male and 3 female individuals (28%), in the Maturus group there were 4 males and 1 female (24%) and in the Senilis group there was one male individual (4%). The male to female ratio (9:4) probably resulted from the partial excavation of the burial site. (Dombay 1960). In 1960, the burial site was paleopathologically examined by Regöly-Mérei.

Zoffmann (1965) also paid attention to the orientation of the skeletons. The Villánykővesd graves have NE–SW, E–W, SE–NW orientations with skeletons lying on their left, and orientations SW–NE, NW–SE with skeletons lying on their right. The orientation of the skeletons lying on their left side does not diverge from the E–W axis by more than 75 degrees. A similar, but reversed, situation is observed in the case of skeletons orientated W–E lying on their right sides.

Further details of the settlement layout remained unknown until 1987, when the archaeologist I. Zalai-Gaál flew a single sortie in the area searching for Neolithic sites. He discovered traces of circular earthwork near Villánykővesd and identified it as a Neolithic rondel (Zalai-Gaál 1990, 1990a).

Based on orthorectified aerial photographs, Bertók and Gáti (2011) set up a grid to survey the rondel with a magnetometer.

The Villánykővesd enclosure turned out to contain several unique features in comparison with other Late Neolithic rondels. Its outer ditch, 300 m in diameter, is interrupted at regular 50 m intervals and the interruptions are blocked by protruding, semi-circular extensions.

The function of these extensions is unknown. Yet, there are some analogies; near the villages of Szemely, Kaposújlak, and Szólád as well as near the town Nagykanisza.

The closest analogy to this type of interrupted ditch with semi-circular extensions is that found at Kaposújlak. Though similar in structure, the Kaposújlak ditch is not circular but linear and blocks the entrance to hilltop the shape of which resembles a promontory. This means that the usual cultic/astronomical interpretation associated with rondels is not plausible here. Due to its linearity and location, the structure at Kaposújlak may be indicative of the defensive nature of these semi-circular extensions, an interpretation that may also apply to Villánykővesd.

3.2.2 PALEOPATHOLOGICAL CHARACTERISTIC OF THE ANALYSED COLLECTION (N = 23)

The finds were paleopathologically reviewed in autumn 2017.

CONGENITAL ANOMALIES

CONGENITAL SKULL DEFECTS
In 4 male individuals 3 skulls were preserved, where in the male, aged 49–58 (grave 13), posterior *plagiocephaly* (figs. 1a, b, c, d) was identified and also in the male, aged 41–45 (grave 24), with prevalence of 50%. In grave 13, the condition was not caused by premature fusion in the lambdoidal suture being a case of nonsynostotic plagiocephaly.

Among the 4 male skulls and 3 female skulls with preserved sagittal sutures (*sutura sagitalis*), *premature closure* was determined in a male aged 49–58 (grave 13) (fig. 1c) with prevalence of 25% and in a female, aged 53–62 (grave 21) with prevalence of 33.3%.

In the 4 male skulls with preserved lambdoidal suture (*sutura lambdoidea*), two instances of *intrasutural bones* were discovered: in the male, aged 49–58 (grave 13; fig. 1b) and male, aged 41–45 (grave 24), with prevalence of 50%.

In seven child skulls the lower jaw was examined. A child aged 12–13 (grave 12; fig. 2a) exhibited an *asymmetrical mandible*, with prevalence of 14.3% and an *artificial deformation* (a cut incisor).

14 skulls (4 male, 3 female and 7 children's) with tooth rotation disorders were examined.

In some individuals multiple rotated teeth were found, e.g. male, aged 41–45 (grave 24), with anomalously rotated upper cuspids, and male, aged 36–43 (grave 22), with a rotated maxillary left second incisor (I2) (fig. 3) and mandibular left cuspid. In the male, aged 49–58 (grave 13) a rotated maxillary right first premolar (P1) was detected.

That is, in three males out of the 4 examined, *anomalous tooth rotation* was determined with prevalence of 75%.

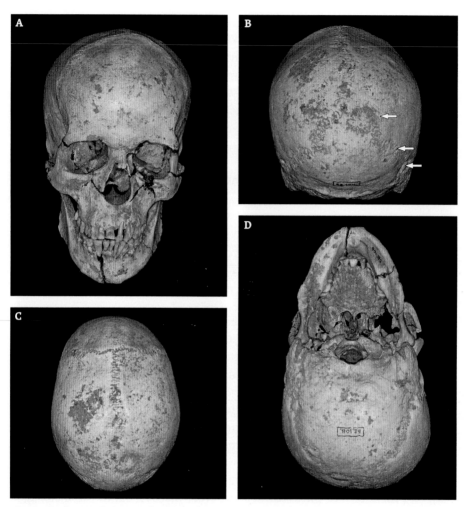

Fig. 1a–d. *Plagiocephaly* in male, aged 49–58, in grave 13, A: frontal, B: occipital, C: superior, D: inferior. Photo: Zdenka Musilová.

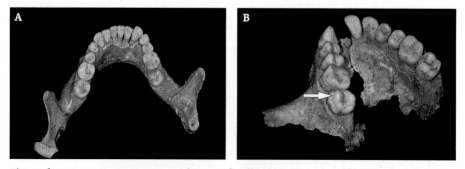

Fig. 2a–b. A: *Lower jaw asymmetry* with an artificially cut incisor in child, aged 12–13, in grave 12. B: Anomalous tubercle on the second molar of a child, aged 12–13, in grave 12. Photo: Zdenka Musilová.

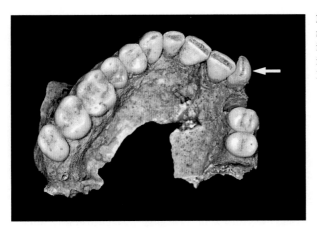

Fig. 3. *Anomalous tooth rotation* of the second left incisor, male aged 36-43, in grave 22.
Photo: Zdenka Musilová.

Of the 3 examined females, in one, aged 23-32 (grave 20), tooth rotation in mandibular cuspids with prevalence of 33.3% was determined.

Out of the 7 examined children, a child of 10-10.5 years of age (grave 14) had bilateral rotation of second molars (M2) in the lower jaw with prevalence of 14.3%.

In one child, aged 12-13 (grave 12), an anomalous tubercle on the second molar (M2) (fig. 2b) in the upper right jaw was identified, with prevalence of 14.3%.

CONGENITAL SPINE DEFECTS

The lumbar spine was examined in 10 individuals (6 male, 3 female and 1 child).

In one female, aged 36-40 (grave 10), spinal fusion was determined in vertebrae L4-L5 with prevalence of 33.3%.

ARTHROSIS

VERTEBRAL OSTEOPHYTOSIS

CERVICAL

9 cervical spines were examined (5 male, 1 female and 3 children's), of these, in one female, aged 36-40 (grave 10), *osteophytes of 1-2 mm* in size were detected with prevalence of 11.1%.

THORACIC

10 thoracic spines were analysed (6 male, 3 female and 1 child). In one female, aged 30-40 (grave 1), 2 *mm osteophytes* were determined, with prevalence of 10%.

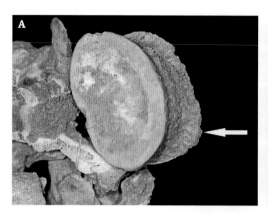
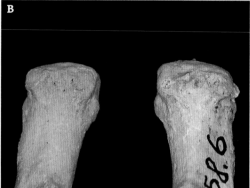

Fig. 4a–b. A: *Lumbar spine osteophytosis* exceeding 3 mm, in male aged 43–52, in grave 8.
B: Thumb *rhizarthrosis* in male, aged 43–52, in grave 8. Photo: Zdenka Musilová.

LUMBAR

The same number of lumbar spines was examined—10 (6 male, 3 female and 1 child). In one male, aged 43–52 (grave 8; fig. 4a), *osteophytes* were found *on L4, L5 up to 3 mm in length*, with prevalence of 16.7%.

In one woman, aged 30–40 (grave 1) the *osteophyte length* even *exceeded 4 mm*, with prevalence of 33.3%.

RHIZARTHROSIS OF THUMBS

Among the inspected phalanges of 6 hands (3 male, 1 female and 2 children's), in one male, aged 43–52 (grave 8) (fig. 4b) probable arthrotic impairment on the heads of phalanges of both thumbs were detected, with prevalence of 33.3%.

NONSPECIFIC INFECTIONS

Among the 14 skulls (4 male, 3 female and 7 children's), in one male's skull, aged 68–80 (grave 5; fig. 5) *ozaena* with prevalence of 25% was identified.

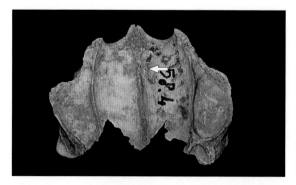

Fig. 5. *Ozaena* in male, aged 68–80, in grave 5. Photo: Zdenka Musilová.

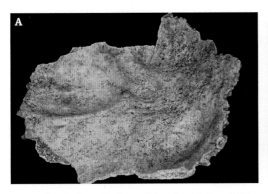
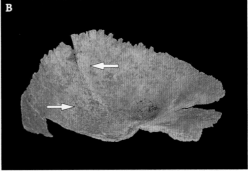

Fig. 6a–b. A: *Endocranial periostitis* in a child, aged 1–1.5, Villánykővesd. The new bone formation is rippled, corresponds to brucellar granulomas in the meninges. B: *Striated periosteal remodelling* in the intracranial part of the occipital bone of an unborn child in grave 10. Photo: Zdenka Musilová.

INTRACRANIAL PERIOSTITIS

Among the 7 inspected child skulls, two instances of *intracranial periostitis* were determined with prevalence of 28%: in child from grave 19 (58.16) of Infans I age group (1–1.5-year-old) with periostitis inside the skull in the occipital area (fig. 6a), and in an unborn infant from grave 10 (fig. 6b).

There were two instances of periostitis in children: the first case was in a child, aged 1–1.5, from grave 19 (fig. 6a—6031; chapter 3). The new bone formation is rippled, which corresponds to the bacterial character of the granuloma type on the meningeal coverings of the brain. It is presumed that it was an occurrence of *brucellar meningitis*.

The second (fig. 6b; chapter 3) in an unborn child in grave 10. Besides striated endocranial new bone formation, the foetus also had periostitis in the pelvis. The foetus suffered a liver disease (see chapter 6), probably of viral origin. In the Slavic female with endocranial periostitis, Parvovirus was dis-

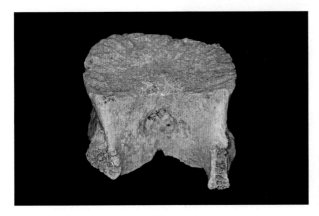

Fig. 7. *Osteomyelitis fistula* in thoracic vertebra of a 14-year-old child, grave 27. Photo: Zdenka Musilová.

covered (Mühlemann et al. 2018a), however considering the affection of liver, it could have also been an instance of hepatitis B (Mühlemann et al. 2018b) or another viral infection.

OSTEOMYELITIS FISTULA

Among the 10 examined thoracic vertebrae (5 male, 3 female, 2 children's), in a 14-year-old child (grave 27), a lesion of the *osteomyelitis fistula* type (fig. 7) with rounded edges 7 × 5 mm was identified, with prevalence of 50%.

SPECIFIC INFECTIONS

A *specific inflammation, probably of tuberculous origin,* was discovered in the *form of rib periostitis* in a child, aged 0–7 (in grave 3) with prevalence of 14.3%. Similar *periostitis* type lesions were detected in a male, aged 30–37 (grave 23) in the following bones: the talus, a thoracic vertebra (where a fistula is apparent, most likely resulting from casein outflow) (fig. 8a, b) and the sacrum (with prevalence of 11.1%).

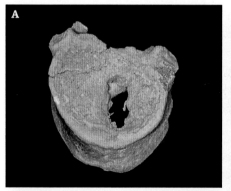
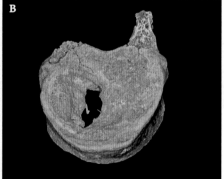

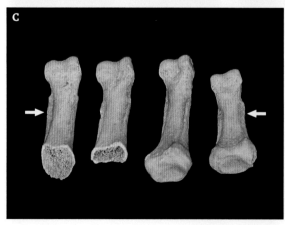

Fig. 8a–c. A: *Tuberculous Fistula* in a thoracic vertebra in a male, aged 30–37, grave 23. B: *Tuberculous Fistula* in a thoracic vertebra in a male, aged 30–37, grave 23. C: *Bone Rims* caused by excessive strain on interosseal muscles on the proximal phalanges of the left hand of a male, aged 30–37, grave 23. Photo: Zdenka Musilová.

TUMOURS

Among the 11 analysed occipital regions (3 male, 4 female, 3 children's), in one male, aged 41–45 (grave 24), an *osteoma* (fig. 9a, b) in the occipital region was detected, with prevalence of 33.3%.

CRIBRA ORBITALIA

At the Villánykővesd burial site a total of 9 orbital regions were examined (5 right and 4 left) in 1 male and 4 children.

Type 1 was detected in a male, aged 23–30 (in grave 17) with both orbits affected. Then in a child aged 12–13 (grave 12), also with bilateral affection; in an 8.5-year-old child (grave 15) only the right orbit was affected while the left one

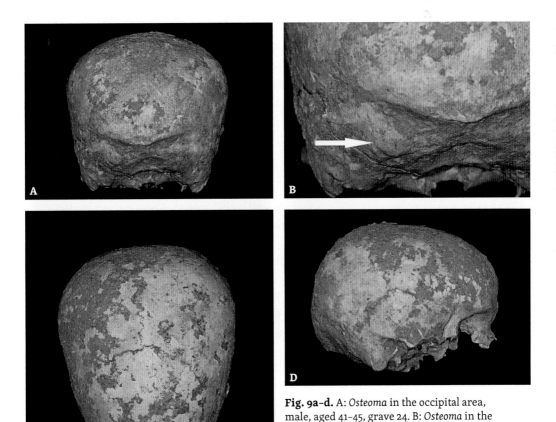

Fig. 9a–d. A: *Osteoma* in the occipital area, male, aged 41–45, grave 24. B: *Osteoma* in the occipital area, male, aged 41–45, grave 24. C: View of a skull with the considered bilateral *posterior plagiocephaly* in adult age. D: View of a skull with the considered hydrocephalus in adult age. Photo: Zdenka Musilová.

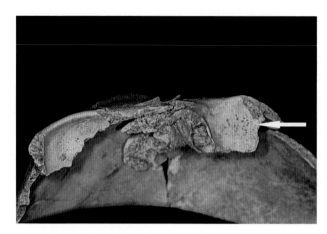

Fig. 10. *Cribra orbitalia* type 2, in the left orbit of an 8-year-old child, in grave 15. Photo: Zdenka Musilová.

was not preserved; and in a 3-year-old child (in grave 16), where orbital cribra was determined in the right orbit while the left orbit was not preserved. The prevalence of right orbital cribra was 80%, left 50%.

Type 2 orbital cribra was identified in an 8-year-old child (in grave 15) (fig. 10) in the left orbit, with prevalence of 25%.

Type 3 of orbital cribra was detected in a 9.5–10-year-old-child (in grave 18) with prevalence of 25%.

TOOTH DEFECTS

TOOTH WEAR
14 jaws were analysed (3 male, 4 female and 7 children's). Among the 3 males, *type 2* tooth wear was identified in a male, aged 36–43 (grave 22), with prevalence of 33%.

Type 3 tooth wear was detected in a male, aged 40–50 (grave 9), with prevalence of 33%.

Type 4–5 tooth wear occurred in a male, aged 68–80 (grave 5) (figs. 5 b, c) with prevalence of 33%. At the same time in this individual, numerous *abscesses* were found—on the right incisors 1 and 2, and the right premolar P1 (fig. 5d) and on the left on P1 and M1.

Abscesses were also identified in the case of a male, aged 49–58 (grave 13), in the upper right M2 and M3 regions with prevalence of 66.7%.

TOOTH DECAY
Among the 14 examined jaws (3 male, 4 female and 4 children's) *tooth decay* was detected in two males: the male, aged 49–58 (grave 13) in maxillary left M3, and in the male, aged 43–52 (grave 8) in maxillary left M1.

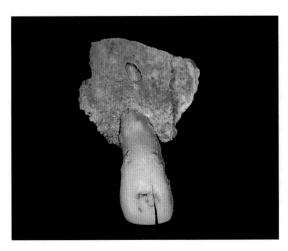

Fig. 11. *Artificial deformation with an incision in a tooth,* female, aged 40-60, in grave 2.
Photo: Zdenka Musilová.

PERIDONTITIS

Was detected in one female, aged 36- 40 (in grave no. 10) with prevalence of 25%.

ARTIFICIAL DEFORMATION

A *cut tooth* (fig. 11) was detected in the case of a woman, aged 40–60 (grave 2) with prevalence 25%.

EXCESSIVE STRAIN, BONE RIMS ON PHALANGES

In 9 males, 3 left hands with phalanges were preserved. In one male, aged 30–37 (grave 23), bone rims on proximal phalanges of the left hand were identified with prevalence of 33.3% (fig. 8c).

DISCUSSION AND CONCLUSION

CONGENITAL DEFECTS

PLAGIOCEPHALY

Plagiocephaly can be defined as an asymmetry of the scull due to one sided synostosis of the lambdoidal or coronal sutures, however, at the same time it also denotes the anterior or posterior deformational molding of the skull with patent sutures (Cohen 2000, 104).

It was the latter case that occurred in the asymmetrical skull of the male, aged 49-58 (in grave 13). When observing the facial region (fig. 1a, front view), it is apparent that the axis of the skull is bulged to the right. The skull is bulged in the right posterior region (fig. 1c, superior view), where, in the lambdoidal suture supernumerary intrasutural bones are present (fig. 1b, in the rear view indicated by arrows). The sagittal suture near the occipital region is partly fused in an instance of early sagittal suture fusion (fig. 1c).

The right mandibular ramus (fig. 1d, bottom view) is also deformed, more teeth are compressed in the left part of both the upper and lower jaw. The deflection, bulging to the right is most prominent in the lower part of the face. The teeth of the upper arch exhibit rotation in maxillary left P1, and also in a mandibular left premolar (fig. 1e).

It is apparent that this posterior nonsynostotic form of plagiocephaly might have arisen from numerous intrauterine factors, which affected the postnatal position of the infant's head (Mulliken et al. 1999). In right-sided molding it has to be presumed that the right ear of the male, aged 49–58 (grave 13), was positioned asymmetrically towards the posterior aspect. (Huang et al. 1996).

Factors such as hypotonia, foetus position, prematurity of delivery could have led to asymmetric flattening of the occipital region, while the infant's position on the back subsequently induced plagiocephaly. The changes and role of the occipital region are also indicated by the irregular shape of the foramen magnum (fig. 1d, bottom view).

BILATERAL POSTERIOR PLAGIOCEPHALY OR HYDROCEPHALUS

In the male, aged 41–45 in grave 24 (inventory no. 58.21) Zoffmann (1968, 30) described a hydrocephalic skull. The increase of the measurements of cranial breadth, concurrently with unaltered longitudinal and vertical dimensions indicate a hydrocephalic skull, while the slightly vaulted state of the skull, and some also increasing breadth measurements of the facial skeleton contradict this assumption (Brothwell 1963, 163–165). The skull and the postcranial bones in this grave were well preserved.

The neurocranium (braincase) is, in norma verticalis (superior aspect) widely rhomboideal, and in norma occipitalis (posterior aspect) wide and low wedge-shaped. In norma lateralis (lateral aspect), the forehead is low and steep, the vertex elongately and flatly arcuate, the occiput is weakly curvooccipital, and lambdoid flatness is slight. The maximum length of the skull is extreme (193 mm) but, owing to the extraordinary breadth (158 mm!) the cranial index indicates a slight brachycrany (81.87). The increase of the maximal breadth of the skull was also concomitant with the widening of the forehead. Thus, the low forehead became wide- metriometopic. Besides the considerable breadth, the other measurements are analogous to those of the other skulls from Villánykővesd.

Hydrocephalus is a condition in which there is an accumulation of cerebrospinal fluid within the brain ventricles. This occurrence must have been a case of Normal Pressure Hydrocephalus (NPH) which developed at a later age. It could have been caused by a stroke, meningitis, tumour or brain injury, but it could have also started idiopathically, without a specific cause. The male in grave 24 probably suffered from the typical triad of symptoms associated with this diagnosis: 1. Dominant walking disorder with very small steps and balance issues, 2. Memory failure and retarded psychomotorical pace, 3. Urinal incontinence with spontaneous urine leakage (Kala 2005).

Diagnostically, we are inclined to believe it was an occurrence of *bilateral posterior plagiocephaly with patent sutures*, however, since it is valid that 4–10% cases of craniostenosis are connected to hydrocephalus, the possibility of hydrocephalus needs to be considered in all patients with craniostenosis, particularly in those with complex synostosis or with syndromic synostosis (Camfield in Cohen et al. 2000, 179). Nevertheless, that does not make a difference to the valuable diagnosis that Zsuzsanna Zoffmann arrived at on the basis of craniometric examination.

LOWER JAW ASYMMETRY

In the 12–13-year-old child (grave 12 in fig. 2a), *lower jaw asymmetry* was determined with prevalence of 14.3% together with *artificial deformation* (a cut incisor). It was a congenital defect, because the right side of the jaw is shorter than the left and the 7th tooth on right is opposite the 6th tooth on the left. In addition to this, an anomalous tubercle on the maxillary right second molar (M2) (fig. 2b) was identified in the same child with prevalence of 14.3%.

DEATH IN CHILDBIRTH AND CONGENITAL SPINE DEFORMITY

In grave 10, among the pelvis of a female, aged 36–40 (inventory no. 58.8), fragments of a foetal skeleton with periostitis inside the skull in the occipital region were discovered (fig. 6).

It is likely that the foetus was affected by meningitis, intracranially, *striated periosteal remodelling* is apparent and the same changes were also identified in the pelvic bones (fig. 12a). Presumably, the foetus might have contracted an infection, but the mother was unable to deliver it. The pelvis of the skeleton is very narrow, the sacrum being more arcuate than the average female sacrum (Zoffmann 1968, 27). According to Dombay's observation (1959, 63) the bones of the infant were partially still within the pelvis of the female skeleton. Therefore, in all probability, the buried individual had a pelvic structure causing her death during delivery (Regöly-Merei 1960, 76–77).

In the lumbar section of the spinal column the vertebrae L4, L5 are in fusion, and since the other vertebrae show no pathological deformation, this fusion is probably congenital (Regöly-Merei 1960, 76, plate v, fig. 21, plate vi, fig. 24).

It needs to be agreed that the fusion is most probably congenital. It is characteristic of the fifth lumbar vertebra that its body is much larger in the anterior aspect than the posterior one (Gray's Anatomy 1977, 43). In this

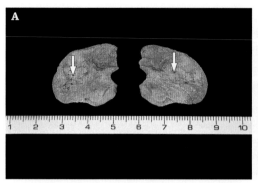
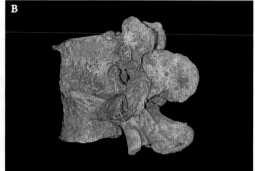

Fig. 12a–b. A: *Striated periosteal remodelling* in pelvic bones of an unborn infant, grave 10. B: *Congenital fusion of lumbar vertebrae L4-L5,* which probably prevented the delivery of the foetus and subsequently caused death Photo: Zdenka Musilová.

instance, from the lateral aspect (fig. 12b) in the compound L4, L5, this is reversed, and the placement of the fusion is difficult to detect, which is also indicative of a congenital defect.

In the Lengyel culture the mortality rate in childbirth was high, in Alsónyék- Bátaszék Köhler discovered two similar occurrences in graves 474 and 4414 (see her entry). She believes the reason for this was the difference in size between the mother's pelvic brim and the foetus's skull.

OZAENA

In the male, aged 68–80 (grave 5) based on unusual broadness of the nasal base and unusual narrowing of the facial cavities an atrophic deformity was described by Regöly-Mérei which he identified with the clinical picture of ozaena (Regöly-Mérei 1960, 76, plate ii, fig. 9, 1962, 138, fig. 116, wrongly cited as a find from Zengővárkony) (Zoffman 1968) to which only the find of periostitis in the crista nasalis region can be added (fig. 5).

TUBERCULOSIS OR BRUCELLOSIS

In a thoracic vertebra of the male, aged 30–37 (grave 23), there is an obvious cavity with a fistula, probably caused by the outflow of casein (fig. 8a, b); the lesion affecting the whole vertebra is bottle-shaped with openings on both plates of the vertebra. Near the upper plate the vertebral body collapsed, with a prolapse of the nucleus pulposus into the cavity narrowing the intervertebral space. The big cavity in the vertebral body was filled with a mass of "caseation," and the spreading of granulation tissue from this saddle cavity (Adler 2000, 146) must have continued even into the lower intervertebral space, probably up to the anterior longitudinal ligament. The formation of a hypostatic abscess can be presumed with further development leading to the formation of a wedge vertebra and subsequently gibbus angularis (hump). It is typical for tuberculous spondylitis and was described for the Lengyel Culture in 2007 at the Alsónyek-Bátaszek site (5th millennium B.C.) (Köhler et al. 2014, figs. 3, 4) in an adult male, aged 30–35, in grave no. 4027, where most characteristic pathologic changes were observed between the 10th thoracic and 4th lumbar vertebrae.

The formation of the vertebral compound which originates through fusion and replacement of the disk with osseous tissue is very strongly aided by circumjacent osteoporosis, however, it is not present in the vertebra from grave 23 in Villánykővesd. From the point of view of differential diagnosis, this leads us to take into consideration the possibility of brucellosis in this instance. That may radiologically imitate tubercular spondylitis in every detail (Adler 2000, 154), however, osteoporosis is exhibited to a much lower extent in brucellosis than in tuberculosis.

TRANSMISSION OF ZOONOSES

The Lengyel Culture (LgC) herds comprised of domesticated cattle, goats, sheep and hogs.

The Neolithic farmers could have contracted contagious zoonoses such as tuberculosis from cows or their milk, or brucellosis from goats and their milk.

The origins of dairying and usage of unpasteurized milk in the diet was an important innovation of the Neolithic, yet, at the same time crucial for the transmission of zoonoses onto the human population.

Zooarchaeological research shows that dairying originated in the Middle East in the 8th millennium B.C., nevertheless, direct evidence of organic remains preserved on pottery dated to the 7th millennium B.C. comes from Anatolia (Evershead 2008).

BRUCELLA MELITENSIS

Mixing of the goat population in a Neolithic village can be presumed. Even though Brucella Melitensis is also found in semen, only female goats are potentially contagious. The infectious material is the vaginal secretion of infected goats in miscarriage or full-term parturition. Goats remain contagious for several months.

The increased mortality rate of he-goats led to their killing and therefore also specialization for meat consumption in Neolithic breeding. Goats were kept for reproduction. However, that is how Brucellosis was maintained among goat populations. The number of female goats increased, and adult female goats were responsible for the transmission of the pathogen.

The disappearance of the pathogen was therefore more likely in small village populations than in great goat populations belonging to large settlements.

Goat breeding grew in the middle of the 7th millennium B.C., when in most Neolithic sites, male goats were being killed. Subsequently, with further development the transmission of brucellosis to the human population increased due to escalated dairying practices (Fourié et al. 2017).

3.3 BELVÁRDGYULA-SZARKAHEGY: ARCHAEOLOGICAL DESCRIPTION AND PALEOPATHOLOGIC ANALYSIS
VÁCLAV SMRČKA AND ZDENKA MUSILOVÁ

Location: on a plateau northwest of Belvárdgyula, 300 m north of the M60 Motorway (Belvárdgyula 601106 70868 (EOV, 11-111).

3.3.1 ARCHAEOLOGICAL DESCRIPTION

In 2006 and 2007, a rescue excavation was carried out on the route of the M60 Motorway on the outskirts of the village of Belvárdgyula. It was already obvious then that the motorway would cut a late Neolithic settlement and cemetery.

Excavation and field-walking data showed that the motorway excavation covered the southern edge of the site while the bulk of the settlement lay to the north.

During an aerial photography sortie aimed at documenting the progression of excavation works along the motorway route Bertók, Gáti and Lóki (2008) a circular enclosure on the northern perimeter of the settlement was detected. In 2008, further field—walking and geophysical—surveys were carried out to acquire dating information and a detailed plan of the site. The results showed that the enclosure was contemporary with the adjacent settlement.

The geophysical survey also indicated that the rondel enclosure had had elaborate gate structures that were destroyed and levelled most probably in the Neolithic, and therefore the detail of their structure could not be discerned in the magnetogram. There are several features showing up as magnetic anomalies. Based on their shape and size, some of these anomalies may be identified as houses. This was the first site in Baranya county where the close relation between a settlement and a rondel could be demonstrated (Bertók and Gáti 2011, 2014).

3.3.2 PALEOPATHOLOGICAL ANALYSIS (N = 21)

The skeletal collection from the Belvárdgyula site was examined in the depositories of the Janus Pannonius Museum in spring 2018. The bone material was highly fragmentary. It comprised of a total of 21 burials (5 male, 8 female, 3 children and 5 unspecified individuals); complete skeletons (No = 7), as well as skull burials (No = 7) and skeletal burials without skulls or their fragments (No = 7) were represented. The feasibility of paleopathological analysis was limited due to the bad condition of the skeletons. The bones were examined macroscopically and along with description of their pathology the intactness of bones was also documented, which allowed for the frequency of individual pathologies in the population to be determined.

WORKLOAD

Traces of workload were discovered both in male and female bones.

RIMS ON PHALANGES

In one male and two females the phalanges of the hands were examined for marks of excessive workload.

The female, aged 40-60 (grave no. 98-292/1529), exhibited *bony rims on the phalanges of both the right and left hand* (with prevalence of 50%) (fig. 1).

Longitudinal osseous rims, about 2 mm high were present on the palmar edge of proximal phalanges with maximum bone "expansion" between the middle and distal thirds of the mentioned phalanges. These are insertion points of short palmar flexors (mm. interossei et lumbricales). The rims originated as the result of long-term work, probably in fibre processing.

CONGENITAL DEFECTS

In the group of 10 skulls examined at the burial site (4 male, 5 female and 1 child) two cases of *metopism* were found, one in a male, aged 20-40 (grave

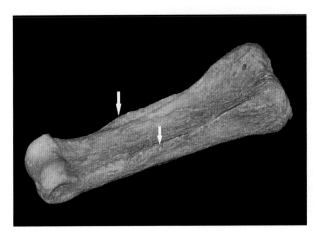

Fig. 1. *Bony rims* on the proximal left hand phalanx of a female, aged 40-60 (grave 98-292/1529) (arrows indicate bone rims caused by excessive action of interosseous muscles). Photo: Zdenka Musilová.

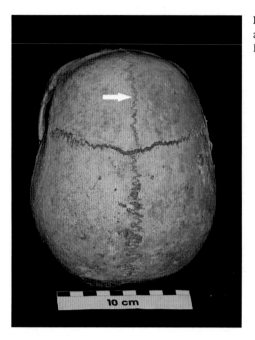

Fig. 2. *Metopism* (arrow) male, aged 20–40 (grave 98-155/622). Photo: Zdenka Musilová.

no. 98-155/622; with prevalence of 25%) (fig. 2), and in a female, aged 20–30 (grave no. 98-42/137; prevalence of 20%).

One instance of a *pentagonal skull* in a male, aged 20–40 (grave no. 98-243/-) with prevalence of 25%, was discovered. The same individual exhibited Wormian bones, which were also found in a male, aged 20–40 (grave no. 98-155/622) with prevalence of 50%.

In the skull of the male from grave no. 98-243/-, Wormian bones were found in the lambdoid suture above processus mastoideus bilaterally, and at the same time, an occipital protuberance was apparent.

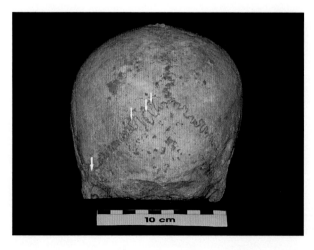

Fig. 3. *Ossa wormiana* (arrows) male, aged 20–40 (grave 98-155/622). Photo: Zdenka Musilová.

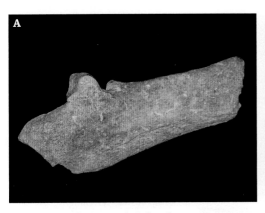
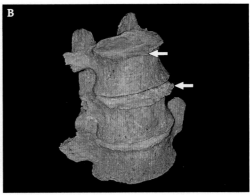

Fig. 4a-b. A: In Belvárdgyula, in grave no. 98-292-1529, of a woman aged 40-60, a long goat's/sheep's bone with *striated periostitis* was found (6975). B: In the lumbar spine region of this female there is a *periosteal reaction with traits of brucellosis* in the region of fixation of the anulus fibrosus. Photo: Zdenka Musilová.

In the second occurrence of Wormian intra-sutural bones, male (grave no. 98-155/622), these would be found along the external part of the lambdoidal sutures, while these sutures were open (fig. 3).

Congenital defects mostly affected the cranial region.

SPINAL OSTEOPHYTOSIS

The lumbar part of the spine was examined in 7 individuals (4 males and 3 females). In a male of undetermined age (grave no. 98-373/2359) spondylar *osteophytes, 1 mm in size*, with prevalence of 25% were identified. (The same individual exhibited soft bones on hip bone sampling for osteoporosis testing). In a female, aged 40-60 (grave no. 98-292/1529) periostal reactions with traits of brucellosis and large osteophytes were observed (fig. 4).

SPINAL AND FEMORAL OSTEOPOROSIS

Deformed vertebrae, L4 and L5, were discovered in the lumbar spine of a 20-40-year-old male (grave no. 98-243/1231). These deformed vertebrae (*Fish Vertebra*) had concavely deformed plates of the vertebral bodies and a narrowed central part of the vertebral body indicating *spinal osteoporosis* (with prevalence of 25%) (figs. 5a, 5b).

The identified "fish vertebrae" in the lumbar spine and their concave shape originated through increased tension in the nucleus pulposus of the vertebral disc, its broadening and pressure exerted on the vertebral body itself. The vertebral body endplate curved inwards because the trabecular pillar structure was weakened.

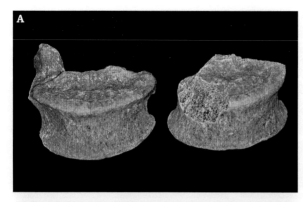

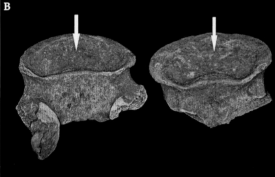

Fig. 5a–c. A: In Belvárdgyula, grave no. 98-243-1231, of a male aged 20-40, the lumbar vertebrae show marks (6952) of *brucellar osteolytic lesions*, an impression of the anulus fibrosus in a layer of compact bone in the superior, frontal aspect of the vertebrae. On the chipped part of the vertebral body there is evidence of new bone formation below the revealed part of the plate. B: *Osteoporosis of vertebral bodies* with concavely deformed lumbar vertebra plates, "Fish Vertebrae" (arrows indicate the location of the nucleus pulposus denting in on the vertebral planes), male, aged 20-40 (grave 98-243/1231). C: *Femoral Osteoporosis* preceding age-related changes in a male, aged 20-40 (grave 98-243/1231) Photo: Zdenka Musilová.

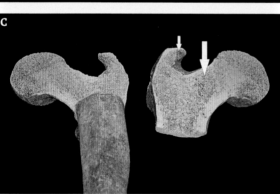

The vertebral body subsequently narrowed in its central part, in which instance, we assume the development of stage 3 osteoporosis (Adler 2000, 68-71).

In grave in Belvárdgyula (no. 98-243-1231), of a male, aged 20-40, in whom osteoporosis with fish vertebra was described, traits (fig. 5a—6952) of osteolytic lesions of the impression of the anulus fibrosus in a layer of compact bone in the superior frontal aspect of lumbar vertebrae were also present. In the chipped-off part on the right, new formation under the uncov-

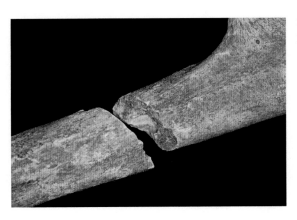

Fig. 6. The *oblique perimortal fracture* of the right femur, male, aged 20–40 (grave 98243/1231). Photo: Zdenka Musilová.

ered segment of the plate is apparent. But these signatures can be associated with *brucellosis*.

In the case of this individual, osteoporotic changes preceded the estimated age of the individual even in the aging of the left femoral neck and the greater trochanter, while the sustentacular spongious trabecula of the head were still well-preserved (fig. 5c).

TRAUMA

16 femurs were examined at the burial site: 9 right (4 male, 3 female and 2 children) and 7 left (4 male, 2 female and 1 child). One instance of an *oblique perimortal fracture of the right femur* was found (in a male, aged 20–40, in grave no. 98-243/1231) with prevalence of 25% (fig. 6). The fracture did not show any signs of healing and there is a high probability that the individual died due to complications. It could also have been a pathological fracture since the opposite femur exhibited osteoporotical changes both in the neck and the greater trochanter (fig. 5c) and at the same time there was spinal osteoporosis in the lumbar spine L4, L5.

INFLAMMATIONS—PERIOSTITIS

In Belvárdgyula, grave 98-292-1529, along with a woman, aged 40-60, a long goat's/sheep's bone with striated new bone formation (fig. 4a—6975; chapter 3) was found. In the lumbar spine region (fig. 4b—6960; chapter 3) of the woman, a periosteal reaction in the superior frontal part of two lumbar vertebrae indicating *symptoms of brucellosis* in the region of anulus fibrosus fixation was present (Capasso 1999). Large osteophytes result from tendon osseous metaplasia. Periostitis found in the goat's bone would also correspond to the symptoms of brucellosis in the woman's spine. This woman also suffered from cribra orbitalia in the left orbit.

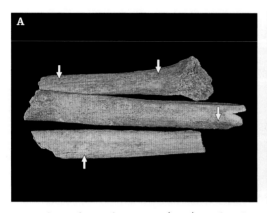
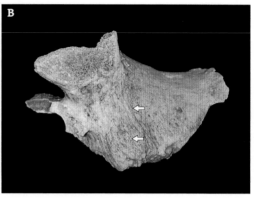

Fig. 7a–b. A: *Rib periostitis* (6922) in a female, aged 40–60, from grave no. 98-83-408, Belvárdgyula, exhibiting multiple periostitis probably of brucellar origin. B: Periostitis was also identified in the pelvic region (6924). Photo: Zdenka Musilová.

13 tibias were examined: 7 right (4 male and 3 female) and 6 left (4 male and 2 female). In one right tibia of a female, aged 20–40 (grave no. 98-447/2941), *periostitis of right tibia* was detected.

At the same time, right tibia periostitis was also identified in a woman, aged 40–60 (grave no. 98-83/408) with prevalence of 66.7% (fig. 7). This female had *multiple periostitis*, with periostitides in both upper and lower limbs as well as the pelvis.

The inflammation of the periosteum may result from various causes and may indicate infection and even tumours (Adler 2000). The bone and the periosteum react in a similar manner to various influences, in cases of infection by striated periostal remodelling, in cases of tumours generally by outgrowths, spicula. It may be a case of generalized periostitis affecting multiple

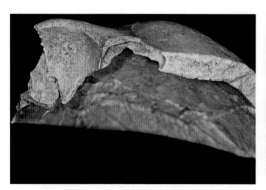
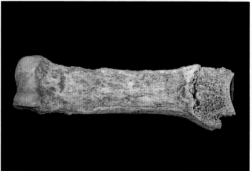

Fig. 8a–b. A: *Cribra orbitalia I-II* in the preserved right orbit of a female, age undetermined (grave 98-73/202). B: In grave no. 98-73/ 202, Belvárdgyula, in an unidentified individual, probably male, *periostitis* was also found in the proximal phalanges of the fingers (6983). Photo: Zdenka Musilová.

bones or limited to a single one (Gladykowska-Rzeczycka 1998). In the case of the female, aged 40-60 (grave no. 98-83/408), it was an instance of *generalized periostitis*. Perhaps an unspecific inflammation, considering the fact that the pelvis was affected, the infection could have originated in the birth canal.

But the female, aged 40-60, from grave no. 98-83-408, who had multiple periostitis in Belvárdgyula probably suffered from brucellosis, as visible in the lower limbs periostitis (fig. 7a—6922) and it also occurred in the pelvic region (fig. 7b—6924).

In grave no. 98-73/202 in Belvárdgyula of an unidentified individual, though probably male, with right orbital cribra (fig. 8a—6983), signs of brucella periostitis in proximal phalanges was also detected (fig. 8b—6983).

CRIBRA ORBITALIA

In Belvárdgyula a total of 14 orbits were examined: 8 right (2 male and 6 female) and 6 left (2 male and 4 female).

Type 1 cribra orbitalia was identified in the case of a male, aged 20-40 (grave no. 98-243), in both preserved orbits (prevalence 50%). In the case of male, aged 20-40 (grave no. 98-379/2387), bilateral *type 2* cribra was determined, with prevalence of 50%.

A female, aged 40-60 (grave no. 292/1529), had both orbits preserved, and *type 1* cribra, with 25% prevalence, was determined in the left one. In the case of a female of undetermined age, only the right orbit was preserved, with *type 1 cribra orbitalia* and prevalence of 16.7% (fig. 8).

RIB POROSITY AND PERIOSTITIS

A detailed rib examination was conducted in eight individuals (3 male, 4 female and 1 child).

In a male, aged 20-40 (grave no. 98-379/2387), *rib porosity* with prevalence of 33.3% was detected. But also signs probably of *brucella periostitis* can also

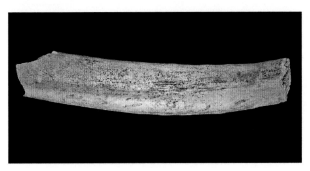

Fig. 9. *Signs of brucellar periostitis* can also be observed on the ribs (6893) of a male, aged 20-40, in grave no. 98-379-2387, Belvárdgyula. There are small oblong neoformations and impressions of the pleura (6886). Photo: Zdenka Musilová.

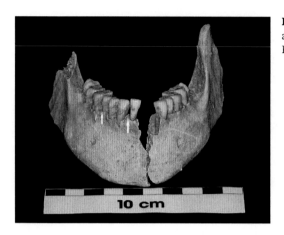

Fig. 10. *Periodontitis* in a male, aged 20-40 (grave 98-155/622). Photo: Zdenka Musilová

be observed in the rib where there are small elongated neoformations and impressions of the pleura (fig. 9—6886). In this male, anaemia manifested through type 2 cribra was also identified.

CHANGES IN TEETH

Teeth were assessed in 13 individuals (4 male, 7 female, 1 child and 1 undetermined individual).

PERIODONTAL DISEASE
In a male, aged 20-40 (grave no. 98-379/2387), then in male, aged 20-40 let (grave no. 98-243) and male, aged 20-40 (grave no. 98-155/622) *gingival recession* with prevalence of 75% was found.

TOOTH DECAY
In female, aged 40-60 (grave no. 98-83/408), coronal caries in M3, lower left, with a prevalence of 28.6% was determined.

DENTAL CALCULUS
In a female, aged 40-60 (grave no. 98-292/1529), *dental calculus* was identified on the lower left second incisor (I2), cuspid (C) and the first premolar (P1) with a prevalence of 14.3% (fig. 11).

TOOTH WEAR IN MALES

Type I
In a male, aged 20-40 (grave no. 98-379/2387), and male, aged 20-40 (grave no. 98-243), *type I tooth wear* with prevalence of 50% was determined.

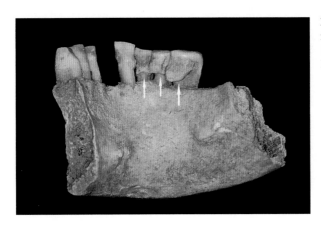

Fig. 11. *Dental calculus* in a female, aged 40–60 (grave 98–292/1529). Photo: Zdenka Musilová.

Type II
In a male, aged 20–40 (grave no. 98–155/622), *type II tooth wear* with prevalence of 25% was present.

Type III
In a male of undetermined age (grave no. 98–373/2359) *type III tooth wear* was identified with a prevalence of 25% (fig. 12).

TOOTH WEAR IN FEMALES

Type I
In a female, aged 20–30 (grave no. 98–42/137), *type I tooth wear* was determined with a prevalence of 14.3%.

Type II
In a female, aged 20–40 (grave no. 98–447/2941), *type II tooth wear* was identified and in a 30-year-old female (grave no. 98–284/1440) the presence of *type II tooth wear* with prevalence of 28.6% was also detected.

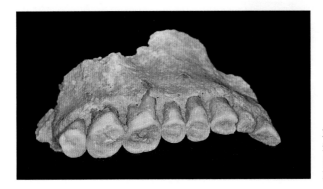

Fig. 12. Type III tooth wear in a male, age undetermined (grave 98–373/2359). Photo: Zdenka Musilová.

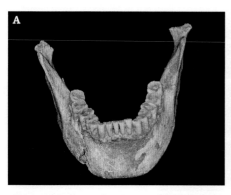
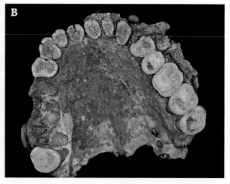

Fig. 13. Type III tooth wear in a female, aged 40–60 (grave 98-83/408), a) lower jaw, b) upper jaw. Photo: Zdenka Musilová.

Type III

In a 20-year-old female (grave no. 98-368/2207), *type III tooth wear* was described, likewise, in a female, aged 40–60 (grave no. 98-83/408) (fig. 13) as well as in a female, aged 40–60 (grave no. 292/1529), *type III tooth wear* was found with prevalence of 42.8%

ARTIFICIAL INCISIONS IN TEETH

In the case of a female, aged 40–60 (grave no. 98-83/408), incisions were discovered in the lower left cuspid and incisor, and in another female, aged 30 (grave no. 98-284/1440), an *artificial incision* was identified in the lower incisor with a prevalence of 28.6% (fig. 14).

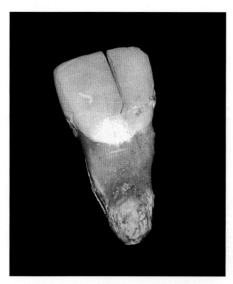

Fig. 14. *Artificial incision* in lower incisor, female, aged 30 (grave 98-284/1440).

CONCLUSION

The described skeletal collection from the Belvárdgyula site shows signs of excessive workload in fibre processing in the case of an elderly female. This is proved by rims on the proximal phalanges. At the same time, in one male and two females, excessive strain is proved by tooth wear probably caused by hide processing. The lumbar spine was affected and exhibited 3 mm osteophytes in the case of one female, and even in this instance, excessive strain, for example in daily preparation of grains on the quern-stone, can be presumed.

The population was afflicted by congenital skull defects with a prevailing suture closure disorder.

In one individual, osteoporosis of the lumbar spine, femoral neck and an unhealed collateral femoral fracture were determined. It could seem to be an isolated case of osteoporosis, however, the histological findings indicate a greater incidence of osteoporosis in the population. Osteoporotic changes will also be indicated in trace element levels (chapter 5) as well as by the incidence of orbital cribra and rib porosity.

In the population, there was one occurrence of multiple periostitis, probably caused by a nonspecific infection.

To sum up, it can be said that the LgC population from the Belvárdgyula collection from the Belvárdgyula suffered from periostitis of the skeleton, of which some cases can be associated with brucellosis, at least in the 5 cases in Belvárdgyula (where periostitis in a goat was identified in grave no. 292).

3.4 BELVÁRDGYULA-SZARKAHEGY: RESULTS OF THE MACROSCOPICAL AND HISTOLOGICAL EXAMINATION
CTIBOR POVÝŠIL AND VÁCLAV SMRČKA

3.4.1 MACROSCOPICAL FINDINGS
VÁCLAV SMRČKA

The analysis of stable strontium isotopes in the remains from Belvárdgyula-Szarkahegy revealed that the population was local. The bone materials were only fragmentary preserved. The main macroscopical pathological findings were as follows:

1. Grave 98-243-1231. A male, aged 20-40, who had Wormian bones in the skull. He suffered from anaemia, manifesting as cribra orbitalia and his lumbar vertebrae were concavely curved (see photos no. 5a, b). He suffered a perimortem fracture of the femur as a result of the fragility of his long bones due to his condition.

2. Grave 98-284-1440. A female, aged 30, without noticeable pathologies. She had type 2 tooth wear and an artificial incision on an anterior incisor.
3. Grave 98-292-1529. A female, aged 40-60, with cribrification in the left orbit, tooth decay and dental plaque deposits, and 3 mm osteophytic rim on the lumbar vertebrae. This woman would have endured strenuous work, evidenced by prominent muscle insertions and rims on phalanges; these are indications of work that would have placed excessive strain on the interosseous muscles of the hands.
4. Grave 98-83-408. A histological sample from the pelvis of a female, aged 40-60, with generalised periostitis.
5. Grave 98-379-2387. A pelvis sample of a male, aged 20-40, with anaemia manifesting as bilateral cribra orbitalia type 2 and rib porosity.
6. Grave 989-447-2941. A pelvis sample of a female, aged 20-40, with periostitis of the right tibia.
7. Grave 98-353-2109. A pelvis sample of a child, aged 8, without noticeable pathologies.
8. Grave 98-368-2205. A pelvis sample of a female, aged 20-40, without noticeable pathologies.
9. Grave 98-373-2359. A pelvis sample of a male of undetermined age with arthrosis of the lumbar vertebrae.

Among the 9 individuals from the aforementioned site, from whom pelvic samples were taken, there were instances of cribra orbitalia and rib porosity (3×), and periostosis, including 2 occurences of generalised periostosis. These would not have been affected by diagenesis of the soil.

A special case is the male, aged 20-40, from grave no. 98-243-1231, whose bone fragility and susceptibility to fractures, as well as his concave vertebrae could point to osteoporosis.

This would correspond to Adler's data (Adler 2000, 54). The female, aged 40-60, from grave no. 98-292-1529 is also of note due to indications of brucellosis on her spine.

3.4.2 HISTOLOGICAL EXAMINATION
CTIBOR POVÝŠIL

MATERIAL AND METHODS

Bone samples from 5 men and 6 women were histologically examined. A sample composed of the medial and lateral cortical bone, including cancellous bone, was removed from the anterior part of the ilium. An anterior iliac crest sample was used, as this site is considered optimal for bone histomorphometric examination. One part of each specimen was processed using standard techniques for histological examination after demineralisation in

EDTA. After fixation in a buffered 10% formaldehyde solution for 2 hours and tissue dehydratation, the samples were embedded in parafin and sectioned into 5 μm sections. Each section was stained with hematoxylin and eosin to evaluate the general morphology and cell organisation of the bone tissue.

The second part of each specimen was fixed in 70% ethanol for 48 hours. Without demineralisation, it was then dehydrated in absolute alcohol and embedded in a methyl metacrylate based resin. Subsequently, non-decalcified thin sections were cut from the sample using a Leica SM microtome and stained using several techniques. 5μm sections were stained with hematoxylin-eosin, Masson's trichrome, Goldner's trichrome method, van Giesson method, von Kossa's impregnation method, Gomorl's method for reticular fibres, toluidine blue, histochemical reactions for Al (aluminoin technique) and Perls' method for iron (Bancroft and Gamble 2002). Qualitative and quantitative analysis of sections using light and polarised light were performed.

The basic quantitative histomorphometric analysis of trabecular bone was carried out using the following calculations: trabecular bone volume (TV/BV) = bone volume (BV/tissue volume (TV) × 100 (%), corresponding to a percentage of the total bone tissue volume; osteoid relative surface (OS/BS) = trabecular surface covered with osteoid (OS/all trabecular surface (BS) × 100 (%), corresponding to a percentage of the trabecular bone surface covered with osteoid (Eriksen et al. 1994; Malluche et al. 1986; Povýšil, Sotorník, and Válek 1990; Povýšil 2017; Vigorita 1999). Trabecular diameter was the shortest distance from one surface to the other. The median value of at least 100 measurements was used to define the trabecular diameter.

Measurements were made by semi-automated image analysis using a Quick photo camera from Olympus and Laboratory Imaging Lucia image analyser. All morphometric measurements were done in the spongy bone of the iliac crest. The field for morphologic evaluation was 30 mm^2.

RESULTS

The samples obtained from iliac bone in the majority of cases (no. 98–243–1231, 98–284–1440, 98–292–1529, 98–83–408, 98–379–2387, 989–447–2941, 98–353–2109, 98–368–2205) had abnormal histological architecture in both main components i.e. in both cortical and trabecular bone (figs. 1–5). It was not possible to identify osteons of the haversian system in cortical bone due to its compact structure. Cortical bone porosity was not increased, and cortical thining was observed.

When studying cortical and trabecular bone in polarised light, a clear lamellar pattern, which is characteristic of normal bone (Eriksen et al. 1994; Povýšil et al. 2017; Vigorita 1999) was not visible. No woven bone structures were observed, which would have been indicative of some metabolic bone

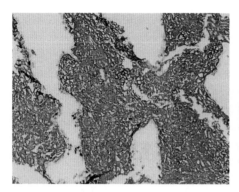

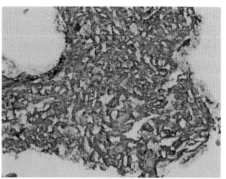

Fig. 1. A histological section from the non-decalcified sample obtained from iliac bone (casse no. 98-243-1231). In this picture is seen cancelous bone with preserved connectivity of bone trabecullae. In the inner structure of trabecullae there were multiple small empty spaces of uncertain origin. Magnification 24×, stained with haematoxylin eosin.

Fig. 2. Detail of the inner structure of bone trabecullae containing multiple empty spaces surrounded with mineralised bone tissue (case no. 98-243-1231). Magnification ×120, stained with hemaoxylin eosin.

disorders. Cancelous bone consists of thick bone trabeculae, that is interconnected in a honeycomb pattern (figs. 1–3). It was not possible to identify deep resorption cavities on the surface of bone trabeculae which occurs in renal or endocrine bone diseases. No osteoid seams on the surface of bone trabeculae were observed when using the von Kossa impregnation method (figs. 3 and 4). However, all examined bone trabeculae had an abnormal inner structure; they contained multiple large, irregualrly distributed empty spaces of the

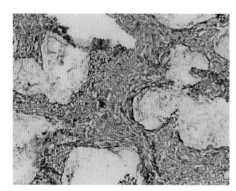

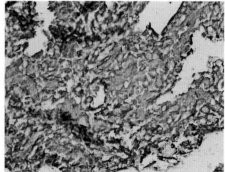

Fig. 3. Histological section from the undecalcified bone tissue after impregnation with von Kossa's technique (case no. 98-284-1440). Mineralised bone is brown or black. Empty spaces remain unstained. Magnification ×120.

Fig. 4. Detail of the inner structure of bone trabeculla after impregnation with von Kossa's technique (case no. 98-284-1440). Mineralised bone is brown or black. Empty spaces remain unstained. Magnification ×250.

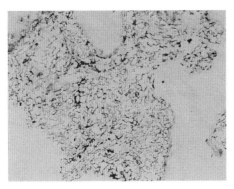 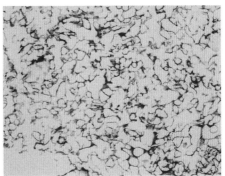

Fig. 5. Histological section from the decalcified bone tissue stained with Masson's technique (case no. 98-243-1231). Bone tissue contained sparce preserved collagen fibers in mineralised parts surrounding empty spaces. Magnification ×120, Masson's trichrom stain

Fig. 6. Detail of the collagen fibers in bone trabeculla from decalcified bone tissue stained with Masson's technique (case no. 98-243-1231). Magnification ×250

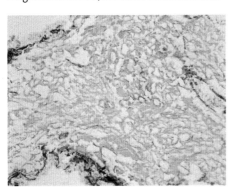

Fig. 7. Histological section from the undecalcified bone tissue stained with alcian blue. In the empty spaces there are residua of alcian blue positive material of the unknown origin (case no. 98-243-1231). Magnification ×120, alcian blue stain

varying shape and size (figs. 1–6). Typical osteocytic lacunae were absent in the vicinity of these large spaces. These empty spaces were surrounded with thin bundles of mineralised bone tissue oriented in different directions (fig. 3). In some small areas of these empty spaces, deposits of amorphous substances without the presence of crystals were identified; this stained with alcian blue (fig. 7) and was slightly positive using the von Kossa impregnation method (fig. 4). Furthermore, no cement lines were present. The reticulin impregnation method showed a delicate pattern of collagen fibers surrounding empty spaces in bone trabeculae. A similar pattern of collagen fibers was also seen using Masson's staining method (fig. 5).

A different microscopic pattern was seen in case no. 98-373-2359. In this case, empty spaces in bone trabeculae were absent, as were microscopical lamellar structures.

Bone biopsy samples reflect past and current bone cellular events in during the life of an individual. Some parameters also remain preserved after

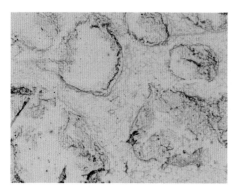

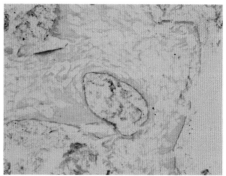

Fig. 8. Histological section from the decalcified bone tissue stained with Perls method for iron (case no. 98–243-1231). Soil material in intertrabecular spaces is intensivelly positive as well as surfaces of bone trabecullae. Positive linear staining of trabecullar surfaces is probably result of diffusion of iron from soil containing the admixture of this metal. Magnification ×120, Perls method

Fig. 9. Detail of Fe positive linear staining of trabecullar surfaces in decalcified bone tissue (case no. 98–243-1231). Magnification ×250, Perls method

death e.g. the bone mass, which is dependent on the balance between bone resorption and formation. In the examined cases, the mineralisation of the bone was preserved within normal parameters (figs. 3 and 4), excluding the non-mineralised, so called empty spaces. The median trabecular volume was increased by ~24% as a result of a thickening of bone trabeculae. The median trabecular diameter was 180 ± 58 µm. The osteoid relative surface was negative as no osteoid seams were observed (figs. 3 and 4). Signs of erosion were absent on bone trabeculae meaning that osteoclastic activity was minimal.

Bone remnants were contaminated with soil from the site where they were deposited. The soil material was seen in intertrabecular spaces, and in some cases also contained mineral crystals. Staining with Perl's method showed the presence of iron in the materials deposited between bone trabecullae. In additon, the surfaces of bone trabecullae were also positive for iron in a linear orientation (figs. 8 and 9), likely as a consequnnce of post mortem impregnation with iron during the diagenetic process.

DISCUSSION

The data derived from exhumed bone tissue samples allow us to assess only some of the static variables: bone volume, trabecular diameter, osteoid surface, and/or osteoid volume. The identification of osteoblasts and osteoclasts was not possible due to postmortem autolytic processes that had destroyed the bone cells, as well the non-mineralised bone tissue in some cases.

Higher values of trabecular bone volume (BV/TV) were shown in the iliac crest when compared with control data (Považil, a control group of Czech men and women, unpublished data). Conditions characterised with focal or generalised increased trabecular bone volume are known as osteoscleroses. They have different aetiopathogenesis, including a variety of dietary, metabolic, endocrine, haematological, and neoplastic disorders. The diffuse forms of osteosclerosis is rare. It occurs in primary and secondary hyperparathyroidism (Vogel et al. 1995), heavy metal poisoning such as strontium and fluorine (Brun et al. 2014; Marie 2006; Vigorita 1999) and as a consequence of ionizing radiation exposure.

In addition, many rare hereditary disorders may also cause primary focal or generalised osteosclerosis (Warman et al. 2011). They constitute a group of disorders conveniently termed 'sclerosing bone dysplasias'. The literature on these conditions has largely been compiled by radiologists as the x-ray findings are often the most predominant feature of these disorders. Our histological findings show that it is possible to presume the presence of generalised osteosclerosis from promoted bone formation and a reduction in bone resorption. As bone samples were limited to those from the iliac crest, a broader analysis is required to verify this conclusion. X-ray analysis of skeletal remains could likely specify the character of these pathological bone disorder in older agricultural populations.

Staining methods were used to enable separation of osteoid from mineralised bone in histological sections prepared from non-decalcified bone samples. No osteoid seams, composed of unmineralised bone matrix, were identified in the examined group. Such finding excludes the presence of disorders such renal osteodystrophy, nutritional osteomalacia, vitamin D and calcium deficiency from malabsorption syndromes, intoxications with certain metals, and phosphate deficiency. Hypophosphatemic syndromes occur in acquired and congenital forms. These are predominantly either a result of a loss of phosphate secondary to mesenchymal tumour, or with an altered renal tubular function as consequence of a primary inborn error of phosphate transport in the proximal nephron. We can also exclude osteomalacic disorder, which occurs as a complication of various renal, endocrine and gastrointestinal diseases, as well as a consequnce of the deposition of some metals e.g. Al and Fe.

It is difficult to evaluate the relative degree of collagen deposited in skeletal remains due to the millenia they have spent buried. Histochemical methods used during histological examination of bone samples e.g. Masson's trichrome, Goldner's trichrome method, van Giesson method and Gomorl's impregnation method are reliable means for the identification of collagen

(Bancroft and Gamble 2002; Jellinghaus et al. 2018) as they yield good results. These staining methods verified sparse collagen fibers in the mineralisied component of bone trabecullae surroundings the empty spaces.

The described histological changes of examined bone tissue with the empty spaces are completely unusual; no similar bone pattern has previously been described. A possible explanation may be that a histological examination of samples from the iliac crest has not been sytematically performed until now. In paleopathological literature, the study of diseases affecting organisms of the past is dominated by descriptions of macroscopic pathological changes, with a shortage of microscopical documentation (Ortner 2011), or it focuses on structural changes occurring in long bones (Caruso et al. 2018; Hackett 1981). These structural changes were associated with focal loss of mineral and bone matrix. These findings were compared with similar findings in Saint Ivan, a Czech hermit, who had likely suffered from chondrocalcinosis (Povýšil et al. 2017). In contrast, these empty spaces in bone tissue contained calcium phosphate and hydroxyapatite crystals. Crystal deposition were positive when stained with alcian blue and were birefrigent in polarized light microscopy. Furthermore, the residua of lamellar bone was locally preserved and easily identifiable in Saint Ivan; this was not discernible in the previously mentioned bone tissues with the empty spaces

These differences are difficult to explain and are a topic for discussion. The possibility that these empty spaces may have contained materials that were dissolved during the samples' millenia buried cannot be excluded. Another hypothesis is that these spaces correspond to osteocytic lacunae that were surrounded with thick osteoid seams, and were subsequently destroyed during autolytic processes. Taphonomic experimental research models, using pig skeletal remains, produce similar post-mortem microstructural changes in skeletal tissues. Kontopoulos et al. (2016) demonstrated that microbial attack caused enlargement of osteocyte lacunae, that later coalesced to constitute larger foci in bone trabeculae. These diagentic changes cannot be excluded as cause of the described empty spaces.

Through staining with Masson's trichrome, van Giesson, and use of Gomorl's impregnation method, it is seen that the decalcified histological sections of mineralised bone tissue contain reduced quantities of collagen fibres (Bancroft and Gamble 2002; Jellinghaus et al. 2018; Povýšil 1990). Surprisingly, only thin interconnected bundles of collagen fibres surrounded originally nonmineralised empty spaces in the bone trabeculae. It is possible that such findings may be explained by the hypermineralization of reduced organic bone matrices, which occur in some genetic skeletal disorders, such as fibrogenesis imperfecta ossiium (Barron et al. 2017) and Nasu-Hakola disease (Shboul et al. 2018). Determing of diagenetic changes as a result of deterioration of bone through microbial activity is difficult.

In fibrogenesis imperfecta ossium, the bone matrix is abnormal. It lacks the normal lamellar birefringence of collagen with polarized light, and is associated with large amounts of incompletely calcified osteoid (Barron et al. 2017). In contrast to osteomalacia, in which the collagen content is normal, the trabeculae with deficient collagen are thickened and contain coarse granular calcifications. Examination with an electron microscopy confirmed that the numbers of collagen fibers are reduced, have a random orientation, are curved and irregular with variable diameters (Barron et al. 2017). It is supposed that the mineral is poorly bound to collagen, which can explain the observed rapid and easy decalcification of bone samples during histological examination. Such patients had widespread bone pain, reduced vertebral body density, and marked sclerosis at the ends of long bones. In the spine, marked osteopenia with central collapse of the endplates that produced a concave appearance was evident. A circulating IgG kappa paraprotein was identified (Barron et al. 2017). Our findings were similiar in many aspects but osteoid seams were absent. Unusual defects of collagen in bone trabeculae may explain the observed apparent speed and ease of decalcification of the bone samples. The additional influence of post morten changes on the bone structure were not determined.

With the exclusion of intraosseous depositon of some metabolic substance, the differential diagosis narrows to disorders that produce nonlamellar bone. This type of bone, known as fibrous bone, occurs in some variants of ostegenesis imperfecta. The most characteristic feature is the abundance of osteocytes. The quantity of the extracellular matrix separating the cells is reduced and the distance between the cells is reduced. This finding is a result of a decrease in the amount of collagen matrix produced by bone cells. In contrast to the iliac crest samples, the bone lamellae are usually thin. An increased number of osteocytes and enlargement of the lacunae also occur in bone fluorosis (Simon et al. 2014; Turner et al. 1996; Vigorita 1999). Hypophosphatasic bone is also composed of immature or woven bone, sometimes with a mosaic pattern (Vigorita 1999).

It is difficult to find any clear term for describing the bone tissue architecture observed in our study. One possibility is to designate such bone tissue as a "bone with perforation"—the perforated bone. Another possibility is to use descriptive terminology: "bone with channel-like pore architecture," "bone with lace-like pattern," or "bone with honeycomb pattern." However, in taphonomic literature, Kontopoulus et al (2016) and Hackett (1981) used the term microscopical focal destruction (tunnels).

It is well known that the post-mortem alterations are investigated by taphonomy. The exposure of a skeleton for prolonged periods of time to the elements, to damage from fauna, and to plant roots, lichens, and algae may detroy the bones in different manners (Kontopoulos et al. 2016). Several dia-genic pathways are recognised as causing alteration of bone: chemical deterioration of the organic and inorganic components, and biological deterioration in the form of microbial attack of the composite. It is supposed that fungi and cyanobacteria create branched tunnels in the bone matrix, while bacteria reorganise the mineral content of bone by creating points of microscopic focal destruction (Kontopoulos et al. 2016, Bell and Elkerton 2008). The initial stages of microscopic focal destruction (tunnels) in exhumed human bones are represented by enlarged osteocyte lacunae. The formation of tunnels (Wedl's) may be associated with focal mineral relocation, characterised with focal mineral and bone matrix loss (Hackett 1981). Such destrcutive, microscopic foci/tunnels can completely obscure the pattern of pathological changes (Hackett 1981).

CONCLUSION

The majority of examined specimens had marked osteosclerosis, documented histologically from the iliac bone samples. These examined skeletons showed diminished collagen content on light microscopy, with reduced collagen birefringence on polarised light microscopy. Cortical and trabecular bone contained multiple small spaces with measurable amounts of alcian blue and Kossa's impregnation positive material, without the presence of collagen fibres. These structures may correspond to residues of metabolite deposits that were dissolved during autolytic, post-mortem changes e.g. crystals of hydroxyapatite and calcium phoshate. Another possibility is that these empty spaces correspond to osteocytic lacunae, exhibiting changes in their dimensions as a consequence of where the osteoid was destroyed by diagenetic changes. There were focal differences in intensity of periosteocytic hematoxylinophilia in bone tissue. Characterisitc osteoid lakes or seams were not identifiable. The described microscopic bone architecture is unusual, but it cannot be determined if these changes developed during the life from autolytic processes or as a result of post-mortem decomposition. A definite conclusion would only be possible through examination of vital bone tissue (Povýšil et al. 2017). Under these circumstances, it is likely that such changes are the result of post-mortem, diagenetic, microstructural processes that occur in buried bones (Hackett 1981; Kontopoulos et al. 2016).

3.5 THE BURIAL OF A WOMAN OF LENGYEL CULTURE WITH PERIMORTEM TRAUMA OF LOWER EXTREMITIES AT BORJÁD-KENDERFÖLD

VÁCLAV SMRČKA, ZDENKA MUSILOVÁ, CSILLA GÁTI

In the autumn of 2010, a local amateur archaeologist donated a more-or-less intact pedestalled vessel to the Department of Archaeology of the Janus Panonius museum Pécs. He reported that the vessel and some other sherd were washed out by a temporary watercourse in the vicinity of the village of Borjád. The vessel was dated to the Late Neolithic Lengyel Culture because of its characteristic shape and porous red paint (Gáti and Bertók 2015-2016).

This led to the discovery of the "Lady of Borjád," the burial of a woman, aged 23-39 (Zoffmann 2015-16), discovered on 5th November 2010 (3. obj. V1-2).

3.5.1 SITE SUMMARY. BASED ON THE ARCHAEOLOGICAL FIND

In the rectangular grave, a contracted skeleton was lying on its left side in an east-west orientation. The bones were preserved in bad condition, and parts of the crushed skull were missing, most probably removed by a burrowing animal. Along the eastern and western wall of the pit there were two trench-like elongated hollows that contained the majority of grave goods. In the corners of the pit, the ends of the "trenches" were further deepened forming four posthole-like cavities. The skeleton was positioned on the central "plateau," slightly off to the south of the west-east axis of the rectangular grave. The head extended beyond the central floor of the grave and, as we found it, lay inclined on the slope of the eastern trench. It seems, though, that originally the head had been supported by an object made of perishable material, e.g. a wooden burial bed or a pillow that decayed over time, thus causing the head to descend onto the steep slope below it.

The grave pit measured 175 × 210 cm. The original depth of the grave cannot be determined because of erosion of the slope. Measured from the present-day surface, the deepest points in the corners were 70–75 cm deep, while the main floor was at a relative depth of 40 cm.

The grave goods consisted of 15 ceramic vessels and a necklace comprising of beads made mainly of copper and seashells. Most of the pottery items were placed into the hollows in the corners. However, three pieces lay on the shallower, central part of the western trench and three pieces were placed on the central floor. One of the latter two vessels was adjacent to and leaning on the south wall ca. 10 cm higher than the skeleton, and two other vessels lay near the knee of the body. Four vessels were found on a second level: below the level of the skeleton, in the SE and SW holes, below other vessels.

3.5.2 OSTEOLOGY

The woman was buried with parts of a sheep/goat, bone fragments of which were preserved, with the lower part of the tibia and part of the ulna (figs. 2–4). The woman was wearing jewels with copper parts, which left some traces on the skeletal remains—on the cervical vertebrae, left collar bone, right scapula, first rib, phalanges of the thumb as well as phalanges of the fingers of the right hand (figs. 5–6).

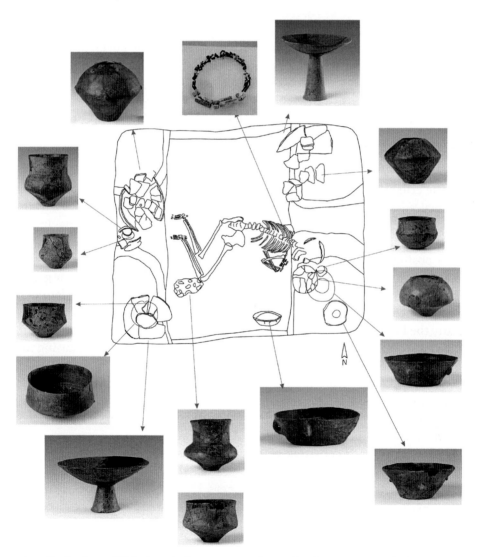

Fig. 1. "Lady of Borjád," the burial of a woman, aged 23–39 (Zoffmann 2015–2016), discovered on 5th November 2010.

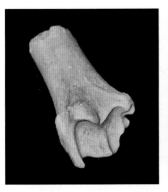 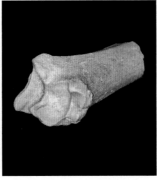 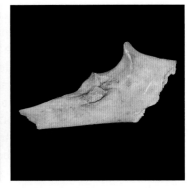

Figs. 2–4. Remains of funerary food, fibiae and ulna of a sheep and goat. Photo: Zdenka Musilová

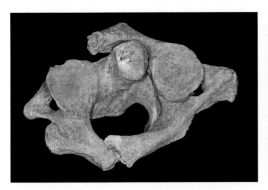 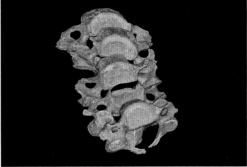

Figs. 5–6. Traces of copper on the cervical vertebrae. Photo: Zdenka Musilová

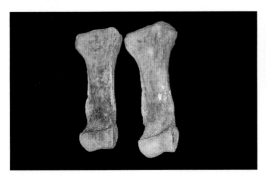 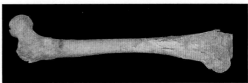

Fig. 7. *Bone rims* on phalanges of the fingers. Photo: Zdenka Musilová

Fig. 8. Right femur, front side, three bone fragments. Photo: Zdenka Musilová

On phalanges of the fingers that had been in contact with the copper object, we found *bone rims* on the borders suggesting excessive strain, probably work load, on interosseous muscles of the hand probably due to weaving (fig. 7). The whole preserved skeleton comprised 74 bone items.

In the lower extremities, knee joints, a perimortem trauma was found, affecting the lower parts of the femurs and upper parts of the tibias.

The trauma was caused by pronounced massive pressure on the lateral side of the lower part of the right femur and right tibia, and at the same time on the medial parts of the left femur and left tibia.

From the above, we deduce that the said pressure from the right acted upon the woman, who was lying on her left side. The distal part of the left femur is affected even more than the lateral part of the right femur. In the left femur, in its proximal third, there is a spiral fracture, communicating with multiple fragments in the distal segment via a crack.

A similar finding can be seen in the area of the tibias, where, however, the pressure acting upon the right tibia was markedly higher. In the mediolateral direction, the tibia is flattened as much as to one third of its original width.

Next to the right femur on the lateral side of the distal segment of the bone there are three fragments (33 × 15 mm, 20 × 15 mm and 100 × 25 mm) with a metaphyseal wedge. Partly, however, a joint fracture in the frontal plane is present here.

In the left femur in the upper third of the diaphysis, there is an *unhealed spiral fracture*. In the distal segment of the left femur there is a *complex me-*

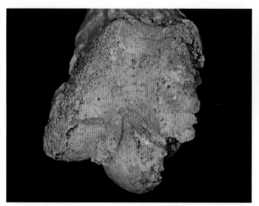

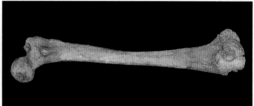

Fig. 9. Right femur, *intra-articular fracture*. Photo: Zdenka Musilová

Fig. 10. Right femur, the back side. Photo: Zdenka Musilová

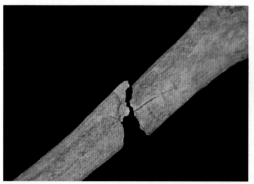

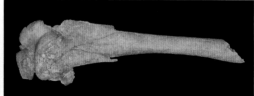

Fig. 11. Left femur, *spiral fracture*. Photo: Zdenka Musilová

Fig. 12. Left femur, front surface with four bone fragments. Photo: Zdenka Musilová

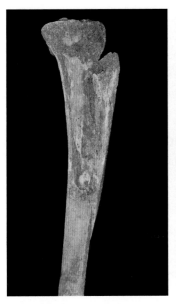
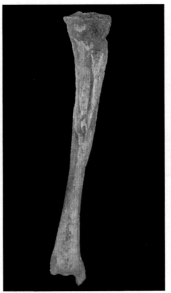
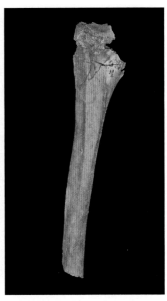

Fig. 13. Right tibia, with four bone fragments at the front side. Photo: Zdenka Musilová

Fig. 14. Left tibia, with four bone fragments at the front side. Photo: Zdenka Musilová

Fig. 15. Left tibia, with four bone fragments at the back side. Photo: Zdenka Musilová

taphyseal extra-articular fracture with six fragments, of which four are found at the front side (60 × 20 mm, 45 × 20 mm, 40 × 10 mm, 35 × 10 mm) and two at the back side (65 × 30 mm and 65 × 20 mm). From this fracture, three cracks run, and the one on the front surface runs as far as the spiral fracture in the proximal part of the diaphysis.

In the right tibia in its proximal part, a metaphyseal extra-articular fracture with six fragments at the back side (80 × 15 mm, 130 × 15 mm, 25 × 8 mm and 120 × 20 mm) is found. The middle of the fracture is at the lateral side.

In the left tibia, in its proximal part, there is a complete joint fracture connected to a metaphyseal fracture with multiple fragments. At the medial side there are four fragments (15 × 10 mm, 15 × 8 mm, 35 × 15 mm and 10 × 15 mm). From the fracture, a 40 mm crack runs distally. At the lateral side four other fragments are found (35 × 25 mm, 10 × 20 mm, 10 × 10 mm and 25 × 15 mm). The tibia is flattened in the mediolateral direction. After the joint fracture, one half of the head is missing. All the fractures described above are *perimortem* and *unhealed ones*.

In conclusion, we can state that the said woman was lying on her left side. Her legs were broken to pieces and crushed by a big round object, a rock or log, either before her death or immediately after it. The said compressive fractures, if inflicted before death, not only rendered the woman immobile but also caused lethal bleeding and subsequent death.

3.5.3 STRONTIUM ANALYSIS

It was discovered through strontium isotope analysis, that the sheep (93-373-2359) was local while the "Lady of Borjád," a woman aged 23-39, had her origins elsewhere (see pp. 181–182).

3.6 ALSÓNYÉK-BÁTASZÉK: PALEOPATHOLOGICAL EXAMINATION OF THE LATE NEOLITHIC SITE EXCAVATED AT ALSÓNYÉK-BÁTASZÉK
KITTI KÖHLER

3.6.1 INTRODUCTION

The Lengyel culture is known since several decades by arhaeologists and anthropologist, too. The paleoanthropological analysis of the most earlier excavated Lengyel cemeteries examination (Villánykővesd, Zengővárkony, Aszód-Papi földek, Mórágy-B.1., Mórágy-B.2 etc.) can be connected to the name of Zsuzsanna, K. Zoffann (Zofmann 1968, 1969–1970, 2004, 2011). She dealt in total in the course of the bone examinations with demographic-, metric and morphological analysis, which based on searching the origin and connection of the population. Moreover she observed the anatomical variations and described the pathology on bones and teeth.

Beside and before her investigations, there were two Hungarian paleopathologists, who published separately the interesting cases from this period (Regöly-Mérei 1960; Regöly-Mérei 1962; Bartucz 1966). So we have a lot of well-written sources, datas about the Lengyel population.

The earlier determination of any disease on the bones was mainly based on macroscophical investigations. But, in the last decades a lot of effective type of observation (X-ray, CT, MR, aDNA, isotopic analysis, microscopic techniques, etc.) help us for better understanding or to define in a more precise way the pathological alterations, which was earlier debated. For example, there is a new article about the re-examination of paleopathological observations of the Zengővárkony cemetery, which modified the earlier results of the investigation (Smrčka et al. 2018).

3.6.2 MATERIAL

Between 2006 and 2009, a large prehistoric settlement and cemetery was excavated at Alsónyék-Bátaszék (south-eastern Transdanubia, Tolna County). The excavation was carried out by the Institute of Archaeology of

HAS-Archeosztráda Ltd., Ásatárs Ltd., Field Service for Cultural Heritage and Wosinsky Mór County Museum (Osztás, Bánffy, et al. 2016).

During the excavation the remains of several Neolithic cultures were discovered (Starčevo-, Central European Linear Pottery-, Sopot- and Lengyel culture). The Lengyel occupation included houses, pits and graves, reaching ca 80 ha extent, perhaps larger. The excavation have been followed by several analysis, some of it is still ongoing. One of them was the collaboration with the European Researh Council-funded project, "The Times of Their Live" (ToTL). This applied formal chronological modelling—explicit, quantified an probababilistic interpretation of radiocarbon dates within the Bayesian statistical framework (Osztás, Bánffy, et al. 2016; Osztás, Zalai-Gaál, et al. 2016; Bayliss et al. 2016).

The site was occupied most intensively by the Late Neolithic Lengyel culture in the first half of fifth millennium B.C. (Gallina et al. 2010; Osztás et al. 2012; Bánffy et al. 2016; Osztás, Zalai-Gaál, et al. 2016).

Since the total size and the correlation of different parts of the cemetery and the settlement at the time of the excavation wasn't clear, the physical anthropological investigation first focused on graves were found on subsite 10/B of the site. From this part a total of 7780 features, within these 862 graves

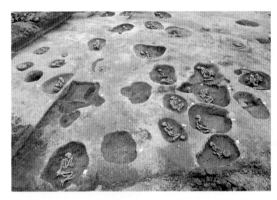
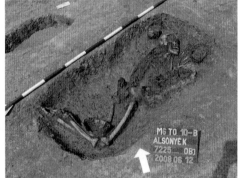
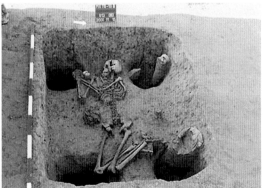

Fig. 1. Burial group in subsite 10B.

Fig. 2. Simple grave. Grave no. 7225.

Fig. 3. Grave of the elite. Grave no. 813.

were recorded (Osztás, Zalai-Gaál, et al. 2016). The anthropological analysis of the them was my PhD dissertation topic. Later the burials of the whole site were investigated, too, but the evaluation of the data of the more than 2300 burials is still in progress.

A large proportion of the burials were found in spatially discrete grave groups, which by some researchers are assumed to somewhat artificial constructs, while others supposed, that these reflects kinship links between the deceased (fig. 1) (Kalicz 1985; Zalai-Gaál 1988; Gallina et al. 2010; Bánffy et al. 2016; Osztás et al. 2012; Osztás, Bánffy, et al. 2016; Osztás, Zalai-Gaál, et al. 2016). In some cases, these groups were compact and clearly separated from the others, but in other cases they were rather diffuse and spatially overlap or merge. Within groups a more or less strict burial rite were observed. They contained usually 25–40 burials. At the part of the subsite 10/B 41 such burial groups were uncovered. With the exception of a few grave groups the orientation of the burials was E–W, with the head to the east, and with faces to the south (fig. 2). But there were a lot of graves out the groups scattered across the site.

Moreover, some of the burials can be considered as graves of the elite, resting on four wooden pillars and contain a large amount of high-quality grave goods (fig. 3). Besides these unique burial phenomena, this site is significant as it is the largest known Late Neolithic Age cemetery excavated in Central-Europe, providing a unique opportunity to study the classical anthropological features and the paleopathological alterations of the population buried here.

So, here we publish primarily the main paleopathological results of the examination of the subsite 10/B.

3.6.3 METHODS

The preservation of the human remains was mainly medium. The skulls were very fragmentary, while the postcranial elements were relatively well preserved.

For the sex determination and the biological age estimation I used the combination of multiple methods (Éry et al. 1963; Kósa and Fazekas 1978; Schour and Massler 1941; Ubelaker 1989; Stloukal and Hanáková 1978; Ferembach et al. 1979; Schincz et al 1952; Nemeskéri et al. 1960; Meindl and Lovejoy 1985; Todd 1920; Lovejoy et al. 1985; Işcan et al. 1984, 1985; Miles 1963; Perizonius 1981). The examination of the pathological changes was conducted systematically in a statistically way, using Bernert' software (Bernert 2005).

The pathological investigation was based on the systematization according to Steinbock (1976), with a little modification (Ortner and Putchar 1985; Ubelker 1989; Roberts and Manchester 2005; Ortner 2003). The skeletons were studied mainly macroscopically. In a few and important cases we used X-ray and aDNA analysis for a better diagnosis.

The skeletal material is stored in the Wosinsky Mór County Museum, Szekszárd, Hungary.

In this study we seek the answer for the following main questions: What was the general state of health of the community settled at Alsónyék? What diseases occurred most frequently within the population? How does it inform us about their lifestyle? Can we see any pathological difference suggesting alternative lifestyle, health, diet between the peoples buried in simple graves and individuals buried in post-framed grave constructions?

3.6.4 RESULTS

DEMOGRAPHY

According to the demographic analysis, the population of the Alsónyék community was blessed with some unrealistic mortality parameters. The proportion of neonates (± 0) was merely 1%, and consequently the life expectancy at birth is 32.6 years. The proportion of the infant I. and infant II. aged group children were low (9.1% and 8.0%). In the meantime, contrary to the expected value, the ratio of adult and mature aged individuals is almost equal (36.7% and 36.8% respectively), while senile aged individuals are practically missing from the cemetery (0.2%).

The ratio of male and female (248:336) is not even, too. Because of the condition of the skeletal material with many fragmentary and incomplete bones, we couldn't determine the sex of 101 individuals (especially from the juvenile age group). As it is usually observed in other Lengyel cemeteries, Alsónyék is also characterized by a female dominance (Zoffmann 2011; Köhler 2012).

Moreover, though it is believed that the archaeologically outlined grave groups formed according to kinship, the demographic analysis didn't verify it. But it's not concluded, that other methods will disprove this demographical data. The age and sex distribution don't correlate with the assumed family relationship.[7]

As for the 68 graves with four-post constructions the demographic characteristic is similar to that observed in the whole cemetery.

PATHOLOGICAL ALTERATIONS

CONGENITAL ANOMALIES

Developmental anomalies are defects that develop in utero and manifest themselves more noticeably at birth or in the infant growth phase. Some of

---

7   Morever we investigated 17 hereditary anatomical variations to help us define the relationship in the grave groups. This investigation again contradicted to the familiar burials.

them cause some kind (e.g. functional or aesthetical) deterioration of quality of life (Barnes 1994).

Fenestratio sterni congenita, which cause no clinical complaints occurred in four cases in the series.

Sacrum bifidum, when the sacral canal is opened. It can extending over the whole sacrum occurred only in a few cases (males: 2.56%, females: 2.38%). Cranial situated sacrum bifidum were detected again rare (males: 1.89%, females: 1.61%), while the caudally situated form were frequent (males: 37.03%, females: 46.15%). These alterations are generally asymptomatic, but in adulthood may cause pain.

Sacralisation, which is the assimilation of the 5th lumbar to the sacrum, showed 13.33% prevalence for males, while 14.28% for females. *Lumbarization*, when the upper sacral vertebrae appear as a separate lumbar vertebra were again rare (male: 1.64%, female: 1.61%).

TRAUMATIC LESIONS

Trauma is shown by bone lesions caused by external physical impacts, which usually is one of the most frequent within anthropological assemblages. However, the macroscopically detected *fractures* were very rare in the Alsónyék cemetery (males: 9.04%, females: 7.29%) (figs. 4, 5). According to age, the lesion affected most often the mature-aged individuals. The number and the ratio of fractures on the different bones is shown in tab. 1.

Tab. 1. The number and the ratio of fractures on the different bones

	Examinable	Occurred	Ratio	Examinable	Occurred	Ratio
Skull	135	2	1.48%	171	2	1.17%
Clavicle	153	2	1.31%	172	1	0.58%
Ribs	207	3	1.45%	251	3	1.20%
Humerus	392	1	0.51%	440	1	0.51%
Ulna	289	5	1.73%	335	6	1.80%
Radius	345	1	0.29%	381	8	2.10%
Femur	312	4	1.28%	360	2	0.56%
Tibia	284	3	1.10%	369	2	0.63%
Fibula	222	1	0.45%	422	2	0.57%

Injuring resulting from blunt or blow on skull occurred in the case of two males and two males. From among these, on left parietal bone a 2.2 × 1.6 cm oval shaped depression were observed in the case of a mature-aged female' skull (grave no. 4132). The left radius and ulna of the female was fractured,

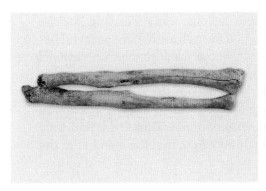
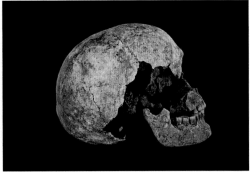

Fig. 4. *Fracture* of the right radius and ulna. Grave no. 369.

Fig. 5. Skull *injury*. Grave no. 1991.

too. Based on it, it can't be exluded that the two injuries arised from the same episode, when the individual defended herself with raising arms againts an attack.

Also classified as a traumatic lesion the *myostitis ossificans*, which etiology is unknown (Ortner and Putschar 1985). Major injury (dislocations, fractures) or minor trauma, is considered as the most frequent cause of it. In the early stage muscle degradation and calcification of muscle, later ossification in or around tendons develop. This alteration occurred in the linea aspera of the femur in the case of a mature-aged male (grave no. 7767). To verify this diagnosis further investigations needing.

At last, another debated or unknown bony defect is the *spondylolysis*. It was earlier believed to be a developmental anomaly. But nowadays it's defined as a defect or stress fracture in the pars interarticularis of the vertebral arch, especially on the lumbar section of the vertebral coloumn (Sarastre 1993). In our serie it occurred in the case of one male and two females on the lumbar part of the spine (fig. 6).

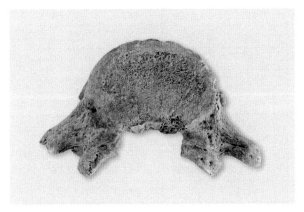

Fig. 6. *Spondylolysis* on a lumbar vertebra. Grave no. 155.

In summary, the number of traumatic lesions, was surprising low. We may assume, that the low number of them may indicate a more peaceful living situation due to the sedentary lifestyle, but we can't conclude occasional or accidental conflict within the community, which was not visible macroscopically and maybe affected only the soft parts of the body. Considering the localisation of the fractures, these may have related to daily activity. In addition, all these traumas were healed with minimal callus formation, only a few with shortness and inflammation. It may sign, that the member of the community knew how to cure.

NONSPECIFIC INFLAMMATIONS

Most infectious diseases produce similar bone responses, such as osteomyelitis and periostitis, which are rather common in archaeological records, and can be caused by different types of microorganisms, or by traumatic events (e.g. inflicted blows or hematomas) (Ortner and Putschar 1985).

Periostitic reactions with new bone formation were rare in the investigated sample and occurred mainly on the bones of the leg. The occurance ratio among adult is shown in tab. 2. Among children it occurs on left tibia with 3.08%, on right tibia with 4.23% prevalence. On fibula it was observed only in one case (fig. 7).

Tab. 2. The occurance ratio among adult

Disease	Occurence		Males		Females	
			Case	%	Case	%
Periostitis	Left tibia	No	133	84.71%	154	89.02%
		Yes	24	15.29%	19	10.98%
		Sum.	157		173	
	Right tibia	No	141	85.45%	175	89.29%
		Yes	24	14,55%	21	10.71%
		Sum.	165		196	
	Left fibula	No	173	94.02%	199	93.87%
		Yes	11	5.98%	13	6.13%
		Sum.	184		212	
	Right fibula	No	174	94.57%	199	94.76%
		Yes	10	5.43%	11	5.24%
		Sum.	184		210	

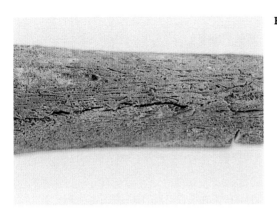

Fig. 7. *Periostitis* on femur. Grave no. 50.

Osteomyelitis, the prevalence of which was very low in our skeletal material, is usually defined as an infection of bone and bone marrow resulting in inflammation, necrosis and new bone formation. The causative agent is mainly *Staphylococcus aureus*, or other microorganisms. Moreover, the pathogens may infect the bones by a traumatic or surgical wound, by adjacent soft tissue infection or via a haematogenous route. Morphologically the bone may increase in size, and drainage channels (cloaca) are formed, through which the pus drains from the bone to the outside (Ortner and Putschar 1985). This alteration was noticed only in the case of three adults.

SPECIFIC INFLAMMATIONS

Tuberculosis is one of the oldest infectious disease, which is caused by a group of the *Mycobacterium tuberculosis* complex (the most common are *M. tuberculosis* and *M. bovis*). The disease usually a *pulmonary TB*, but in a few cases the bacteria spread from the initial site and then affected the skeletal system (Ortner 2003; Donoghue 2009).

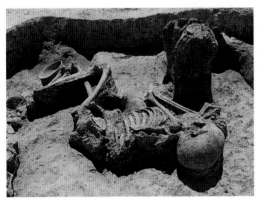

Fig. 8. In situ excavation photo. Grave no. 4027.

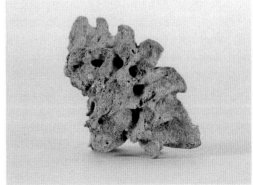

Fig. 9. The affected vertebra with TB (*Pott's disease, gibbus*). Grave no. 4027.

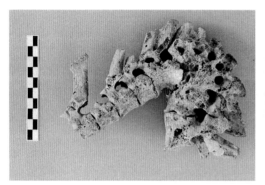

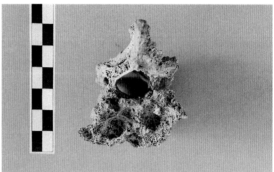

Fig. 10. The vertebral section with TB (*gibbus*). Grave no. 4027.

Fig. 11. The affected 8th thoracic vertebra. Grave no. 4027.

In the Alsónyék series a skeleton of an adult, 30–35 years old male (grave no. 4027) showed the classic, advanced staged TB symptoms. This individual has a typical form of *chronical tuberculosa* (*Pott's disease* with *gibbus formation*), with serious deformity and ankylosis, which was clearly visible at the excavation, too (fig. 8). The most characteristic pathological changes can be observed between the 10th thoracic and the 4th lumbar vertebrae. Pathological remodelling involves the central and anterior portions of them, which results in collapse and fusion of the affected vertebrae. The unequal collapse results in a sharp kyphosis (fig. 9, fig. 10).

Another ankylosis developed between the 8th and the 9th thoracic vertebrae. The body of the 8th thoracic vertebra is collapsed. Multiple lytic destructions can be observed on the lower surface of the 9th thoracic vertebral body (fig. 11). The pathological process destroyed almost half of this affected vertebrae (Köhler et al. 2012; Köhler et al. 2013).

Since, the male belong to a grave group with 38 individuals all were investigated to find early stage/atypical symptoms at the Biological Anthropology Department of Szeged University. From among these on the skeleton of the male from grave no. 4027 the following atypical pathological alterations were observed: hypervascularisation or lytic lesions on vertebrae, periostal remodelling on long bones and on vertebrae and cribra orbitalia. In further 16 cases in this group these atypical symptoms were observed, too. After macro-morphological and radiological observations, aDNA analysis was conducted by A. Pósa in the EURAC Institute for Mummies and the Iceman (Bolzano). In total, four individual showed positive molecular results for TB (interestingly one of them hadn't any typical or atypical skeletal alterations!) (Pósa et al. 2013).

Due to the limitations of the article, we have no possibility to present all the earliest TB cases found in Europe and in the Near-East. Let me, just mention from the territory of recent Hungary, the earliest cases, which was founded at the Late Neolithic site (Tisza culture) of Hódmezővásárhely-Gorzsa (Masson et al. 2015a, 2015b). Anonther TB have been discovered recently at the site of Vésztő-Mágor from the Tisza culture, too. Here the palaeomicrobial analysis of the dental pulp region in the teeth of one of the cases confirmed the presence of *M. tuberculosis* aDNA (Spekker et al. 2012; Pósa et al. 2012; Pósa et al. 2013).

Besides, V. Smrčka and his colleagues re-examined the cemetery of Zengővárkony and they found specific tuberculous inflammation with fistulae in the calcaneus and tarsal bones of a male (Smrčka et al. 2018). It was earlier presumed arthritic changes (Regöly-Mérei 1960, Zoffmann 1969–1970).

So the number of the earliest TB cases in the Carpathian Basin is growing and we may assume, that it spreaded due to the sedentary lifestyle and the population explosion in this period.

CRIBRA ORBITALIA/CRIBRA CRANII (OR POROTIC HYPEROSTOSIS)

Cribra orbitalia on the orbital roof and cribra cranii (porotic hyperostosis) on the flat bones of the skull vault are characteristically "coral like" or "sieve-like" alteration, which are among the most frequent pathological lesion in ancient human skeletal collections. This bone lesions usually bilateral in distribution.

Since the 1950s, this condition was widely accepted as these are mainly result of living condition. The formation of this alteration was tracked back to iron deficienct dietary, iron malabsorption, and iron loss from both diarrheal disease and intestinal parasites (Angel 1966).

But more recent studies take into consideration much more factors, and they suggests, that these two types of the alteration have different etiolo-

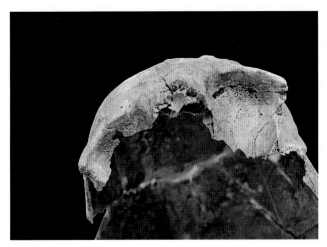

Fig. 12. *Cribra orbitalia.*
Grave no. 813.

gies. Furthermore, due to recent haematological and paleopathological re-
searches, the hypothesis of the only "iron-deficiency-anemia hypothesis" can
no longer be maintained (Ortner 2003; Walker et al. 2009). The appearance
of cribra orbitalia beside the anemia can be caused by bony inflammation,
pressure-induced bony atrophy, hypervascularization, dietary deficiency,
minor trauma (which can cause subperiosteal bleeding and trigger bone deposition, etc.) (Wapler et al. 2004; Walker et al. 2009).

In our series among males cribra orbitalia on the left orbital roof showed
a frequency of 12.32% (17/138), on the right side 11.76% (12/102). For females on
the left side it occurred in 15.78% (24/152), and on the right side 15,88% (20/126)
(fig. 12). In the case of the children there was a 47.83% (24/46) percentage on
the left side and 58.35% (21/36) on the right.

On the external surface of the skulls among males it appeared in 3.02%
(5/166) on the left-, and 3.14% (5/159) on the right side. For female on the left
side it showed a 6.11% (13/213), and 5.92% (12/203) on the right side. In the case
of children the prevalence on the left side was 3.59% (3/82), and 2.50% (2/80)
on the right side.

In summary we can see that this alteration in the orbital roof appeared
with a higher frequency among the children, which phenomenon was commonly seen in other prehistoric and historic populations (Ubelaker et al.
2006). The etiology of the symptoms in the Alsónyék population maybe can
be traced back to nutritional deficiency or infections, but it needs much more
investigations.

JOINT DISEASES ON THE SPINE

Joint diseases are one of the common disorders observable in paleopathology
(Roberts-Manchester 2007). The grouping of them is not uniform in paleopathological literature. The most general type of them is the *Degenerative Joint
Disease* (DID), which affected the vertebral coloumn and the the hand, feet
and large weight-bearing joints. Eburnation, porosity, osteophyte formation
and joint contour change are the main diagnostic features in DJD (Rogers and
Waldron 1987). The appearing and severity of DJD depend on factors such as
strong mechanic stress, macro- or microtraumatic effects, genetic predisposition, infections, age, sex, weight, climate, etc. (Steinbock 1976; Roberts and
Manchester 2007).

The so-called *spondylosis deformans*, which appear on the vertebral
coloumn, was the most frequent and the most severe on the lumbal spine
section. Spondylosis occurs as a result of new bone formation (osteophytes)
on the superior and inferior margins of vertebral bodies. The finding were
classified into three groups according to the character or severity of the morphological changes. In sum, in our series among males its frequency on the
cervical section was 24.7% (45/182), on the thoracic vertebrae 28.6% (59/206),

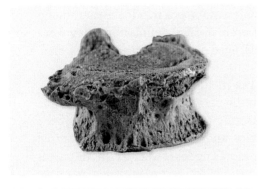

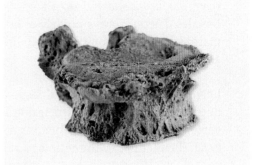

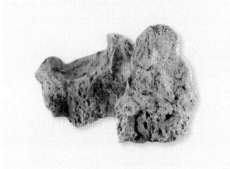

Fig. 13. *Spondylosis deformans* on a lumbar vertebra. Grave no. 50.

Fig. 14. *Spondylosis deformans* on a lumbar vertebra. Grave no. 144.

Fig. 15. *Spondylarthrosis* on a fragmented cervical vertebra. Grave no. 262.

while on the lumbar section was 37.7% (75/199). In the case of females it appeared with a 15.3% (36/235) on the cervical-, with 13.5% (36/237) on the thoracal-, and with 33.3% (84/252) frequency rate on the lumbar section.

With regard to severity of the lesion, we could observe the mild osteophyte formation in the majority of cases, but of course the expressed formation also occurred, mainly on the lumbar vertebrae, which is exposed to a higher load (figs. 13, 14).

The severity of spondylosis deformans can be very advanced, when the bone projections on the margins of the vertebrae fuse and form a bone-bridge. Due to it the height of the intervertebral disc decreases. It affects the joints by changes their function and by deformation, which is the so-called *spondylarthrosis* (fig. 15).

This alteration in both sexes occured most frequently in the cervical part of the vertebral coloumn. In the case of males its rate on the cervical section was 22.62% (38/106), on the thoracic vertebrae was 8.63% (17/197), while on the lumbar section was 16.15% (31/192). In the case of females the incidence rate was 10.0% (19/190) on the cervical-, 4.90% (12/245) on the thoracal-, and 5.83% (13/223) on the lumbar vertebrae.

In sum, both degenerative changes affected mainly the males. The *spondylosis deformans* were 42.86% for males and 32.75% for females. While the *spondylarthrosis* showed 26.54% among males and 11.45% incidence rate among females. Furtermore, similarly to other prehistorical populations they were mainly detected among elder individuals, aged over 40 years (Ubelaker et al. 2006).

The degenerative lesions of the spine include *Schmorl-hernia*, too. The herniation of the nucleus pulposus into the vertebral body produce ectopic deposit of disc material. The lesion is usually localized in the middle of the vertebral body surface by forming a cavity, and less frequently in the spinal canal (Bender 1999). The aetiology of Schmorl's nodes is unclear. In the paleo-pathological literature their presence is usually connected with degenerative joint disease or osteoarthritic changes on the vertebral bodies. Moreover, it is regarded as a stress indicator suggestive for hard physical activity performed by the individual in the course of his/her lifetime (Ortner 2003).

In the case of males its frequency on the cervical section was 0.57% (1/175), on the thoracal section 18.50% (37/200) and 18.32% (35/191) on the lumbal vertebrae. Among females the occurence from the cervical to the lumbar section was as follows: 2.20% (5/227), 14.90% (38/255) and 12.40% (30/242).

As we can see, it was slightly more common among males (25.59%), than among females (18.21%). Moreover, there is no significant difference in the frequency between the younger and the older aged individuals. All this verify Saluja et al. (1986) conclusions, that there is no correlation between the alteration and the aging.

Reviewing the results of the above, the occurrence of spinal degenerative disorders among the population of Alsónyék is not too large compared to the literature data (Ubelaker et al. 2006). The occurance proportion was somewhat higher in the case of males. Hereinafter, while spondylosis deformans and spondylarthrosis were more commonly observed in older individuals, Schmorl-hernia could be detected in the case of the younger age group, too.

JOINT DISEASES ON POSTCRANIAL BONES

Similarly to the vertebral coloumn, joint diseases occur in extravertebral positions as well. The so-called *osteoarthrosis deformans* (OA) is an abnormal condition of the joints, which is paleopathologicaly characterized by grooving or extensions on the articular surface, eburnation and peripheral exostoses. In the formation of the disease are the harms of certain lifestyle and genetic factors are important (Ortner 2003).

Due to the fragmentation of proximal and distal epiphyses of long bones in our material, there was very little chance to exam this alteration. We observed the traces of OA, among males with a 15.13% prevalence (33/218) and with 10.42% (27/259) among females. The gender distribution showed a minimal male surplus occurance. Furthermore, similar to today's- (Bender 1999) and prehistorical human-age data (Ubelaker et al. 2006) the occurrence of

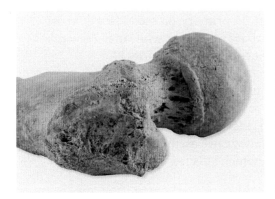

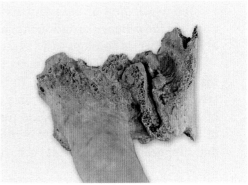

Fig. 16. *Osteoarthrosis* on the femur neck. Grave no. 262.

Fig. 17. *Coxarthrosis*. Grave no. 808.

OA increased with age. Our data, however, don't permit any conclusions to be drawn about the OA, because the number of observations is inadequate.

Hereinafter, in the case of both gender the elbow joint are affected in most cases, however, it is less than 10%. This is followed in the case of males by degenerative lesions of the knee, ankle and hip, while among females the ankle and hip joints. Multiple OA was characteristic of males (fig. 16).

Severe hip arthrosis (*coxarthrosis*) occurred in the case of a mature aged male (grave no. 808). In the course of the disease the cartilage covering the proximal epiphysis of femur and the acetabulum became thinner, lost its smooth glitter and on its surface fissures developed. As the process progressed, the cartilage surface gradually destroyed. In our case the lesion is unilateral. In addition of the typical alteration the angle of the femur neck reduced, too (fig. 17).

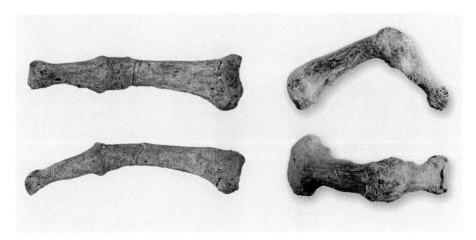

Fig. 18. *Ankylosis* on head phalanges. Grave no. 5115.

The developing of coxarthrosis can be primary or secondary (Ortner 2003). In the primary variation the causes are unknown, while in the secondary coxarthrosis develops as a consequence of several diseases.

Ankylosis of the hand phalanges occurred in the case of two mature aged males (grave no. 5115 and 7654). In the case of the male from the grave no. 5115 the phalanges totally fused, in a direction of the tension side at an angle of 109 degrees. In both cases the fused phalanges caused disability or loss of hand function. The etiology is still unclear, we assume that joint damage and suppuration (with fistula) occured, which affected the bones (fig. 18).

INFLAMMATION OF THE VERTEBRAE

Spondylodiscitis is an inflammation disease of the spine, affecting the intervertebral disc and the adjacent vertebral bodies. Inflammation is most commonly caused by bacteria, which by haematogen way reach and destroy the vertebral disc (Tóth 2006).

The alteration occurred in the case of 28 males and 13 females. Among males the frequency rate on the cervical vertebrae was 13.74% (25/182), on the thoracal section 5.05% (10/198) and on the lumbar section 7.69% (15/198). In the case of females it showed 3.18% (7/220) on the cervical-, 1.92% (5/261) on the thoracal- and 3.24% (8/246) on the lumbar vertebrae. Most of the lesions were mild, but severe forms also occurred (fig. 19).

To sum, the frequency of the lesion was slightly higher among males, moreover it appeared in the adult-mature and mature aged group individuals and don't affected the younger, grown-up peoples.

METABOLIC AND HAEMATOLOGICAL DISORDERS

Metabolic diseases of bone cause disruption of normal bone formation, remodelling, mineralization or some combination of these. Such are vitamin

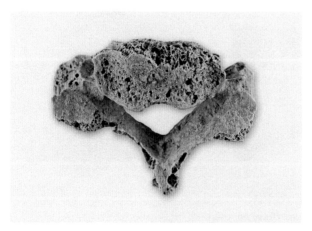

Fig. 19. *Spondylodiscitis* on cervical vertebra. Grave no. 335.

D deficiency disease (ricket, osteomalacia), vitamin C deficiency disorder (scurvy), starvation (which cause protein deficiency), osteoporosis, generalized hyperostosis, etc. In addition, the endocrine glands disorders may also affect the skeletal system (Steinbock 1976; Ortner-Putchar 1985; Ortner 2003).

OSTEOPOROSIS

Osteoporosis (OP) is the most frequent metabolic pathological condition, a complex and heterogeneous disorder. The risk factors are sex, age, hormone levels, dietary factors (low calcium or protein intake, eating disorder), vitamin C and D deficiency, lifestyle, genetic factors, etc. Bone fractures, particularly in the spine or in the hip, are the most serious complication of osteoporosis, especially among elder individuals and females.

The consequence of OP is the thinning of the trabecular structure and the increasing of the porosity of the vertebra. As a result of it the vertebral body crush under pressure. Due to it, the vertebral coloumn had a compression fracture and collapse, which results the gradual decrease of the body height and the deterioration of the spinal statics and bearing capacity (fig. 20). In our materia two males and six females were affected, all belonged to the elder age groups.

On the parietal bone of the skull OP occurred in the case of two mature-aged females, and one undeterminated sex, mature-aged individual. Here the diploë, or spongy tissue within the bones of the cranium, swells and the tissue of the outer surface becomes thinner and more porous in appearance (Angel 1966; Walker 2009).

There is very few evidences of osteoporosis in human history, which nowadays is endemic. The frequency of osteoporosis probably was only a fraction of today's occurrence, in which nutrition, more active lifestyle and

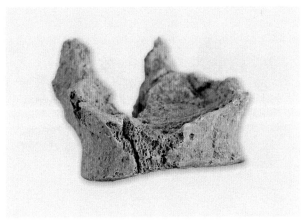

Fig. 20. Collapse due to *osteoporosis* on a lumbar vertebra. Grave no. 713.

possibly the earlier death could have played a primary role (Regöly-Mérei 1961, 1962).

DISH

Among the metabolic disorders are the *Diffuse Idiopathic Skeletal Hyperostosis* (DISH) is a common but often unrecognized systemic disorder observed mainly among elderly individuals. DISH is diagnosed when the anterior longitudinal ligament of the spine is ossified on at least three contiguous spinal levels and when multiple peripheral enthesopathies are present. Moreover there are more minor requirements (retention of the intervertebral disc space and lack of fusion or there a no any changes on the zygapophyseal and sacroiliac joint) (Resnick and Niwayama 1976; Ortner 2003; Waldron 2009).

The etiology of DISH is unknown but previous studies have shown a strong association with obesity, insulin-independent diabetes mellitus, genetic factors, metabolic disorders, physical inactivity, etc. (Rogers and Waldron 2001).

The recognition of DISH is not difficult, but in paleopathology, the osteo-archeological series' different or bad state of preservation may cause diagnostical uncertainty. In our material we assume the occurance of the disease in the case of two females.

In one case (grave no. 5196) on two lumbal vertebrae of a mature aged female the anterior longitudinal ligamentum ossified, but the intervertebral spaces were not affected (fig. 21).

Other extra-spinal alterations were bilateral enthesopathies on calcanei and patellae, which important to distinguish in latter discussed and mainly mechanical origined entheses. Thought our diagnosis is based on few diagnostic criteria (because tha lack of more vertebrae and the fragmentation state of the postcranial bone elements), we assume, that this alterations can be separated from degenerative vertebral diseases or from spondylathrophy.

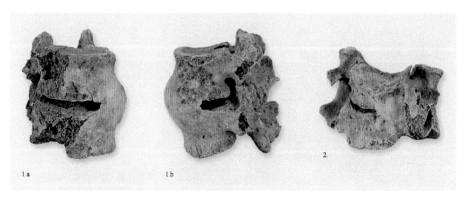

Fig. 21. Possible case of *DISH*. Grave no. 5196.

In the other case (grave no. 2959) the anterior longitudinal ligament ossified on two cervical vertebrae of an adult-mature aged male. Here the joints and the space of the intervertebral disc again aren't affected. Other alterations were spondylarthrosis on the lumbar vertebrae and enthesopathy on both calcanei. The diagnosis in this case also uncertain, but furher examinations can justify or invalidate our hypothesis.

Some other metabolic disorders, in a few cases well recognizable, but some cause such bone changes (such as thinnig and curving of long bones or the lossing of the bone matrix), which have unknown etiologic background (Steinbock 1976). In the Alsónyék serie the long bones thinning and curving, which most commonly occurred on the tibia affected eleven males, five females, and an unidentifiable sexed grown-up individual.

The most interesting lesions occurred in a case of an adult male (grave no. 552). Expressed enthesopathies occured on both sides's ulnae, tibias, patellas and on the right sided calcaneus. Moreover significant deformation and periostitis were visible on calcaneus. Beside it the tuberculum laterale of the same sided talus enlarged and inflammation were detected. All these alterations may indicate two diseases. One of them is an ossification disorder, which could have happened in childhood. We assume, that this is the so-called Blencke syndrome (other names are osteochondrosis calcanei, epyphytis calcanei), which with symptoms are a lesser or bigger defomation and osteodistrophy of the calcaneum. The other possible cause of the alteration is an osteochondral fracture, which also happened during childhood. What is certain is that the deformity could have happened many years before the individual's death, maybe he didn't use his right leg, which indicates on the other side of the calcaneus, with formation of advanced enthesopathy. Other alteration were also detected on the bones of this individual. On both ilium of the hip bone bone loss and on the lateral side of them depression were visible. And finally, on the cervical and lumbar vertebrae spondylosis deformans and on the latter Schmorl-hernia were also visible (Józsa 2006).[8]

OTHER DISEASES

ENTHESOPATHIES

The pathologies of tendon and muscle insertions are called *enthesopathies* (*insertion tendinopathy, insertion osteopathy*). Enthesopathy develops as an adaptation to repeated traumatic effects or increased burden. The burden-dependent adaptation develops slowly. The symptoms depend on the range of burden, and if the burden stops, the alterations may regress.

---

8   Here I would like to thank for László Józsa, who helped me to search the etiology of these alterations.

The frequency of enthesopathy is 2.0–4.0% nowadays. The lesions appear mainly at sportsmen, e.g. longdistance runners, walkers, ski-runners (Smart et al. 1980). Contrary to this fact, enthesopathy could be recognized more frequently in osteoarcheological samples, where its incidence may reach 50% in certain populations (Dutour 1986).

The development and localisation of enthesopathy may inform us about the way of life and the activities of the examined population. Alterations in the upper limbs may refer to overuse of the trunk (e.g. in the case of smiths, fismermans, etc.), while the lesion in the lower limbs and girdle may occur in walkers, runners, agricultural workers, etc. (Józsa 2006).

The paleopathological literature (Dutour 1986) only those listed basically in this hyperthropic alterations, when enthesopathy isn't linked to other disease (e.g. DISH or other diffuse pathological alteration (e.g. spondyloarthropathy). So our statistical data information take into account only those lesions, which have a sure mechanical origin.

In the observed material the enthesopathies were the most freqent pathological alterations (especially on the bones of calcanei and patellae). It was detected among 308 individuals. In the case of males the occurance was 71.49% (153/214), while among females is was 57.40% (155/270).

Among males on the left calcaneum it occurred with a 74.68% (115/154) prevalence, while on the other side it was 71.71% (109/152). Among females this occurance were 60.92% (106/174) on the left, and 63.31% (107/169) on the right (fig. 22).

On the basis of the patella, due to the burden of the muscle—and tendon quadriceps, among males the occurrence ratio was on the left side 42.34% (47/131), while on the right side 46.21% (61/132). Among females it showed on the left 26.40% (47/131), and 27.91% (48/17) incidence rate on the right side.

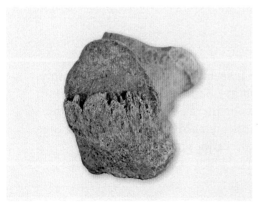

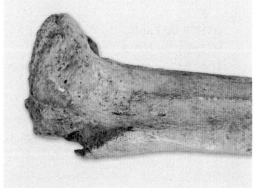

Fig. 22. *Enthesopathy on calcaneus. Grave no. 500.*   **Fig. 23.** *Enthesopathy on tibia. Grave no. 552.*

On the bones of the upper limbs we detected it rarely, while on the lower limb bones it occurred, with a significant higher frequency (fig. 23).

All in all, enthesopathy were more typical among males and occurred much more in the adultus-maturus-, and mature-aged groups. Because this alteration was typical on the lower limb bones, it can be related to that the people in the Neolithic had a locomotive lifestyle, and carried out activ agricultural activity beside the animal husbandry. Based on the fact, that it appeared most often among males, we may conclude, that there existed a sex-realted division of work, assumed that, the hardest physical work was done primarily by males.

TUMOURS

According to our current knowledge, tumors are the same age as mankind itself. The prevalence of tumorous diseases, however, was seemingly relatively low in the past. One of the most important reasons for this is that people who lived in the past died earlier. Hovever, it's not a neglicable factor, that such carcinogenic factors (like environmental pollution, radiation damage, etc.) didn't existe in the past.

The grouping of the tumours is varied. We can classify them as primer or seconder-, as bening or malignant, etc. (Ortner and Putschar 1985; Ortner 2003).

In our serie two **benign tumour** occurred and there were no malignant type.

On the frontal bone of the cranial vault of a mature-aged female (grave no. 617), near to the coronal suture, sized ca. 1.5 × 1.5 cm, distinct, round shaped osseous lesion, with smooth, well-defined thickness appear. It can be diagnosed on the basis of the morphological appearance as an *osteoma* (fig. 24).

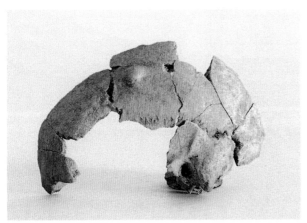

Fig. 24. Possible case of *osteoma* on the skull. Grave no. 617.

In the other case of an adult female (grave no. 6244), on the dorsal side of the right humerus diaphysis, ca. 1.2 × 0.6 cm oval shaped protrusion occurred, which could be diagnosed as osteoma, too.

Osteoma is one of the most common bening tumour, which is asymptomatic in a lot of case. It can occur on the cranium and on the long bones, too. They're usually small and well-defined, shaped bony growing and can be formed on the outher or the inner surface of the bone. If they're appearing example in the sinuses of the cranium, they can cause narrowing and obstruction. **Malignant** tumour in the population of the Lengyel culture occurred only at the site of Mauer (Austria), which was diagnosed as *myeloma multiplex* (Strouhal and Kritscher 1990).

PATHOLOGICAL BIRTH

In the paleopathological literature very few cases can be found, which dealing with death during or sortly after the childbirth. In ancient times, obstetric knowledge were more rudimentary. Complications during birth or death shortly after the birth may have occurred much more, but because of diagnostic difficulties deriving from the poorly preserved, smallbones their fragile skeletons could not survive due to taphonomic process (Regöly-Mérei 1960; Regöly-Mérei 1962).

The few known cases is mainly due to the-so called narrow pelvis, when there is no match between the diameters of the foetal head and the maternal birth canal. This can cause death during childbirth.

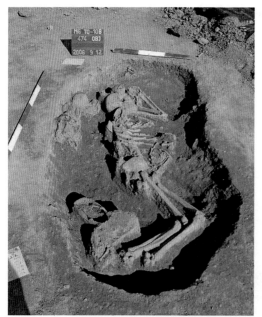

Fig. 25. *Pathological birth.* Grave no. 474.

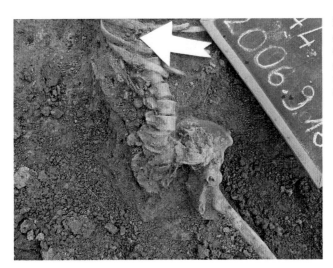

Fig. 26. Close picture of the *pathological birth* case showing the head of the neonate in the mother's pelvic bone. Grave no. 474.

In the Alsónyék serie it was observed in two cases. In grave no. 474, a relatively well preserved adult age female skeleton were found. The female were in a contracted position on her left side and with an E-W orientation. Her arms and hands were in front of her head, which is a realtively rare phenomenon in the burial customs at Alsónyék. Before her ribs and pelvis were the most of the *skeleton of the neonate* (fig. 25).

H skull parts were in the maternal pelvis (fig. 26). The pelvis of the female were fragmentary, both os iliums were preserved, but the os ischiums and the sacrum were in a very fragmentary state, while the os pubis weren't preserved. So we couldn't reconstruct the shape and the size of the pelvis. There were no visible deviation on the os iliums, but they were remarkably small. We measured the bones of the neonate, based on it she or he could be 39–40 weeks, which is the final period of the pregnancy.

In grave no. 4414 again a well preserved mature age female were found. She were in a contacted position, on the left side, with an E-W orientation, too. The skull of the fetus was in the mother's birth canal. In this case the age of the fetus couldn't be estimated, because the bones remained in a fragmentary state, but based on the excavation photo, we may assume that the age of him or her was about the same, as in the other case. The female's pelvis shape an size in this case was normal.

To sum, in the first case the we may assume, that the death of the foetus and her mother is due to narrow pelvis. Moreover, it both cases it could be possible that the babies was born bottom first instead of head first (pathological birth) and the skull of the foetuses couldn't pass throught the birth canal of the pelvis. That could be caused by the difference in size of pelvic of the mothers and the skull of the neonate.

CONCLUSIONS

The detailed paleopathological analysis of the skeletal population of the cemetery-part at the site of Alsónyék showed a relatively low ratio of traumatic deformations, nonspecific inflammations and degenerative articular diseases.

As for the haematological disorders, cribra orbitalia occurred with a high incidence among children, which likely reflects malnutrition and it's consequencies. At the same time, among the adults the most frequent alterations were the enthesopathic deformities, primarily on the calcaneus and on the patella, which are generally considered to be markers of more active lifestyle.

Beside these above mentioned alterations some rare or significant diseases occurred, too. These included the cases of bening tumor and the so-called pathological birth. Two cases of deformities affecting the frontal ligaments of the spinal column suggesting DISH-syndrome, which needs more investigations.

The most important pathological alteration occurred in the case of an individual buried in a post-framed grave construction. On the vertebral column of this person very typical morphological lesions (Pott's gibbus) caused by tuberculosis could be observed. The observation of atypical sign of the inflammation and the aDNA analysis confirmed the diagnosis, moreover detected TB occurrence in other cases.

I had the opportunity to analyze 68 individuals, who were buried in post-framed grave constructions (they're titulated as the elite of the Lengyel society). The demographic, or the morphometric characteristics of them showed similarities to the rest of the Alsónyék population. The frequency of different pathological alterations and dental diseases was also similar to that of the rest of the individuals buried in simple graves. Based on these, the archaeologically manifested socio-economic differentiation couln't be supported by the physical anthropological characteristics and by the lifestyle among the members of the Alsónyék community.

In this work, I didn't publicate the detailed results of the investigations of oral pathology, but have to make a few words about it, too. The general low frequency of carious lesions, alveolar abscesses, cysts and ante mortem teeth loss suggests a relatively adequate dental hygiene. In most cases, caries appeared on the cementum-enamel border (it is a general phenomenon in the Neolithic). This might have been caused by the lifestyle and special nutrition habit in this period, as a result of which the teeth are characterized by great extent of abrasion, exposure of the dental collar and, as a consequence, collar caries on the cementum–enamel border (Schranz and Huszár 1962). However, the dental hypoplasia occured with a relatively high frequency, which suggests unpredictable food supply in the childhood.

The above outlined results and interpretations, the clarification of unanswered questions will be possible only through the physical anthropological analysis of the full population of the Alsónyék cemetery. But the paleopathological investigation of the 862 graves from the cemetery helped us to reconstruct to some extent the lifestyle and health status of this population.

3.7 ARTIFICIAL DEFORMATION OF TEETH IN LENGYEL CULTURE

VÁCLAV SMRČKA, ZDENKA MUSILOVÁ, ŠTEFAN RÁSTOČNÝ, DAVID DICK

On examination of the health state of the dentition from skeletal remains at three burial sites in the county of Baranya-Zengővárkony, Villánykővesd and Belvárdgula (N 95), signs of artificial deformation of the teeth were detected.

On teeth of men, women, and also children, very fine incisions were found. Some were visible with naked eye, while others could be observed using a magnifying glass or in enlarged photographs.

In total, 16 types of incisions were identified, which were repeated in a variety of combinations. We allocated each type letter(s), and described them as follows:

H—a *horizontal type of incision* visible on the cusp (see diagram of tooth, and fig. 1).

C—a *cross-shaped incision* visible on the cusp of the tooth (see diagram of tooth, and fig. 2).

LY—a *Y-shaped incision*, open to the left (left capital upsilon) visible on the cusp (see diagram of tooth, and fig. 3).

PT—a T-shaped incision on the cusp, turned in the lingual direction (*posterior T*) (see diagram of tooth, and fig. 4).

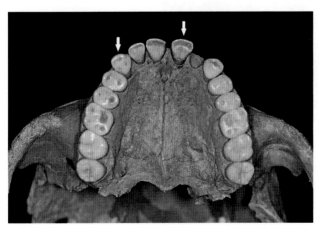

Fig. 1. *Horizontal incisions* visible on the first left incisor and the right cuspid in the upper jaw of a female, aged 40–80, in grave no. 286, Zengővárkony. Incidentally, the woman probably used her upper incisors as work tools (visible grooves at the bottom of which there is the incision). Photo: Zdenka Musilová.

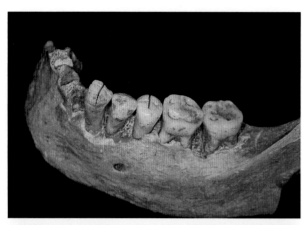

Fig. 2. *A cross-shaped incision* in the lower left cuspid of a woman, aged 33–39, in grave no. 336, Zengővárkony. Photo: Zdenka Musilová.

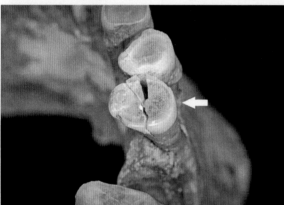

Fig. 3. *Left capital upsilon incision* in the tooth of a man, aged 68–80, in grave no. 5, Villánykővesd. Photo: Zdenka Musilová.

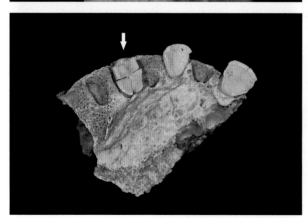

Fig. 4. *Posterior T-shaped incision* in the second right premolar in the upper jaw of a woman, aged 50–70, in grave no. 101, Zengővárkony. Photo: Zdenka Musilová.

AI—an *anterior incision*, visible on the labial side of the tooth, passing only partially the tooth (see diagram of tooth, and fig. 5).

RY—a Y-shaped incision, open to the right (*right capital upsilon*) on the cusp of the tooth (see diagram of tooth, and fig. 6).

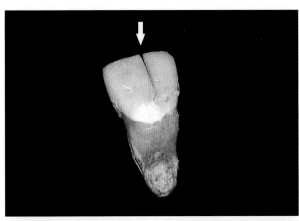

Fig. 5. *Anterior incision* visible on the labial side of the incisor of a woman, aged 30, in grave no. 284, Belvárdgyula.
Photo: Zdenka Musilová.

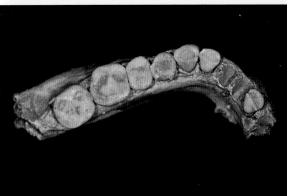

Fig. 6. *Right upsilon incision* in the lower incisor of a woman, aged 50-70, in grave no. 101, Zengővárkony.
Photo: Zdenka Musilová.

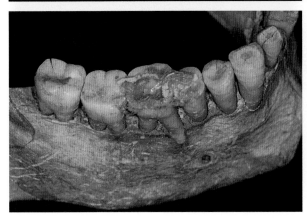

Fig. 7. *Posterior incision* on the lingual surface of the lower right molar of a man, aged 29-33, in grave no. 104, Zengővárkony.
Photo: Zdenka Musilová.

PI—an incision on the lingual surface of the tooth (*posterior incision*) (see diagram of tooth, and fig. 7).

SI—a *sagittal incision*, passing along the entire tooth or the best part of the axis of the tooth (see diagram of tooth, and fig. 8).

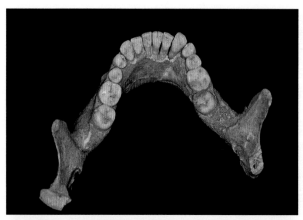

Fig. 8. *Sagittal incisions* in the cuspids and incisor of a 12–13-year-old child in grave 12, Villánykővesd. Photo: Zdenka Musilová.

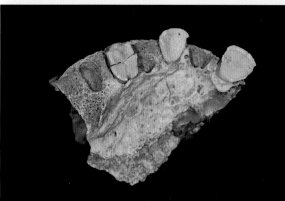

Fig. 9. *An anterior T-shaped incision* in the upper right premolar of a woman, aged 50–70, in grave 101, Zengővárkony. Photo: Zdenka Musilová.

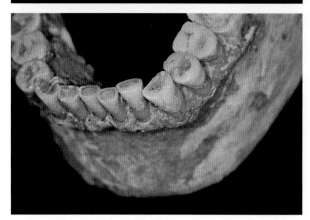

Fig. 10. *Anterior and posterior incisions* in the lower left cuspid of a woman, aged 40–60, in grave no. 83, Belvárdgyula. Photo: Zdenka Musilová.

AT—a T-shaped incision turned in the labial direction on the cusp (*anterior T*) (see diagram of tooth, and fig. 9).

AP—an anterior incision, visible on the labial side of the tooth and accompanied by the posterior incision visible on the lingual side of the tooth (*anterior and posterior incision*) (see diagram of tooth, and fig. 10).

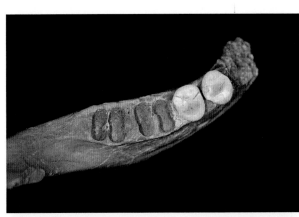

Fig. 11. *Posterior V-shaped incision* in a premolar in the lower jaw of a woman, aged 50–70, in grave no. 101, Zengővárkony.
Photo: Zdenka Musilová.

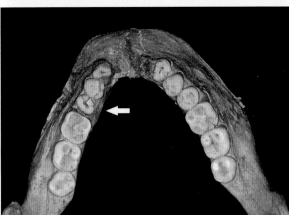

Fig. 12. *Right V-shaped incision* in a premolar in the lower jaw of a man, aged 40–80, in grave no. 238, Zengővárkony.
Photo: Zdenka Musilová.

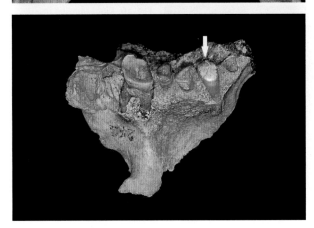

Fig. 13. *Left V-shaped incision* in an upper cuspid of a man, aged 54–66, in grave no. 272, Zengővárkony.
Photo: Zdenka Musilová.

PV—a V-shaped incision, open in the lingual direction (*posterior V*) (see diagram of tooth, and fig. 11).

RV—a *V-shaped incision*, open to the right (*right V*), in a mesial direction to the interdental space (see diagram of tooth, and fig. 12).

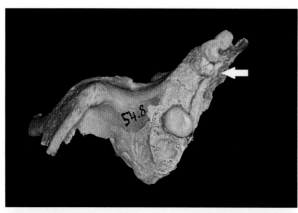

Fig. 14. *Left incision* in an upper right premolar of a woman, aged 39–45, in grave no. 34, Zengővárkony. Photo: Zdenka Musilová.

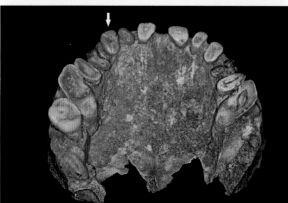

Fig. 15. *Anterior capital upsilon incision* in the upper right cuspid of a man, aged 68–80, Villánykővesd. Photo: Zdenka Musilová.

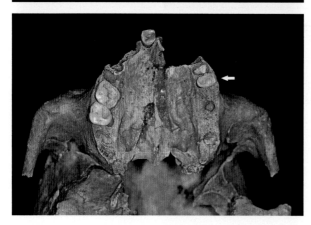

Fig. 16. *Right incision* in an upper left premolar of a woman, aged 50–56, in grave no. 337, Zengővárkony. Photo: Zdenka Musilová.

LV—a V-shaped incision, open to the left (*left V*), in the mesial direction to the interdental space (see diagram of tooth, and fig. 13).

LI—an incision on the part of the tooth directed mesially into the interdental space and towards the left side of the jaw (*left incision*) (see diagram of tooth, and fig. 14).

AY—a Y-shaped incision, open in the labial direction (*anterior capital upsilon*) on the cusp of the tooth (see diagram of tooth, and fig. 15).

RI—an incision affecting the part of the tooth directed mesially into the interdental space and towards the right side of the jaw (*right incision*) (see diagram of tooth, and fig. 16).

Artificial incisions on teeth of 7 men and 12 women were found in 19 graves of the Zengővárkony burial site as follows: 6, 34, 45, 90, 99, 101, 104, 120, 125, 238, 272, 286, 299, 320, 336, 337, 341, 355, and 366.

In Villánykővesd, incisions were detected on the teeth of 3 men, 1 woman and 1 child in 5 graves. The youngest individual with artificial deformation of teeth was a child, aged 12–13, found in grave no. 12. At this burial site, incisions in teeth were also detected in graves 22, 9, 5, and 2.

At the burial site of Belvárdguyla, incisions were found on the teeth of 1 man and 3 women from graves: 83, 284, 379, and 447.

Incisions on teeth were identified at three sites of the Lengyel culture in 28 graves in the teeth of 11 males, 16 females and 1 child.

We assume that these incisions were carved into teeth during initiation rituals. Considering the age of the youngest individual in whose teeth these incisions were detected, we may presume that such interventions were being performed at an age of 12–13.

From the shape of the fracture of the enamel we do not suppose that all the 16 described shapes were incised entirely during the ritual. Various shapes could have originated through incisions in different parts of the tooth with the subsequent effects of age and mechanical wear of the tooth.

4. CARBON AND NITROGEN ANALYSIS: ZENGŐVÁRKONY AND VILLÁNYKŐVESD

VÁCLAV SMRČKA, JAKUB TRUBAČ, MARTIN HILL, ZDENKA MUSILOVÁ,
LENKA PŮTOVÁ, SYLVA DRTIKOLOVÁ KAUPOVÁ, ŠTEFAN RÁSTOČNÝ

4.1 ZENGŐVÁRKONY

In Zengővárkony, 6 individuals (1 male, 3 females, and 2 children) were available for sampling, representing approximately 10% of the total number of skeletons analysed (6/59).

The younger child from grave no. 340 was aged between 1 and 5 ($\delta^{15}N = 14.27 \pm 0.02$ ‰; $\delta^{13}C = -18.94 \pm 0.03$ ‰). Its increased carbon and nitrogen isotopic values in comparison with the other individuals may have been caused by breastfeeding (Fogel et al. 1989, Fuller et al. 2006).

The values for the other child, infans aged 4–5 (in grave 331), ($\delta^{15}N = 9.27$ ‰; $\delta^{13}C = -19.75$ ‰) are already clustered together with the adults and it is probable that he or she was not breastfed anymore. From the aforesaid data it may be suggested that in the Lengyel Culture children were habitually weaned before the age of 4. However, it should be kept in mind that this finding is based at the very small number of samples.

From the placement of the group of 3 females and 1 male it can be clearly seen that there are no differences in $\delta^{13}C$ and $\delta^{15}N$ values between males and females and that the diet was based on plants of the C3 photosynthetic cycle (DeNiro and Epstein 1978, Lee-Thorp 2008), like wheat.

The youngest female, aged 33–39 (grave 336) ($\delta^{15}N = 9.48 \pm 0.03$ ‰; $\delta^{13}C = -20.02 \pm 0.03$ ‰), was in her reproductive age. Her $\delta^{15}N$ values are very similar to those of the 4–5-year-old child from grave 331 and therefore it is highly probable that she sustained herself on a similar diet, for instance on soft wheat-based foods.

Different results were observed in the older female, aged 50–56 from grave 337 ($\delta^{15}N = 10.47 \pm 0.02$ ‰; $\delta^{13}C = -20.10 \pm 0.01$ ‰), in terms of $\delta^{15}N$ a higher proportion of animal protein was detected in her than in the female from grave no. 336 (DeNiro and Epstein 1981, Lee-Thorp 2008).

In the oldest female, aged 62–75 from grave no. 341 ($\delta^{15}N = 10.10 \pm 0.02$ ‰; $\delta^{13}C = -19.69 \pm 0.04$ ‰), the $\delta^{15}N$ value, which is an indicator of animal products in the diet, is in decline again.

Even though the number of females in our collection is small, it is evident that values of $\delta^{15}N$ and the proportion of animal products in the diet of females of the Lengyel Culture correlated with age. However, female variation

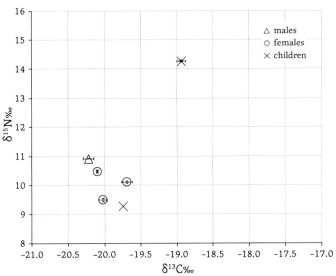

Fig. 1. Zengővárkony: carbon and nitrogen isotope ratios (‰) in humans.

in δ¹⁵N is not high (cca 1‰), suggesting only moderate differences in animal protein consumption.

However, this correlation with age might have applied not only to LgC but also to LPC and SPC. To support our claim, Zn/Ca values relative to age in females in the graph in Chapter 12 should be noted. The graph is based on Zn concentration in femoral bones of 13 females of all the Neolithic Cultures and is indicative of the representation of animal protein with age. The highest level is found in the new-born infant, up to the age of 10 there is a slight decline; up to age 20, it is stabilized; between 20 and 40 years of age, there is a more marked decline; however, in the age group 40–60 the level rises again. Trace element analysis was not conducted for the age group of over 60.

The similarity between the Zn/Ca Graph and δ¹⁵N values throughout the aging of Neolithic females is evident.

In the only analysed male, aged 52–55 from grave no. 338 (δ¹⁵N = 10.91 ± 0.01 ‰; δ¹³C = −20.22 ± 0.04 ‰) there is an slightly higher δ¹⁵N value than in the aforementioned females, the source of which could have based at terrestrial animals and/or freshwater fish.

4.2 VILLÁNYKŐVESD

In Villánykővesd, 9 individuals (3 males, 2 females, and 4 children) were available for sampling, representing approximately 39% of the total number of skeletons analysed (9/23).

The youngest of the group of children was the child from grave no. 19, aged 1–1.5 years ($\delta^{15}N$ = 12.98 ± 0.04 ‰; $\delta^{13}C$ = −18.97 ± 0.01 ‰), holds an eccentric position in graph 2. It is presumed that the child was breast fed.

Completely different $\delta^{15}N$ and $\delta^{13}C$ values are observed in the next child, aged 8.5 years from grave no. 15 ($\delta^{15}N$ = 9,11 ± 0,01 ‰; $\delta^{13}C$ = −20,56 ± 0,01 ‰). Similar carbon and nitrogen isotope values were also observed in the child from grave no. 12, aged 12–13 ($\delta^{15}N$ = 9.64 ± 0.00 ‰; $\delta^{13}C$ = −20.26 = ± 0.01 ‰). It is likely that this type of diet was fed to children from the age of 4 when they were weaned up to the age of 12–13. Decreased nitrogen isotopic values during childhood are commonly observed in agricultural populations, probably as a result of specific child feeding practices (Tsutaya et al. 2017).

The diet could have changed after initiation rituals, which were performed on teeth, as was elaborated in Chapter 3. However, similar values of $\delta^{15}N$ and $\delta^{13}C$ to those of both the children were also detected in a female, aged 53–62 (grave no. 21) ($\delta^{15}N$ = 9.54 ‰; $\delta^{13}C$ = −20.65 ‰).

Another female, aged 36–40, in grave no. 10 ($\delta^{15}N$ = 11.10 ‰; $\delta^{13}C$ = −20.49 ‰), was not local, and her $\delta^{15}N$ values indicate sources of animal protein from terrestrial animals and/or fish. This female was a mother of a fetus from the grave no. 10, who showed similar isotopic values ($\delta^{15}N$ = 10.75 ± 0.03 ‰; $\delta^{13}C$ = −20.07 ± 0.06 ‰) as he or she was nourished through its mother's placenta. The foetus suffered from a liver disease, which was evidenced by trace element analyses (chapter 6) and by the macroscopic find of pelvic and intracranial periostitis (chapter 3).

A special carbon and nitrogen isotopic values were observed in the case of the male, aged 41–45 from grave no. 24 ($\delta^{15}N$ °= 12.01 ± 0.03 ‰; $\delta^{13}C$ = −17.50

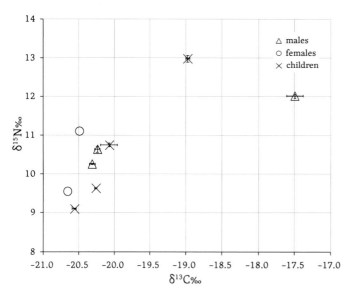

Fig. 2. Villánykővesd: carbon and nitrogen isotope ratios (‰) in humans

± 0.06 ‰). His $\delta^{13}C$ values point to food sources of plants of the C4 photosynthetic cycle, most likely millet. However, millet is in general not supposed to be a staple food in the Neolithic Europe (Miller et al. 2016, Motuzaite-Matuzeviciute et al. 2013). Moreover, due to the relatively high $\delta^{15}N$ accompanying the increased $\delta^{13}C$, the consumption of certain amount of marine or (due to the inland location of the site much more probably) anadromous and/or catadromous fish (such as salmon and eel) cannot be excluded (DeNiro and Epstein 1978 and 1982, Lee-Thorp 2008).

This individual probably suffered from hydrocephalus acquired in adulthood or posterior plagiocephaly. He would have shuffled around the settlement with small steps, been mentally retarded, and suffered from urinal incontinence (chapter 3). Thus, whatever was the real base of his specific diet, it can be speculated that special type of food may be reserved as the food for the ill.

METHODS

The same analytical methods were used for all the sites. After mechanically removing the adhering dirt, bone samples were ultrasonically cleaned in demineralised water. Collagen extract were prepared using the Longin (1971) method modified by Bocherens (1992). Powdered samples were demineralised in 1 M HCl for 20 minutes, followed by removal of humic acids with 0,125 M NaOH (for 18–20 hours), and gelatinisation in 0,01 M HCl at 100°C for 17 hours. Sample were then freeze-dried for approximately 72 hours.

5. STRONTIUM ANALYSIS: ZENGŐVÁRKONY, VILLÁNYKŐVESD, BELVÁRDGYULA, BORJÁD-KENDERFÖLD

VÁCLAV SMRČKA, JAKUB TRUBAČ, ZDENKA MUSILOVÁ,
MARTIN HILL, LENKA PŮTOVÁ, ŠTEFAN RÁSTOČNÝ

The method is based on the principle that the ratio of Sr isotopes in the tissues reflects the isotopic ratio in the diet at the time of their origin. Dental enamel is formed in early childhood and it is not renewed, while bone tissue is renewed continuously over the course of the life. Hence, if dental enamel and compact bone have different strontium isotopes ratio values, it can be

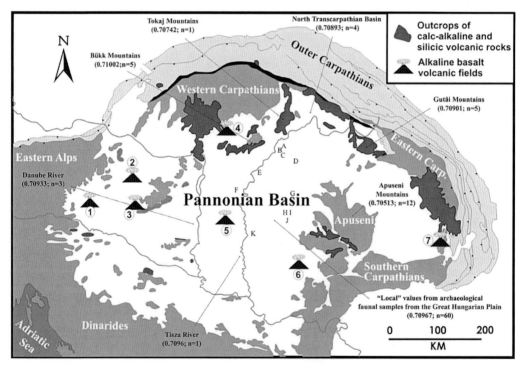

Fig. 1. Geological sketch map of the Carpathiane-Pannonian Region showing 87Sr/86Sr isotope variability and archaeological site locations (Giblin et al. 2013). Archaeological sites: A (Tiszapolgár-Basatanya), B (Polgár-Piócási-dűlő), C (Polgár-Csőszhalom), D (Hajdúböszörmény-Ficsori-tó), E (Kisköre-Gát), F (Abony 36), G (Magyarhomorog), H (Vésztő-Bikeri, Körösladány-Bikeri, Vésztő-Mágor), I (Okány 6), J (Gyula 114), K (Hódmezővásárhely-Gorzsa).

supposed that the examined person spent their childhood and the years preceding their death in different geochemical ambients (Hillson 1997; Price et al. 2002). The strontium isotopes ratio from bedrock, mineral water, and soil also provide important information. The ratios of $^{87/86}Sr$ may show the variability of migration of individuals in a study area (see e.g. Voerkelius et al. 2010; Giblin et al. 2013; Gerling 2014; Hoogewerff et al. 2019; fig. 1).

5.1 ZENGŐVÁRKONY

In Zengővárkony, 11 individuals (4 males, 4 females and 3 children) were available for sampling, representing approximately 19% of the total number of skeletons analysed at the site (11/59).

The minimum $^{87}Sr/^{86}Sr$ isotopic ratio at the site was 0.7095 ± 2.52E-05 and the maximum was 0.7114 ± 1.97E-05.

Individuals, whose isotope average in dental enamel surpassed the average isotopic femoral ratio by more than 2SD, were classified as migrants (nonlocals). The ratio is dependent on local conditions, but also on the tooth used for analysis. In our research, the first molar (M1) was used in six instances. It mineralizes by approximately 2 years of age, while the child would have been breast fed, and thus reflects the mother's mobility. In the other five instances, second molars (M2), which mineralizes between 2 and 8 years of age, and a third molar (M3) which mineralizes between 6 and 16 years of age, were analysed. However alternative sources of Sr isotopes cannot be excluded during this period. 6 individuals (3 males, 2 females, 1 child) were identified as nonlocal:

MALES

The 1st migrant is a male, aged 48–58 (grave no. 5). His M1 (lower right) was extracted and the maximum range was 0.7114 ± 1.97E-05 in dental enamel. The isotopic range in his femur was 0.7095 ± 2.15E-05. He suffered from *spondylosis* of the whole spine with 3–5 mm osteophytes, suggestive of a physically demanding working lifestyle

The 2nd migrant is a man, aged 40–80 (grave no. 99). His M3 (lower left) was extracted and his isotopic ratio in dental enamel was found to be 0.7111 ± 1.64E-05, and 0.7099 ± 2.06E-05 in his femur. He suffered from anaemia, had cribra orbitalia in his right orbit, and rims on the proximal phalanges of his hands. The latter is indicative of strain on the interosseous muscles, possibly from making fishing nets.

The 3rd migrant is a man, aged 38–48 (grave 325). His M1 (lower left) was extracted and the isotopic ratio in his dental enamel was found to be 0.7106 ±

2.47E-05, and 0.7096 ± 1.64 E-05 in his femur. He suffered from tuberculosis in his calcaneus and talus, as well as spina bifida of the sacrum.

FEMALES

The 1st migrant is a woman, aged 33–39 (grave no. 336). Her first molar (M1) was extracted, and the isotopic ratio in dental enamel was found to be 0.7108 ± 2.62E-05. The ratio in her femur was 0.7098 ± 1.65E-05.

The 2nd migrant is a woman, aged 26–32 (grave no. 320). Her second molar (M2) was extracted and the isotopic ratio in dental enamel was found to be 0.7107 ± 1.65E-05. The ratio in her femur was 0.7099 ± 1,56E-05.

CHILDREN

The only nonlocal child was aged 4–5. Its isotopic ratio in dental enamel was 0.7110 ± 2.45E-05, and 0.7098 ± 2.51 E-05 in its femur.

In Zengővárkony, 6 out of 11 analysed individuals were found to be nonlocal, therefore it can be supposed that mobility at this site was 55%.

5.2 VILLÁNYKŐVESD

In Villánykővesd, 9 individuals (3 males, 2 females, 3 children, and 1 foetus) were available for sampling, representing approximately 39% of the total number of skeletons analysed at the site (10/23).

The group of nonlocals consisted of 5 individuals (2 males, 1 female, and 2 children).

MALES

The 1st migrant is a man, aged 36–43 (grave no. 22). His M1 was extracted and the isotopic ratio in his dental enamel was found to be 0.7108 ± 2.32E-05. The ratio in his femur was 0.7104 ± 1.82E-05.

The 2nd migrant is a man, aged 41–45 (grave no. 24). His M2 was extracted and the isotopic ratio in his dental enamel was found to be 0.7102 ± 3.10E-05. The ratio in his femur was 0.7102 ± 2.17E-05. He showed signs of posterior plagiocephaly.

FEMALES

The woman, aged 36–40 (grave no. 10), exhibited an isotopic ratio of 0.7115 ± 2.17E-05 in her dental enamel (and 0.7101 ± 2.25E-05 in her femur). She likely died during childbirth as there was also a baby buried with her.

CHILDREN

The 1st child was 12–13 years old (grave no. 12). Its M2 was extracted and the isotopic ratio in its dental enamel was found to be 0.7096 ± 2.13E-05. The ratio in the femur was 0.7105 ± 2.49E-05.

The 2nd child was 1–1.5 years old (grave no. 19). Its M1 was extracted. The child was likely being breastfed so its values, de facto, illustrate that its mother was a migrant. Its isotopic ratio in dental enamel was found to be 0.7111 ± 2.18E-05. The ratio in the femur 0.7102 ± 1.56E-05.

In Villánykővesd, 5 out of 8 individuals who were analysed for stable strontium isotopes (5/8) were determined to be nonlocal, therefore it can be supposed that mobility at this site was 62.5%.

5.3 BELVÁRDGYULA

Determing the isotopic ratio of Sr typical for the local population iscrucially important; the isotopic ratio $^{87}Sr/^{86}Sr$ in the tissues reflects the isotopic composition of local water sources, for which the dominant source of strontium would be bed rock. Since the majority of rocks are composed of several minerals of various isotopic composition, and, more importantly, since these weather out and release their components into water at various rates, the information about the composition of rocks, in many cases, cannot be used for the purpose of determing mobility. Due to the variability of hydrological and hydrogeological conditions, direct measuring of water sources is also problematic. The skeletons of minor rodents or domestic animals, especially pigs, which are close to humans in the trophic chain (Bentley 2002; Bentley and Knipper 2005; Price et al. 2002), prove to be the best indicators of the local isotopic signal.

At the site, a sheep in grave 98-292/1529 was identified. It was proved to be not local. In contrast, the man aged 20–40 (grave 98243-2006) and the woman, aged 40–60 (grave 98 -292/15929) found in the same grave as the sheep were local

On analysis of randomly selected individuals, it was discovered that the population at the Belárdgyula site was likely local.

5.4 BORJÁD-KENDERFÖLD

The rich woman of Borjád, aged 20–40, was a migrant with the isotopic ratio in her dental enamel of 0.7198 ± 2.20E-05. In her grave, a sheep (98-373-2359) was also found; it was from local stock.

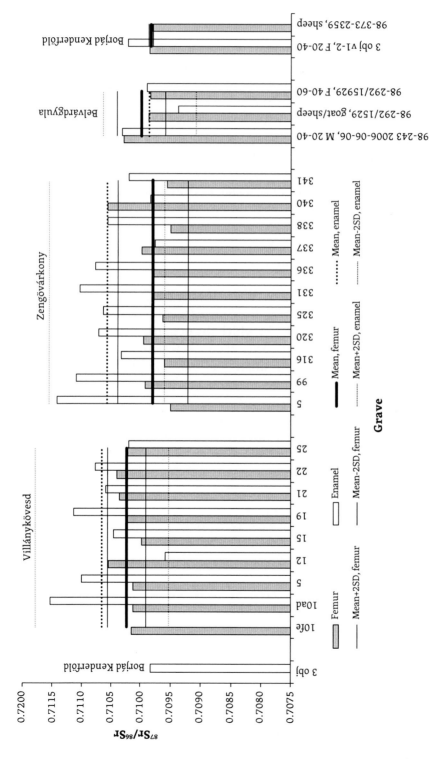

Fig.2. A bar (or dot) chart illustrating pairs of samples from tooth enamel and femoral bones clarifying the isotopic ratio of Sr isotopes in both substrates. The thick line marks the average isotope content in femurs (with 2SD limits).

DISCUSSION AND CONCLUSIONS

Borič and Price (2013) unequivocally proved that in earliest phases of the Neolithic in southern Europe farming communities were paradoxically more mobile than the local foraging populations.

There is greater variance of Sr ratios among the females of this time in comparison with males, suggesting that woman came to these sites from other Neolithic communities as part of ongoing social exchange. The Neolithic communities of south-eastern Europe spread across Eruope in a northerly and northwesterly direction.

In several LgC settlements, migration was 55–60%, while at others there was no evidence of mobility.

In Zengővárkony, 6 out of 11 individuals analysed for strontium isotopes (6/11) were determined to have been mobile, therefore it can be supposed that mobility at this site was 55%.

In Villánykővesd, 5 out of 8 individuals analysed for stable strontium isotopes (5/8) were determined as mobile, therefore it can be supposed that mobility at this site was 62.5%.

On analysis of randomly selected individuals, it was discovered that the population at the Belárdgyula site was likely local (fig. 2).

6. VILLÁNYKŐVESD AND ZENGŐVÁRKONY: TRACE ELEMENTS IN TOOTH ENAMEL AND FEMURS OF THE LENGYEL CULTURE

VÁCLAV SMRČKA, MARTIN MIHALJEVIČ, JAKUB TRUBAČ,
ZDENKA MUSILOVÁ, MARTIN HILL, LENKA PŮTOVÁ, ŠTEFAN RÁSTOČNÝ,
IVO NĚMEC

Our aim was to compare the concentrations of trace elements in the distribution compartments of the upper femoral bone and tooth enamel in samples from Neolithic burial sites of the Lengyel Culture (LgC). It was presumed that the comparison could partially reveal dietary trends of the Lengyel Culture (LgC) settlements and clarify tooth diseases of the Neolithic age, including the low caries incidence.

Trace element concentrations in tooth enamel were investigated for their role in caries rates (Curzon and Crocker 1978) and it was found, that the presence of F, Al, Fe, Se and Sr is associated with a low risk of tooth caries, while Mn, Cu, Cd are associated with a high risk of tooth caries (Curzon and Crocker 1978).

The protective layer of teeth, tooth enamel, is composed of an organic and an inorganic component.

The basic constituents of the organic component are proteins, amelogenin, ameloblastin and tuftelin with small amounts of proteoglycans and lipids. The inorganic component of tooth enamel consists of calcium phosphate apatite (HA) nanocrystals with a small quantity of integrated trace elements where Cr, Mo, Co and Sb have the lowest concentration in tooth enamel compared with other trace elements while Zn, Na and S have the highest one. The greatest difference in concentration of trace elements between tooth enamel and the rest of the body is found in Ni, where Ni is nearly 3500 times more abundant in tooth enamel than in the rest of the body (Ghadimi et al. 2013). In 1936 Noddack came up with the theory of the presence of trace elements including bone and dental tissue in sufficiently sensitive method. Nickel can be absorbed by the body through water, air or food but also via diagenesis from soil (Kampa and Castanas 2008).

We present the contents of the elements in the fetus's and mother's bones from the unique grave 10 in Villánykővesd. In 8 individuals from Villánykővesd (3 males, 2 females, 3 children) and 11 individuals from Zengővárkony (4 males, 4 females, 3 children), 19 trace elements were analysed using ICP and atomic absorption.

Trace elements that were analysed: Aluminium (Al); Barium (Ba); Cadmium (Cd); Cobalt (Co); Chromium (Cr); Copper (Cu); Lead (Pb); Nickel (Ni).

ALUMINIUM (*Al*)

Aluminium can be absorbed by the body from air, food, and water (Maienthal and Taylor, 1968). The concentration in the body is increased with age and in higher amounts it can lead to brain and skeleton disorders (Alfrey et al. 1976).

This element exhibits an interesting interaction with fluorine (F), which is important for the human metabolism also in relation to teeth. It was discovered by Ondreicka et al. (1971) that soluble compounds are formed through

Tab. 1. Concentrations of trace elements in bone and enamel, mean ± SD [ppm].

Element	Bone		Enamel	
	Villánykővesd	Zengővárkony	Villánykővesd	Zengővárkony
Ca	305495 ± 19176	306536 ± 14866	308420 ± 14630	315573 ± 17521
Fe	699 ± 617	821 ± 1382	4.31 ± 1.93	9 ± 15.5
K	79 ± 30.7	80.9 ± 35.7	118 ± 34	134 ± 34
Mg	1327 ± 72	1335 ± 79	2519 ± 434	2340 ± 353
Mn	132 ± 301	26.9 ± 20.7	3.12 ± 3.22	5.17 ± 4.02
Na	1790 ± 263	1790 ± 279	4397 ± 538	4554 ± 697
P	126509 ± 7681	130761 ± 7476	141086 ± 8434	144769 ± 10079
Al	140 ± 117	106 ± 70	16.2 ± 0	16.2 ± 0
V	8.8 ± 3.1	14.1 ± 3.6	4.38 ± 1.89	3.77 ± 4.19
Cr	17.5 ± 3.5	12.8 ± 3.7	4.03 ± 4.55	2.1 ± 2.34
Mn	100 ± 224	22 ± 17	3.82 ± 3.14	3.71 ± 3.89
Co	2.87 ± 1	2.54 ± 0.13	2.35 ± 0.17	2.39 ± 0.3
Ni	61.2 ± 7.3	63.9 ± 13.5	56.4 ± 3.7	58.2 ± 7.5
Cu	11.5 ± 3.1	11.3 ± 5.2	2.3 ± 0.3	2.2 ± 0.2
Zn	145 ± 91	145 ± 55	90.7 ± 14.2	90.9 ± 13.5
Rb	0.135 ± 0.158	0.097 ± 0.088	0.0126 ± 0.0075	0.0173 ± 0.0122
Sr	180 ± 32	217 ± 22	99 ± 27	92 ± 19
Y	0.496 ± 0.765	0.213 ± 0.366	0.025 ± 0.0524	0.0331 ± 0.0479
Zr	1.45 ± 1.22	1.48 ± 0.68	0.0326 ± 0	0.034 ± 0.0047
Cd	0.213 ± 0.23	0.292 ± 0.175	0.0244 ± 0	0.0244 ± 0
Sb	0.062 ± 0.059	0.441 ± 0.178	0.00611 ± 0	0.00611 ± 0
Ba	95.6 ± 32.7	100.1 ± 19.9	21.1 ± 12.4	20.3 ± 14.4
La	0.379 ± 0.578	0.142 ± 0.194	0.0161 ± 0.0299	0.0174 ± 0.0274
Ce	0.385 ± 0.52	0.151 ± 0.154	0.00398 ± 0.0017	0.0096 ± 0.0116
Pb	1.5 ± 2.13	0.74 ± 0.91	0.385 ± 0.594	0.264 ± 0.359
U	1.35 ± 0.59	0.85 ± 0.22	0.12 ± 0.172	0.076 ± 0.116

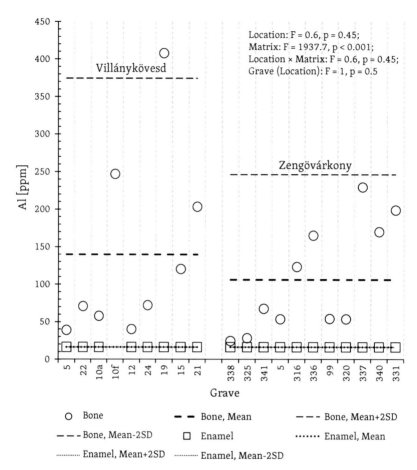

Fig. 1. Aluminium concentrations (Al in ppm) in femurs and tooth enamel at the Villánykövesd and Zengővárkony settlements.

the interaction of Al and F. This compound is significantly more soluble than the common CaF salts. Aluminium is removed from the body when the intake of fluoride is increased.

In both of the Lengyel burial sites, it was discovered that the concentration of aluminium (Al) in bone was higher than in tooth enamel (tab. 1). In Villánykövesd (N = 8), there was greater concentration of aluminium (Al) in femoral bones (p < 0.503) than in Zengővárkony. In the individual from grave no. 19, Villánykövesd, the aluminium concentration in bone was determined to be 400 µg Al/g of bone over 2 SD, while in Zengővárkony, the aluminium concentrations in bone did not exceed 250 µg Al/g of bone (fig. 1). The foetus from grave no. 10, Villánykövesd, contained five times as much aluminium (250 ppm) than its mother (50 ppm).

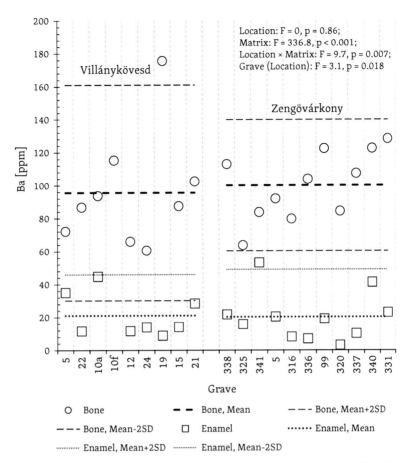

Fig. 2. Barium concentrations (Ba in ppm) in femurs and tooth enamel at the Villánykövesd and Zengővárkony settlements.

BARIUM (*Ba*)

In LgC, the barium (Ba) concentration in bone from Villánykővesd exhibits a greater dispersion of values while being insignificantly lower than in Zengővárkony (tab. 1).

Barium concentration in tooth enamel is approximately the same in both burial sites, yet, it is almost five times lower (p < 0.001) than in femurs (fig. 2).

CADMIUM (*Cd*)

In both LgC burial sites, the cadmium (Cd) concentration in bone is higher than in tooth enamel (p < 0.001), where the cadmium concentration is ten times lower (tab. 1).

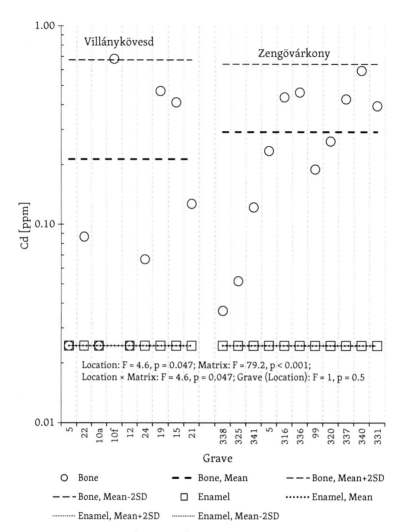

Fig. 3. Cadmium concentrations (Cd in ppm) in femurs and tooth enamel at the Villánykövesd and Zengővárkony settlements.

The concentration of cadmium in bones is higher in Zengővárkony than in Villánykövesd (p = 0.047).

The cadmium concentration in bones of the foetus (0.68 ppm) is higher than that of its mother (lower than LOD) (fig. 3).

It was discovered by Noel et al. (2004) that increased values of Cu, Zn and Mn in the liver may lead to an increase in Cd levels in the bone. It may therefore be speculated, that the aforementioned foetus suffered from a liver disease.

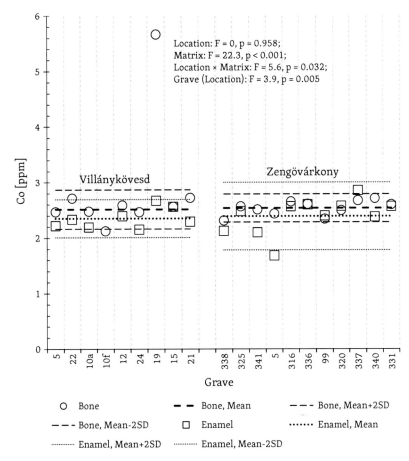

Fig. 4. Cobalt concentrations (Co in ppm) in femurs and tooth enamel at the Villánykővesd and Zengővárkony settlements.

COBALT (Co)

Cobalt (Co) can enter the body through water, air and food (Duruibe et al. 2007).

In both the LgC burial sites, the cobalt (Co) concentrations in bone were higher than in tooth enamel (p < 0.001).

The Co concentration in bone of the mother from grave 10, Villánykővesd, was higher than that of the foetus in the same grave.

In both LgC burial sites, the Co concentrations in bone and in tooth enamel ranged between 2 and 3 ppm Co per gram of bone (fig. 4). The average in bones was 2.68 ± 0.7 ppm Co, and in tooth enamel 2.37 ± 0.26 ppm Co.

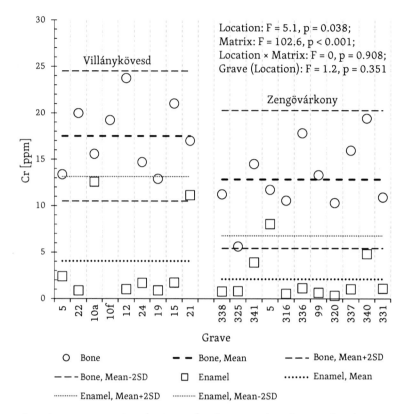

Fig. 5. Chromium concentrations (Cr in ppm) in femurs and tooth enamel at the Villánykövesd and Zengővárkony settlements.

CHROMIUM (Cr)

Chromium is a heavy metal that is essential for the body in small amounts. It can enter the human body through water, air and food (Kampa and Castanas 2008).

Ghadimi (2013) observed a significant association between the concentration of Cr and cell lattice parameter along the c-axis in tooth enamel (Mabilleau et al. 2010).

In both LgC burial sites, the chromium (Cr) concentration in bone is higher than in tooth enamel (tab. 1, $p < 0.001$, fig. 5).

The average chromium concentration in tooth enamel is 4 ppm in Villánykövesd and 2 ppm in Zengővárkony.

The average Cr concentration is higher in Villánykövesd (17.5 ppm) than in Zengővárkony (13 ppm) ($p = 0.027$).

The chromium concentration in bones of the foetus (19 ppm) in grave 10, Villánykövesd, was higher than that of its mother (15 ppm).

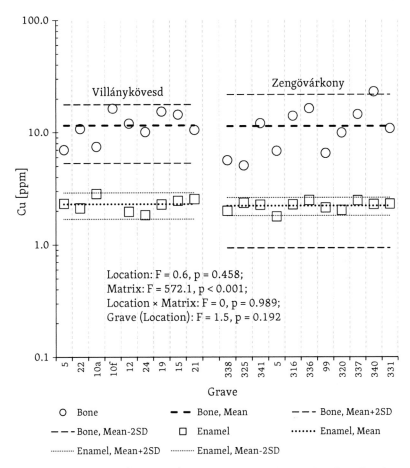

Fig. 6. Copper concentrations (Cu in ppm) in femurs and tooth enamel at the Villánykővesd and Zengővárkony settlements.

COPPER (Cu)

Human studies point to Cu as a caries promoting element. Animal studies have been equivocal. Plaque and oral bacterial metabolism studies would indicate a Cu effect to reduce acidogenicity. There is an indication that Cu may play a role in influencing periodontal disease and alveolar bone resorption (Curzon and Cutress 1983, 263).

In both the LgC burial sites (N = 20) the copper concentrations in bone (average 11.4 ± 4.4 ppm) are approximately five times higher (N = 20) than in tooth enamel (average 2.3 ± 0.3 ppm) (p < 0.001) (tab. 1, fig. 6).

The Cu concentration in bones of the foetus in grave no. 10, Villánykővesd (16.34 ppm) is higher than in the mother (7.46 ppm).

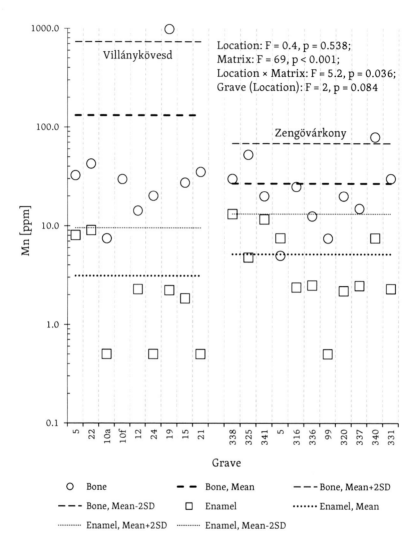

Fig. 7. Manganese concentrations (Mn in ppm) in femurs and tooth enamel at the Villánykövesd and Zengővárkony settlements.

MANGANESE (Mn)

Manganese is associated with a high risk of caries (Curzon and Crocker 1978).

In the LgC, manganese (Mn) concentrations in bone are higher than in tooth enamel ($p < 0.001$). The averages of Mn concentrations in bone are five times higher in Villánykövesd than in Zengővárkony, while the averages of concentrations in tooth enamel are the same (tab. 1, fig. 7).

The Mn concentration in the bones of the foetus (grave no. 10, Villánykövesd) at (23.14 ppm) is higher than that of its mother (5.47 ppm).

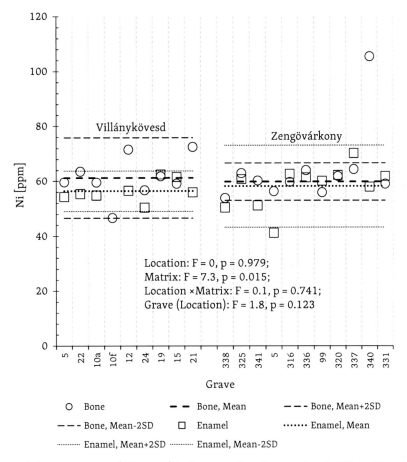

Fig. 8. Nickel concentrations (Ni in ppm) in femurs and tooth enamel at the Villánykövesd and Zengővárkony settlements.

NICKEL (*Ni*)

In LgC, the nickel (Ni) concentrations in bone are higher than in tooth enamel (p = 0.015) (tab. 1, fig. 8). The nickel concentration in the bones of the foetus (grave no. 10, Villánykövesd) is lower (46.6 ppm) than that of the mother (59.5 ppm).

Ghadimi et al. 2013, discovered that substitution of Ni in tooth enamel had a strong positive association with the presence of type B carbonate.

LEAD (*Pb*)

Lead (Pb) can enter the body through water, air or food (Kampa and Castanas 2008). In hydroxyapatite (HA), at low concentrations, Pb^{2+}ions replace

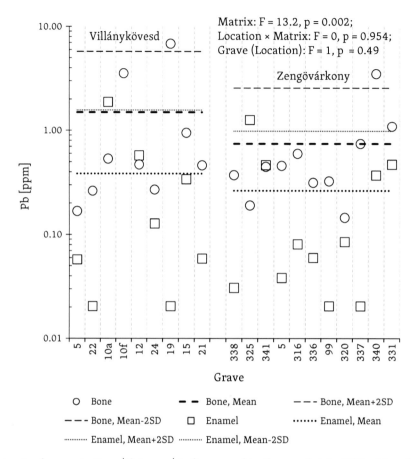

Fig. 9. Lead concentrations (Pb in ppm) in femurs and tooth enamel at the Villánykövesd and Zengővárkony settlements.

Ca²⁺ ions (Mavropoulos et al. 2002). Ghadimi et al. (2013) found that the presence of lead has a negative correlation with the size of enamel apatite crystals.

In LgC, the lead (Pb) concentration in bone is higher than in tooth enamel (p = 0.002) (fig. 9, tab. 1). The Pb concentration in the bones of the foetus (grave no. 10, Villánykövesd) (3.5 ppm) is higher than that of the mother (0.3 ppm).

In foetus skeletons lead is accumulated. However, it causes growth retardation, bone loss and may lead to osteoporosis. Even though chondrogenesis is stimulated by lead, it is not beneficial (Dermience et al. 2015).

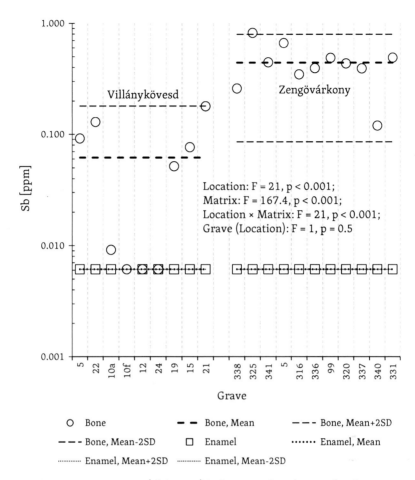

Fig. 10. Antimony concentrations (Sb in ppm) in femurs and tooth enamel at the Villánykővesd and Zengővárkony settlements.

ANTIMONY (Sb)

The antimony (Sb) concentration in bone is higher than in tooth enamel (p < 0.001, tab. 1, fig. 10). In terms of the sites, the Sb concentration in bone was higher in Zengővárkony than in Villánykővesd (p < 0.001).

This points to the character of Zengővárkony as a production centre. Antimony (Sb) is the first impurity to flow off during the process of copper ore roasting.

The foetus from grave no. 10, Villánykővesd, has no antimony contained in its bones and its mother has one of the lowest antimony concentrations in bone at the settlement.

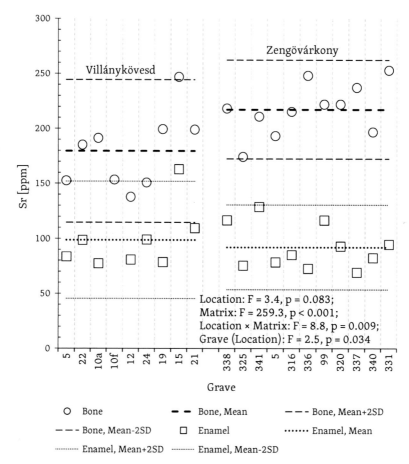

Fig. 11. Strontium concentrations (Sr in ppm) in femurs and tooth enamel at the Villánykővesd and Zengővárkony settlements.

STRONTIUM (*Sr*)

At both burial sites, the strontium concentration in bone is higher than in tooth enamel (N = 19) (200 ± 33 ppm) (95 ± 23 ppm) (p < 0.001, fig. 11).

The foetus from grave no. 10, Villánykővesd, has a lower Sr concentration in bone (150 ppm) than its mother (180 ppm).

URANIUM (*U*)

At both burial sites, the uranium (U) concentration in bone (N = 19) (200 ± 33 ppm) is higher (1.08 ± 0.49 ppm) than in tooth enamel (0.095 ± 0.144 ppm) (p < 0.001). In Villánykővesd, the uranium concentration both in bone and tooth enamel is higher than in Zengővárkony (tab. 1, fig. 12) (p = 0.012).

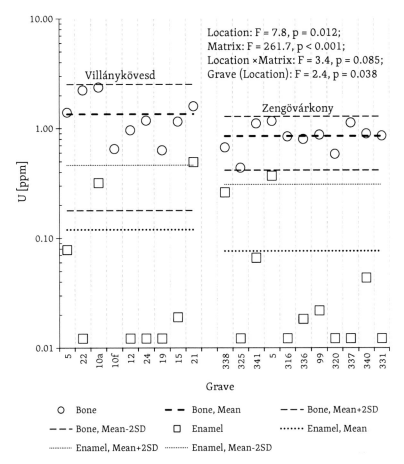

Fig. 12. Uranium concentrations (U in ppm) in femurs and tooth enamel at the Villánykövesd and Zengővárkony settlements.

The higher uranium concentrations in Villánykövesd originate from forest foods (forest fruits), as it was proved at the Těšětice in Moravia settlement.

VANADIUM (V)

The vanadium (V) concentration in bone at both burial sites (N = 19) is higher than in tooth enamel (p < 0.001). The vanadium concentration in bone is higher at the Zengővárkony site (tab 1, fig. 13) than in Villánykövesd. However, the situation is reversed in terms of tooth enamel (significant interaction Location × Matrix, p = 0.001).

The vanadium concentration in the bones of the foetus (grave 10, Villánykövesd) was identical to that of the mother.

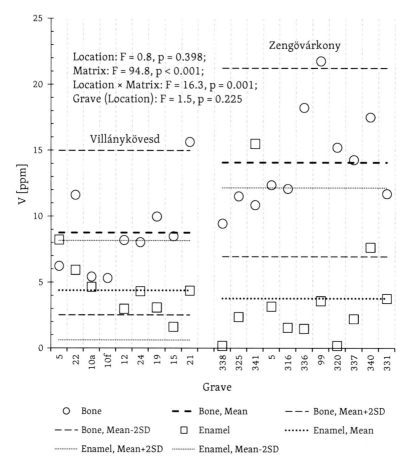

Fig. 13. Vanadium concentrations (V in ppm) in femurs and tooth enamel at the Villánykövesd and Zengővárkony settlements.

ZINC (*Zn*)

The zinc (Zn) concentration in bone is higher than in tooth enamel (p < 0.001). The zinc concentrations in bone are approximately the same both for Zengővárkony (tab. 1, fig. 14) and Villánykővesd; and so is the zinc concentration in tooth enamel (p = 0.53). The zinc concentration in the bones of the foetus (grave 10, Villánykővesd) is four times higher (400 ppm) than that of its mother (p = 0.009).

MAGNESIUM (*Mg*)

The magnesium concentration in tooth enamel is higher than in bone (p < 0.001). In Villánykővesd, the magnesium concentration is insignificantly

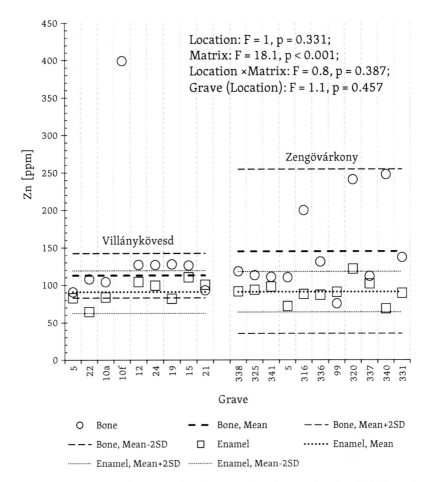

Fig. 14. Zinc concentrations (Zn in ppm) in femurs and tooth enamel at the Villánykővesd and Zengővárkony settlements.

higher than in Zengővárkony (tab. 1, fig. 15). The Mg concentration in bones of the foetus in grave 10, Villánykővesd, is identical to that of its mother.

Magnesium creates positive correlations with sodium (Na), lead (Pb) and sulphur (S) in tooth enamel (Ghadimi et al. 2013).

SODIUM (Na)

The sodium (Na) concentrations in tooth enamel are higher than in bone (p < 0.001) (tab. 1, fig. 16). The foetus in grave no. 10, Villánykővesd, exhibits a higher concentration of sodium in the bone than its mother.

Sodium (Na) creates positive correlations with Mg and K in tooth enamel (Ghadimi et al., 2013).

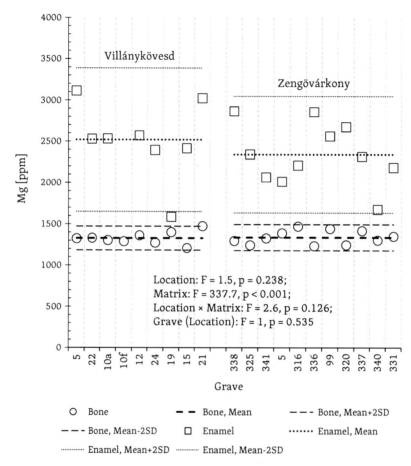

Fig. 15. Magnesium concentrations (Mg in ppm) in femurs and tooth enamel at the Villánykövesd and Zengővárkony settlements.

POTASSIUM (*K*)

In both burial sites, the concentrations of potassium (K) in tooth enamel are higher than its concentrations in bone (tab. 1, p < 0.001, fig. 17).

The foetus in grave 10, Villánykövesd, has higher potassium (K) concentrations than its mother.

PHOSPHORUS (*P*)

Concentrations of phosphorus (P) are higher in tooth enamel than in bone (tab. 1, fig. 18, p < 0.001).

The concentration of phosphorus in bone is higher in the mother than in the foetus in grave no. 10 in Villánykövesd.

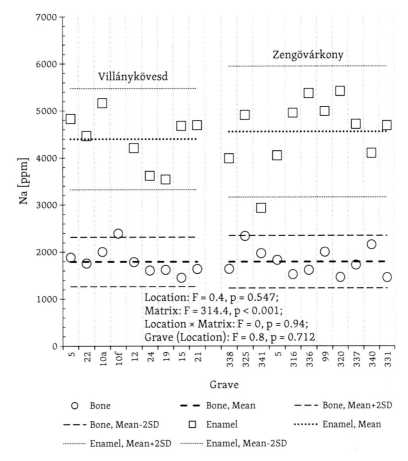

Fig. 16. Sodium concentrations (Na in ppm) in femurs and tooth enamel at the Villánykővesd and Zengővárkony settlements.

CALCIUM (Ca)

The concentrations of calcium (Ca) in bone and in tooth enamel are similar (p = 0.407, fig. 19).

The concentration of calcium in bone is higher in the mother than in the foetus in grave no. 10 in Villánykővesd.

IRON (Fe)

In the LgC, the iron (Fe) concentration in bone is higher than in tooth enamel (tab. 1, fig. 20, p < 0.001).

The foetus in grave 10, Villánykővesd, contains a higher concentration of Fe than its mother.

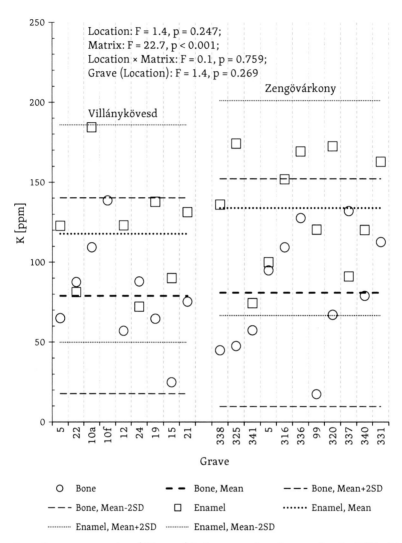

Fig. 17. Potassium concentrations (K in ppm) in femurs and tooth enamel at the Villánykövesd and Zengővárkony settlements.

The mother exhibited raised concentrations of the following elements: Co, Ni, Sr, U, and V.

In the foetus, increased concentrations of these elements were found: Al, Ba, Cd, Cr, Cu, Mn, Pb, Zn, and Zr. For augmented acceleration of bone metabolism, the foetus needed the following elements: Zn, Mn, Cu, Cr. For the transformation of cartilage to bone tissue, lead (Pb) was used. The cadmium (Cd) concentration in the foetus (0.68 ppm) is higher than in the mother (lower than LOD) (fig. 3). The three times higher Cd concentration in com-

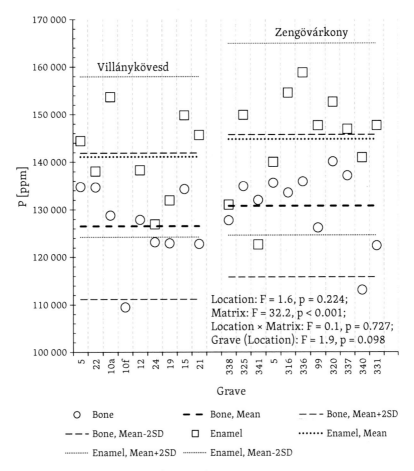

Fig. 18. Phosphorus concentrations (P in ppm) in femurs and tooth enamel at the Villánykővesd and Zengővárkony settlements.

parison with the rest of the burials (tab. 1) needs to be associated with an organ deficiency of the foetus itself.

Periostitis is indicative of viral or bacterial disease, however, it does not reveal which particular organs were affected. It was discovered by Noel et al. (2004) that increased concentrations of Cu, Zn and Mn in the liver may lead to an increase in Cd levels in the bone. It may therefore be speculated, that the aforementioned foetus suffered from a liver disease, probably of viral origin, which can only be proved through genomic analysis of the DNA.

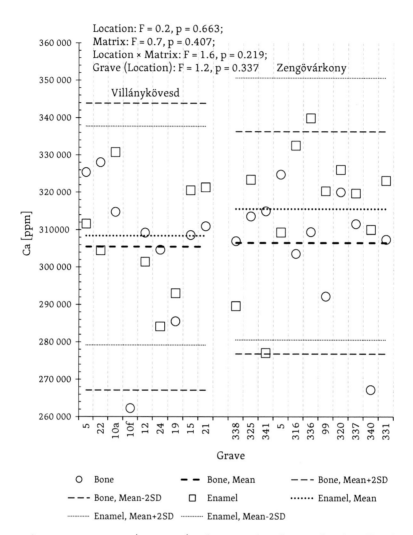

Fig. 19. Calcium concentrations (Ca in ppm) in femurs and tooth enamel at the Villánykővesd and Zengővárkony settlements.

CONCLUSION

ELEMENTS IN BONE AND IN TOOTH ENAMEL

In femoral bones, higher concentrations of these elements are found: Al, Ba, Cd, Ce, Co, Cr, Cu, La, Mn, Ni, Pb, Rb, Sb, Sr, U, V, Y, Zn, and Zr.

The majority of elements exhibits higher concentrations in bone than in tooth enamel. The distribution compartments for bones and tooth enamel differ.

In tooth enamel, raised concentrations are observed for these elements: Ca, K, Mg, Na, and P.

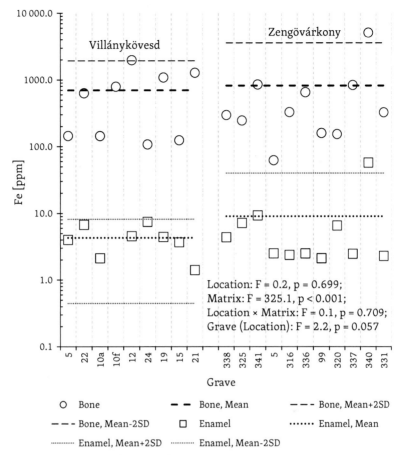

Fig. 20. Iron concentrations (Fe in ppm) in femurs and tooth enamel at the Villánykövesd and Zengővárkony settlements.

A correlation analysis was conducted among the trace elements in tooth enamel.

DISTRIBUTION OF TRACE ELEMENTS IN FEMORAL BONES OF THE HUNGARIAN BURIAL SITES

In Zengővárkony, increased concentrations of the following elements were identified: Cd, Sb, V, Sr, and Zn.

This proves the character of the settlement to be that of a production centre, which was, according to Dombay (1960), a place of distribution of copper and obsidian. It is antimony (Sb) that flows off as an impurity in roasting copper ore. In a similar manner the presence of cadmium (Cd) and vanadium (V) could be explained.

In Villánykővesd, increased concentrations of these elements were detected: Al, Ba, Cr, La, Pb, Rb, U, and Y.

TRACE ELEMENT IN THE LENGYEL CULTURE AND TOOTH CARIES INCIDENCE

Trace elements promote crystal formation and thus determine the physical quality of tooth enamel (Ghadimi et al. 2013). Results of the research in the Lengyel Culture (LgC) burial sites of Villánykővesd and Zengővárkony indicate the presence of elements associated with low caries incidence: Al, Fe, and Sr. According to Curzon and Crocker (1978), F and Se are also employed in this manner, however these were not analysed.

Contrarily, elements with high risk of caries: Mn, Cu, and Cd were found in low concentrations, particularly Cu.

7. LENGYEL CULTURE IN MORAVIA

ZDENĚK HÁJEK, ALŽBĚTA ČEREVKOVÁ

Although potsherds decorated with characteristic colourful patterns must have been encountered by archaeologists in the last quarter of the 19th century at the latest (Podborský 1993, 108), formally the Moravian Painted Ware Culture (hereinafter also "LgC," for Lengyel Culture) was not brought to the attention of the scholarly public until 1888. Its discovery is inseparably connected with the name Jaroslav Palliardi (1861–1922), one of the most prominent scholars and explorers at the turn of the 20th century. Through his studies of the Neolithic and Eneolithic (Chalcolithic) periods in Moravia, he won the respect of his colleagues at home as well as abroad. He was also one of the most influential personalities in the archaeology of the Znojmo region and whole Moravia as well (Kovárník 2008, 4; Sklenář 2013, 79). His

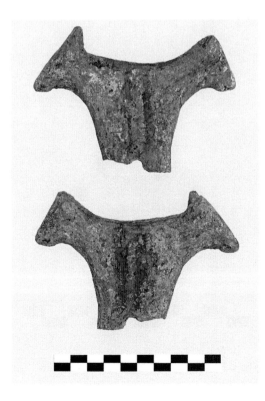

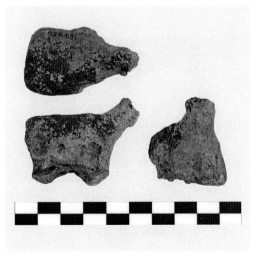

Fig. 1. Fragment of zoomorphic lid from Brno-Komín.

Fig. 2. Fragment of zoomorphic figurine from Brno-Líšeň (the upland site Staré Zámky).

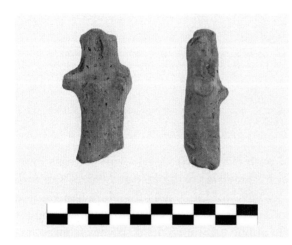

Fig. 3. Fragment of anthropomorphic figurine from Brno-Líšeň (the upland site Staré Zámky).

work was highly appreciated by I. L. Červinka as early as the beginning of the 20th century (Červinka 1902, 14).

By his first trade, Jaroslav Palliardi was a notarial assistant and later a public notary. The seat of his office was Moravské Budějovice. His interest in antiquities began to absorb him in early childhood when the Palliardi family

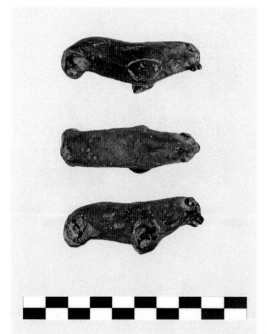

Fig. 4. Fragment of zoomorphic figurine from Brno-Líšeň.

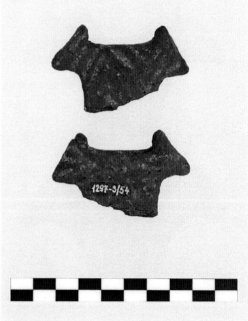

Fig. 5. Fragment of zoomorphic lid from Brno-Žebětín.

lived in Telč, a town packed with great architectural and historical sights. He went in for the same hobby during his grammar school studies in Znojmo, Mladá Boleslav (?) and Kroměříž, where he completed his secondary education. Then he enrolled to study at Charles-Ferdinand University (nowadays Charles University) in Prague. Already, even during his university studies, he showed a keen interest in sites and artefacts of prehistoric cultures. The early 1880s was the time when he started gaining experience in archaeological field research, which he tried to widen continuously. Apart from the discovery of the Moravian Painted Ware Culture, his remarkable activities included research at the Eneolithic fortified site Starý Zámek near Jevišovice and at the sites of the Bronze Age, the Hallstatt culture and La Tène culture periods in the surroundings of Těšetice-Kyjovice (Palliardi 1888; 1894; Podborský et al. 2005, 13-14; Podborský and Kovárník 2012, 12-15).

His enthusiasm for collecting ancient artefacts and his expertise in prehistoric issues caught the eye of the professor (and later Czechoslovak president) T. G. Masaryk, who J. Palliardi kept in contact with through correspondence for a long time. In 1920 Masaryk even visited Palliardi's collection of archaeological finds in Moravské Budějovice. In 1883 J. Palliardi took up the position of a notarial assistant and candidate in Jan Vlk's office in Znojmo. The setting of Vlk's bureau provided J. Palliardi with a favourable environment for his further research. Soon after he came to Znojmo, he took up active archaeological field research and was also active in culture and popular education, carrying on collecting prehistoric artefacts. Pursuing his archaeological activities, he established contacts with prominent scholars in Moravia, such as Karel Jaroslav Maška (1851-1916), Jan Havelka (1839-1886; Jindřich Wankel's son-in-law), František Černý (1867-1918), Jan Knies (1860-1937), Karel Absolon (1877-1860), Inocenc Ladislav Červinka (1869-1952) and others. Soon the circle of his colleagues and friends widened by foreign scholars as well (Kovárník 1995, 23-30; 2008, 4; Podborský, 1995, 19-22; Podborský and Kovárník 2012, 15, 28-29).

Jaroslav Palliardi was the first to describe the artefacts of the Moravian Painted Ware Culture, using the finds from the site at Znojmo-Novosady (Palliardi 1897). The remnants of Neolithic population sites were found during the construction of the provincial workhouse and the municipal almshouse. The performance of the archaeological research was complicated by inevitable negotiations with the respective authorities. For this reason, the site was not explored as thoroughly as required in view of the richness of the location. In spite of that, J. Palliardi managed to save some of the material, including in particular animal bones, stone artefacts and pottery (Čižmář and Hájek 2008, 12).

The ornaments on the pottery, which were made with yellow, red and white pigments, were classified by J. Palliardi as being artefacts of the Mora-

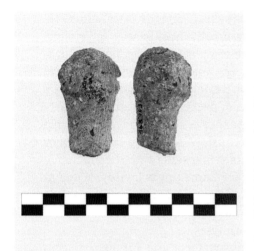

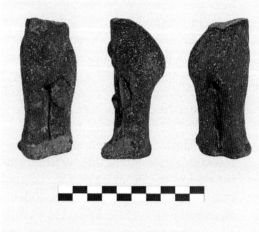

Fig. 6. Fragment (the head)
of anthropomorphic figurine from Brno-Líšeň
(the upland site Staré Zámky).

Fig. 7. Fragment (the bottom part of body)
of anthropomorphic figurine from Hluboké Mašůvky.

vian Painted Pottery Culture. However, some other terms for the material were coined by other authors, such as "Znojmo-style pottery" or "Novosady pottery," and Hermann Müller-Karpe suggested to name the culture "Střelice group" after the site Střelice u Znojma, one of the most prominent sites of the given culture. These terms, however, did not take hold. In connection with the virtually contemporary discovery of similar finds at the fortified high settlement at Lengyel in South Hungary (by Mór Wosinsky), also the term Lengyel Culture (hereinafter "LgC") or Lengyel Cultural Complex came into use. This term denotes the circle of Late Neolithic cultures with similar mate-

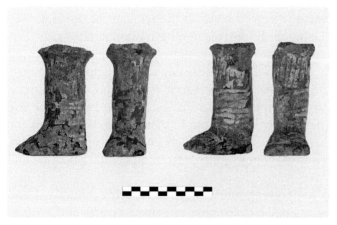

Fig. 8. The fragments
of anthropomorphic
figurines
(or vessels?) from
Hluboké Mašůvky.

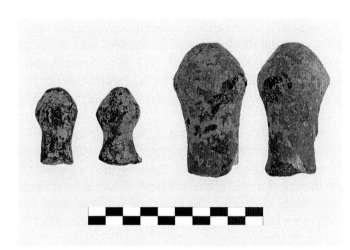

Fig. 9. The fragments of anthropomorphic figurines (the heads) from Hluboké Mašůvky.

rial possessions in the regions close to Moravia, i.e. Lower Austria, Burgenland, Pannonia and West Slovakia (Podborský 1993, 109; Kovárník 2008, 4).

Jaroslav Palliardi was also the man behind the creation of the first system of the relative chronology of the LgC. Based on the finds from several locations near Boskovštejn ("Výhon," "Smoha," Písařovic's field above the pond), he defined three phases. The main criterion he adopted was the ornament of the pottery, above all the colour of the painting, or also the nature of the patterns when appropriate (Palliardi 1911). According to Palliardi, the earliest phase was characterized by the typical red and yellow painting, the middle phase by the occurrence of white colour and the later phase by the absence of colour motifs. Nowadays this way of division into periods may appear somewhat awkward, although J. Palliardi meticulously checked on his new knowledge at many sites of the Znojmo and Moravské Budějovice regions.

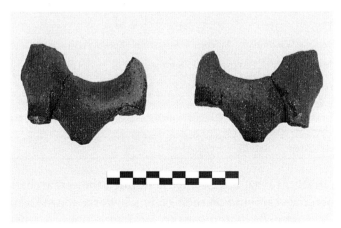

Fig. 10. Fragment of zoomorphic lid from Hluboké Mašůvky.

During his research, he gathered an extensive collection of archaeological finds, which contained a considerable quantity of artefacts, and many of them from the LgC period, in particular (Červinka 1902, 19). Several years later, he also separated the phase IIc within the late stage. His asset to the research of LgC is invaluable (Podborský 1970, 253; 1995, 19-22; Kovárník 1995, 23-30; Kovárník 2008, 4).

During his active life in the region of Znojmo, J. Palliardi established a close scientific co-operation with F. Vildomec (1878-1975). František Vildomec worked as a teacher in the village of Hostim, where the two scholars met in 1898. From 1906, they performed archaeological research together at many sites in the surroundings of Znojmo, the most important of them being Boskovštejn, Jaroměřice nad Rokytnou, Štěpánovice, Jevišovice, Střelice, Bojanovice, Grešlové Mýto, Horní Dunajovice, Hodonice or Těšetice. Soon their research activity spread further to the region of Třebíč. Apart from Jaroměřice nad Rokytnou, they also frequented the surroundings of Lesůňky, Hrotovice etc. Later the settlement at Jaroměřice provided the main basis for the separation of phase Ib (Šimek 1935, 33; Kovárník 1995, 23-30; 2001, 108-112; 2008, 4; Podborský 2005, 40-44).

In 1929, F. Vildomec further divided the LgC into periods. In either of the earlier and later groups (cp. degrees), he identified three degrees (cp. phases). He formulated his conclusions, above all, based on the analysis of pottery finds from Střelice, Jaroměřice nad Rokytnou, Ctidružice, Štěpánovice and Boskovštejn. Nevertheless, apart from the shapes and ornaments of pottery vessels he also noticed the other utensils (particularly the sets of stone artefacts) and also speculated over the funeral rite of the culture and its relations to other Neolithic cultures (Vildomec 1928/1929, 1-38; Čižmář et al. 2008, 76).

Tab. 1. Division of LgC according to F. Vildomec

Group	Degree		Site
Earlier	1.		Střelice - "Kloboušek," Střelice - "Bukovina," Boskovštejn - "Výhon"
	2.		Střelice - "Sklep", Boskovštejn - "Smoha"
	3.		Jaroměřice nad Rokytnou
Later		1.	Střelice - "Sklep"
		2.	Ctidružice, Štěpánovice
		3.	Boskovštejn - "Rybník"

After J. Palliardi's death in 1922, F. Vildomec continued the research of settlements of LgC, therefore carrying on their common work, above all in Střelice and Hluboké Mašůvky. The latter was the site where in 1934 he discovered the famous "Venus," unique for its elaborateness and state of preservation. Figurine sculptures of the culture were dealt with by F. Vildomec with considerable attention (Vildomec 1949). These artefacts, together with vessels, constitute the best part of his extensive collection. He glued and reconstructed these vessels himself. Some of his other important archaeological assets include, in particular, the research of the fortified settlement Starý Zámek near Jevišovice, burial mounds near Suchohrdly and exploration of St. Hippolytus settlement in Znojmo. After World War 2, the research of the settlement at Hluboké Mašůvky was overtaken by the State Archaeological Institute and shortly after that by the prehistorical department of the National Museum in Prague under Jiří Neustupný (1905–1981), who in particular documented the oval ditch that surrounded the settlement (Podborský et al. 2005, 16–18; Kovárník 2001a, 95; 2008, 4; Podborský 2005, 44–49, 54–60; Podborský and Kovárník 2012, 93–94). In connection with research into LgC in South-West Moravia, we must mention another prominent Moravian prehistorian Josef Skutil (1904–1965). The main focus of his scholarly interest was the Palaeolithic period and, among other merits, he took credit in the discovery of many Palaeolithic sites in Moravia. J. Skutil's knowledge of LgC was ascertained in cooperation with F. Vildomec following studies on pottery sculptures and the processing of material of important finds of a mass grave at Džbánice, which was discovered by the teacher J. Horňanský (Horňanský and Skutil 1950; Kovárník 2001a, 97).

In the first half of the 20th century, particularly before archaeology became a well-established branch of science that could be studied at schools, Moravia witnessed a good number of amateur researchers, enthusiastic lovers of history, who above all actively gathered archaeological finds and information about said acquisitions. These finds, commonly accompanied with more or less detailed documentation, are often the only and thus invaluable source of information about the given original situation at the site of the find. In this connection, we must notice Vilém Gross (1894–1977), who had discovered many Neolithic sites in the Oslavany area and close surroundings to his credits. He also explored the remarkable polycultural site at "Kopaniny" near Nová Ves u Oslavan. He often co-operated with a considerable number of prominent scholars and visited archaeological sites and excavations, e.g. Těšetice-Kyjovice (Koštuřík 1994, 391–392).

After World War 2, the study of the Moravian Neolithic archaeology was already under the control of archaeologists with specialist education. In the Znojmo region, these were primarily the staff of the South Moravian Museum in Znojmo as well as expeditions from Masaryk University in Brno. The main objective of their activity was an exploration of the sites at risk—emergency excavations and preliminary research. The research in Křepice was of great importance for LgC considering the discovery of the rare torso of a female statuette, which had been found by V. Vildomec. The Brno branch of the Archaeological Institute of the Czechoslovak Academy of Sciences charged Rudolf Tichý with the task of performing emergency excavations, which also unearthed traces of ditches and palisades—a relic of the then not yet recognized rondel enclosure (Kovárník 2001a, 97–98; Podborský et al. 2005, 18).

A remarkable new stage in the exploration of LgC began in 1964, near Těšetice-Kyjovice in the Znojmo region. Under Vladimír Podborský's guidance, research of the settlement with a circular ditch—rondel enclosure—was performed at the location called "Sutny" between 1968 and 1978. This was the first comprehensive research of a rondel enclosure within all Central Europe (Podborský 1988). Since that time, the excavations have been systematically performed until now. Up to the present, several hundreds of prehistoric structures of varying ages and types have been uncovered. The most important structures of LgC include silo pits, two houses partially recessed into the ground and claypits containing a large quantity of material (Podborský et al. 2005, 32, 43–45). In 2012, re-examination research of the filling in the rondel ditch was done in order to apply modern geo-information technology and collect specimens for geochemical and micromorphological analysis which could not be employed in the previous research in the 1970s. During this research, the location of the north entry into the rondel enclosure was specified more precisely, and so was the width of the ditch at the site of the control profile. Next year, the soil samples from the filling of the ditch were floated and gradually analysed geochemically (Válek et al. 2013a, b; 2016).

In Těšetice-Kyjovice, a team of researchers was gradually established and soon became one of the leading agents of research into LgC, or into the Neolithic period in Moravia. V. Podborský can be pinpointed as the central personality in the team. Besides being the long-standing leader in the exploration of the site, he paid intensive attention to material items of the culture, mainly to figurine sculptures (Podborský 1985). In connection with the discovery and research of the rondel enclosure at Těšetice he also concentrated on the issues of socio-ritual architecture ("rondel archaeology"; Podborský et al. 1999) and other aspects of religious perception in prehistoric societies (Kazdová and Podborský 2007; Podborský 2006). In the meantime, he observed and collected information about the development of the prehistoric population in the Znojmo region, assisted by V. Vildomec, F. Vildomec's son (Podborský and Vildomec 1972). At present, the main focus of his activity is the history of archaeology in Moravia in the context of Central Europe.

Another archaeologist whose name may be connected with the issues of rondel archaeology is Jaromír Kovárník. He became one of the pioneers of aerial archaeology in Moravia, whose development he promoted from the beginning of the 1980s. Developing aerial prospecting, he was the man behind the discovery of many Late Neolithic rondel enclosures, e.g. at Vedrovice and

Rašovice (Kovárník 1985; 1996; 1998; 2001b; 2004). Furthermore, he also explored many sites in South and Southwest Moravia, as well as participated in the research of the site at Těšetice-Kyjovice.

The Těšetice team also included one of the renowned specialists in Moravian Neolithic and Eneolithic period, Pavel Koštuřík (1946-1998). The main focus of his interest was the last stage of the Neolithic period, or rather the issues of the beginning of the Eneolithic period (Koštuřík 1973; 1983a). He performed the extensive emergency excavations to save the site Hradisko u Kramolína (Koštuřík 1975-1976; 1981) and dealt with the LgC population in Jaroměřice n. Rokytnou as well (Koštuřík 1974, 18-20; 1980a). In Těšetice-Kyjovice he worked for nearly thirty years, and from 1985 as the team leader. Under his leadership, the research was focused in particular on the immediate surroundings of the rondel enclosure and its closest background (Kazdová 1999, 10-11; Koštuřík 1972; 1980b; 1983b). In addition, he published a fair number of studies about the Late Neolithic period in South and Southwest Moravia (e.g. Koštuřík 1977-1978; in summary Palátová 1999, 13-20).

One of P. Koštuřík's coevals and close colleagues was Ivo Rakovský (1952-1992). He, too, ranked among the most prominent scholars of the 1980s who dealt with LgC. He was mainly focused on the later phase of development of the Lengyel complex and its transition into the earliest Eneolithic phase (however he, regretfully, did not live to see his study on the Jordanov culture). Basing on the analysis of the material from Brno-Bystrc and Jezeřany-Maršovice, he defined the phase Ic within the relative chronology (Rakovský 1985; Rakovský and Čižmářová 1988). His assets in the sphere of research of LgC also include the leadership in the research of two significant settlements, first at Jezeřany-Maršovice in 1976 and further, for example, in Pavlov between 1982 and 1988 (Sklenář 2005, 474).

An active member of the Těšetice team has been Eliška Kazdová, who is still engaged in the leadership of exploration at that site. She deals with the Neolithic period in Moravia, in particular with the Stroked Pottery Culture (hereinafter "SPC") and LgC and their mutual relations. Within the LgC she focuses her attention, above all, on the earlier stage of the culture and, in terms of geography, on the sites in the regions of Brno and Znojmo (Kazdová 1994a, b; 1998; 2001a, b, c; Kazdová and Čižmář 2004; Kazdová and Přichystal 1994; Kuča, Kazdová, and Přichystal 2004).

Of the younger generation, Martin Kuča may be classified as a prominent researcher. He continued the topics of P. Koštuřík and I. Rakovský's studies and deals, apart from the LgC itself, with the issue of origins of the Neolithic period as well. Above all, he focuses on stone artefacts, in the aspects of both technology and material (e.g. Kuča 2008; Kuča and Bartík 2013). Thanks to his prospecting activity, a good number of Late Neolithic (and other) sites were found in the regions of Brno, Uherské Hradiště and South-West Moravia

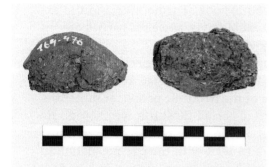

Fig. 11. Fragment of anthropomorphic figurine (the buttock part) from Horákov.

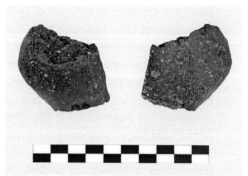

Fig. 12. Fragment of anthropomorphic figurine (the buttock part) from Horákov.

(např. Kuča 2009), and under his supervision, the exploration of an important site of phase Ic in Mokrá u Horákova was carried out. He also worked in Těšetice-Kyjovice, where he processed the information on the part of the settlement between the ditch and the outer palisade of the rondel enclosure (Kuča et al. 2010).

Considering the continuing systematic research of the Těšetice rondel enclosure and settlement structures in other sites, the necessity in a more accurate division and definition of the subject matter of the particular phases arose. The knowledge last applied by F. Vildomec had to be validated, particularly so because of newly obtained data of material culture of the LgC. Considerable attention was also paid to the separation of particular sub-phases. The

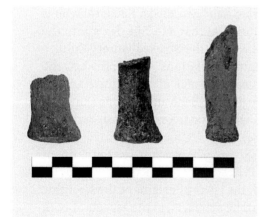

Fig. 13. The fragments (the legs) of anthropomorphic figurines (or vessels?) from Horákov.

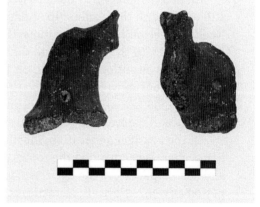

Fig. 14. Fragment of anthropomorphic element (the arm) from Horákov.

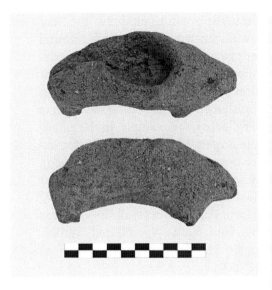

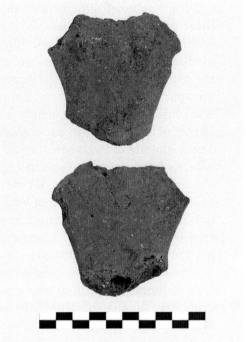

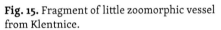

Fig. 15. Fragment of little zoomorphic vessel from Klentnice.

Fig. 16. Fragment of anthropomorphic figurine (the trunk) from Radostice.

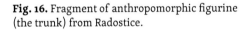

information summarized in Numeric Code MMK originated predominantly from the research base at Těšetice-Kyjovice (Podborský et al. 1977). In the 1980s, the knowledge base about the LgC was further widened and specified through the separation of sub-phase Ic (Rakovský 1985), which defined the transition between the earlier and the later degree. Further, some distinctive regional features were recognized (Podborský 1985). Another issue discussed was continuity of the LgC into the early Eneolithic period. The final stage of the culture is thus included in the late Stone Age (Čižmář et al. 2004).

SETTLEMENTS

Settlements are still one of the primary sources of information on the life of the LgC population. When founding their settlements, people chose sunny locations on loess grounds near rivers or streams. Often they occupied the same sites as their predecessors from the early and middle Neolithic periods. Inhabiting of similar areas within the life of particular Neolithic cultures is a well-known phenomenon (e.g. Kazdová 2004, 56–57). This fact is mainly due to the state of research, as an overwhelming majority of settlements were only explored in a fragmentary way. In many cases, we assume the existence of a settlement when one or several structures have been explored.

The number of settlements compared to the previous phases of the Neolithic period grew considerably, and several settlements were often found within the cadastre area of one village or town. Even though all these settlements may or may not have been contemporary, we can say that the density of the population increased. The information available currently suggests that the appearance of the Lengyel Culture settlement in the setting of Moravia was considerably variable, which is also reflected, for example, in the extent of the inhabited area. In our opinion, the large settlements include, for example, the site of Pavlov-Horní Pole (Geislerová, Rakovský, and Tichý 1989), where a total area of up to 20 ha (nearly 50 acres) can be presumed. Similar situations have been known, for example, from Svodín or Aszód (Kalicz 1985; Podborský 1993, 124). In case of Pavlov-Horní Pole, however, all the area was not built up at the same time but rather continuously populated. Similar considerations may apply to some other sites too, e.g. Těšetice-Kyjovice, or Jezeřany-Maršovice (Podborský 1993, 124–128).

The settlements were usually open; however, some evidence of the presence of fences or fortifications around the settlement can be found, especially from the phase Ib. One of the best-explored sites of this type is Hluboké Mašůvky (Hájek 2014).

Unlike in the case of the Linear Pottery Culture (hereinafter "LPC"), there are considerably less residential structures of the LgC found in Moravia. In the all-European aspect, the ration is much better. And it is the all-European view that allows us to state that the residential architecture of the Lengyel complex was considerably variable. Differences between particular types of residential structures are sometimes believed to be related to the geography-dependent cultural situation (Podborský 1984a). Typology of Lengyel houses was attempted by Ján Vladár and Jan Lichardus, based on the finds from Branč (Vladár and Lichardus 1968). They divided the structures at that site into five types:

A = long rectangular houses supported with poles, with antae on both sides, divided into halves by a partition;
B = long rectangular houses with a foundation trench, with antae on both sides, divided into halves by a partition;
C = small rectangular houses with a foundation trench;
D = small rectangular houses, outlined with 4, 6 or 8 timber postholes;
E = small houses partially or fully recessed into the ground.

Their classification was adopted by V. Podborský, who extended it in order to comprise the diverse scope of residential structures across the whole Lengyel complex. Both said typologies are based on the spatial nature of the building (shape and size) on the one hand, and on the construction elements used on the other hand. V. Podborský's typology includes eight types in total:

Long, big rectangular houses with an internal partition
Medium-sized, one-space, rectangular houses
Long houses on trapezium ground plan
Houses with apse
Smaller megaron and plain rectangular houses
Small two-nave house
Small one-nave house
Small houses fully or partially recessed into the ground

In all the types, V. Podborský also discriminated varieties A and B. Variety A meaning that the ground plan is preserved in the form of rows of postholes, while variety B denotes ground plans defined by a foundation trench.

Houses are not very sensitive in terms of chronology, but still, some trend can be traced. For the earlier degree, smaller structures built with poles on the area of 20-30 m² seem to be typical, while larger structures are expected in the later degree (Čižmář et al. 2008, 77-79).

One special phenomenon is the structure whose floor was recessed below the level of the contemporary ground. According to their floor levels, these dugouts can be referred to as earth-houses or semi-earth-houses. They were usually rather small (5-10 m² as a rule) and more often we associate them with the earlier degree. Specifically, two structures partially recessed into the ground in Těšetice-Kyjovice are well-datable in phase Ia. They rank among the most well-known and best-analysed structures of the given type in Moravia. Nevertheless, despite careful analysis of the material, the function of these structures cannot be established. In some cases, researchers are inclined to believe in their residential purpose while in other cases they tend to interpret the dugouts with the construction of poles as roofed grain silos (Rakovský 1985, 23-26; Kuča et al. 2010, 90-95). We presume the existence of similar structures already in the early Neolithic period.

The appearance of Lengyel buildings is also witnessed by the finds of pottery models or rather their fragments sporadically found at the archaeological sites. Perhaps the most famous model of a house originates from the site Střelice-"Sklep." Other similar artefacts were discovered, for example, in Boskovštejn or Těšetice-Kyjovice and elsewhere. The question is, however, to what extent these finds reflect the true appearance of the residential structures. It is possible that the images are idealized or stylized, and the possibility that the models depict a specific building, e.g. one of sacral nature, cannot be excluded (Podborský 1984a, 50).

Apart from residential buildings, there are other structures found at LgC sites that allow us to get an idea of the appearance of the settlement. These mainly include pits, dug out for various purposes, most commonly claypits and storage pits. Many Lengyel claypits are characterized by their considerable size, with a large area and depth of up to several metres. One of the recent finds is an extensive claypit (300 m²) in the settlement in Vídeňská Street in Brno-Štýřice, dated to phase Ib (Černá and Sedláčková 2017, 150–153). Also typical of these claypits is the conspicuously broken ground plan and the irregular bottom. Actually, it is a superposition of many pits that occurred gradually as the need for more clay arose. Apart from giving an idea of the amount of the clay dug out, the claypits often provide a considerable quantity of archaeological material if they had been secondarily used as refuse pits.

The storage pits of LgC are often characterized by their specific sac shape. Their depth may even exceed 2 m, which was detected, for example, at the settlement in Havřice, district Uherské Hradiště (Geisler and Kohoutek 1997, 117). Storage pits, too, were often secondarily used as refuse pits and a number of fragments of common house utensils can be found in them.

Further, kilns can be encountered in settlement settings. They were—without any exceptions—situated outside the living quarters, i.e. in the utility part of the settlement. Sometimes they were built in partially filled claypits, e.g. in Těšetice-Kyjovice (Podborský 1988, 104). Mostly they were simple kilns with a dome of clay, reinforced with wickerwork (Podborský ed. 1993, 128), which occurred quite commonly in the settlements. Recently, kilns were discovered, for example, in Borotice, district Znojmo (Stuchlík 1997, 115) or Mohelnice, district Šumperk (Zeman 2013, 147). A unique case is a kiln discovered in Kramolín, which chronologically, however, falls into the very end of LgC, i.e. into the beginning of the Eneolithic period. It is a more sophisticated type of two-chamber kiln with a grate, which served for firing pottery vessels (Koštuřík 1975/76, 106). This hypothesis has been verified through work experiments dealing with the issues of Neolithic agriculture, pottery and construction (Podborský 1984b, 225; Podborský 2005, 117, 124–127). Besides kilns, most probably also open fireplaces, simple hearths etc. could commonly be found within the backgrounds of the settlement. Recently, one hearth was discovered in Pasohlávky; this structure was situated in superposition with the field hospital of a Roman fortified camp. Within the settlement pit, the hearth was outlined by a layer of baked clay, with fragments of pottery and burnt animal bones nearby (Komoróczy et al. 2010, 321). Other sites providing proof of the existence of the hearth include, for example, Bánov, district Uherské Hradiště (Vaškových 2010, 305).

Taking some research that has not been published yet into consideration, it seems that the internal build-up of the settlements was highly variable and that it, apart from culture specifications, reflected the local geographical conditions. This verifies V. Podborský's hypothesis of the breakdown of the codified model of settlements, known from the early Neolithic period, which was more oriented towards the extended family community, and new orientation towards the nuclear family, i.e. a couple unit (Podborský 1984a, 28). Besides the above "standard" structures at the LgC settlements, there are also various atypical structures, whose function cannot be conclusively identified. These are mostly classified as structures with a religious function.

RONDEL ENCLOSURES

Circular areas enclosed by a ditch, or rondel enclosures, are a specific phenomenon of the middle and later Neolithic period. The first rondel enclosures occur in Central Europe as early as in the LPC period (in summary, Řídký et al. 2011, 20). They were most abundant in the area of the spread of the earlier degree of the Lengyel complex to Western Slovakia, South Moravia, Lower and partly Upper Austria, Burgenland and Western Hungary. In the region of Bohemia and lower Bavaria, these structures are connected with even later phases of SPC (Řídký et al. 2011, 12). Sporadically this phenomenon can be observed in Moravia and Lower Austria (Kovárník 2004, 28–29).

The first comprehensive research of a Lengyel rondel enclosure was performed in Těšetice-Kyjovice (location called "Sutny") under supervision of V. Podborský (see above). Soon, similar structures started to be discovered and explored over the whole of Central Europe (Podborský 1999, 7). Rondel enclosures can be divided into several types according to the nature of their basic elements (shape and number of ditches, entrances, palisades, etc.). Another criterion is the size of the rondel enclosures, varying from ca 40 up to 200 metres (Podborský 1993). Combination of various parameters in particular architectural elements and dimensions gives each rondel enclosure its unique appearance but probably meaning as well. Furthermore, the function of rondel enclosures is still regarded as an open question that can only be partially answered with a hypothesis on their changing role in space and time. This hypothesis can be verified only to some extent based on archaeological finds obtained in connection with a rondel enclosure, such as the filling of the ditches, structures in the background or immediate surroundings of the rondel enclosure etc. (Řídký et al. 2011, 13–16). Nevertheless, five basic potential functions of rondel enclosures have been defined, which can be held as generally valid: economic, social, military, astronomical, sacral (Podborský 2001, 209-212; 2006). This classification, including various combinations and other possible functions, has been dealt with in detail by János Makkay (Makkay 2001).

HIGH SETTLEMENTS

Inhabitation of high locations is known already from the early Neolithic period. In many cases, however, we can hardly describe them literarily as "high locations" in terms of the altitude, but perhaps we can call them "strategic positions." Settlements at strategic positions are particularly typical of the earlier degree of LPC (e.g. Žádovice, Spytihněv). One of the possible explanations of the existence of sites located like that is the pursuit of control over the populated area in a so far little explored countryside (Vaškových 2006, 22–25; Schenk et al. 2008, 285; Čerevková 2015, 116–117). In the later degree of the LPC, in turn, we can observe the typical settlements located on mild slopes.

In the period of the LgC, high locations are mainly bound with the later degree. During the earlier degree, we tend to describe them as fortified or fenced sites in lowland locations. Only a few high location sites are known from the earlier degree, such as Brno-Maloměřice-Holý kopec, Znojmo-Hradiště, Luleč (Podborský 1993, 130).

The spread of the high settlements corresponds with the spread of the whole culture. The missing information from some regions seems to be due to the state of research rather than the real absence of this type of settlement. Before, high locations were concentrated mainly in the Znojmo and Brno regions, which corresponded with the state of archaeological research. Recently, above all thanks to the increasing prospection activities and rescue explorations, other new sites have been discovered in the area of South-West Moravia adjacent to the Bohemian-Moravian Highlands (Bartík 2015), in Central Moravia or the region of Uherské Hradiště.

According to I. Rakovský (1990), high locations were populated continuously until the end of the Eneolithic period, but in many cases, this assumption does not apply. Some sites in South-West Moravia, explored by J. Bartík, showed monocultural nature. This, applies to the whole microregion, as the remarkable increase in population here can only be connected with the later Jevišovice culture (Bartík 2015, 265).

A specific phenomenon, concerning the high settlements, is their interaction with lowland settlements, which were found in their vicinity and sometimes quite abundant. It seems that the said settlements were founded systematically so that their location related to each other would be as convenient as possible. Of course, the question is whether particular sites of these agglomerations really were contemporary. Their general dating with the later degree is, naturally, insufficient in these cases. Another interesting question is the function of particular sites. In the case of high locations, we most often consider their centralization role, and further, they may have played some strategic-military or social-religious role. The adjacent lowland locations, however, cannot be denied potentially the same functions either, but it is possible that particular sites performed more than one function at a time. Virtually the only available guide is the material sources, often collected through surface gathering, and therefore lacking in the site context of the find. It must be borne in mind, then, that the given archaeological material can only provide very limited information. What we know so far is that high locations provide some finds suggesting common settlement life activities, such as the production of stone tools, pottery or processing of foods (Bartík 2015).

Apart from South-West Moravia, where the issues of agglomerations are dealt with by Jaroslav Bartík (Bartík 2015; Bartík and Bíško 2013), a similar phenomenon was identified in Central Moravia as well, e.g. the site Luleč (Kalábková 2008; 2009). The questions concerning the mutual interaction of these locations, however, still stay open.

Despite the increasing number of high locations, the lowland settlement still prevails remarkably, of course, if we consider the whole Moravia. In South-West Moravia, 29 high locations have been recorded by now, and the number will likely increase in the future. At present, this area is being explored intensively, using predictive models and their subsequent verification by field research (Bartík and Bíško 2013). The number of high locations also increased thanks to M. Kuča's prospection in the Uherské Hradiště region (see above).

Another question that can be linked with high locations is their fencing or fortification. The very positioning of the site in the specific relief of the landscape alone secures that its strategic function will be fulfilled, and by the construction of elements of fortification, this function could be remarkably promoted. The end of the Neolithic and turn of the Eneolithic period are connected with social changes which may have been the cause (or perhaps the effect too) of the changing pattern of the settlements. Fortified high location settlements of the later Lengyel degree are demonstrably found in Lower Austria (Neugebauer and Neugebauer 1977; Neugebauer-Maresch 1983-1984; Lenneis et al. 1995, 30), while in the adjacent area of South-West Moravia J. Bartík recorded only one location (Velký Újezd-"Na Volských") where the presence of fencing or fortification may be considered. Otherwise, no high location of the LgC was found in Moravia that would show such features. The situation at some sites is complicated by their polycultural nature. In most cases, however, fencing or fortification can only be related to late Eneolithic populations, Bronze Age or the period of the Hallstatt culture.

The issue of high locations will require more exploration in the scale of all Moravia, as the nature of the settlements is likely to vary depending on the region.

FUNERAL RITE

Regarding the arrangement of funerals in the people of LgC we can learn from isolated individual (or sometimes multiple) burials, which do not show any signs of uniformity. The situation of the findings known so far are remarkably variable, as are the hypothesises that argue whether they document specific ways of handling the dead bodies or an established way of burial. A codified funeral rite at that time either did not exist or did not leave any traces that could be identifiable with our contemporary methods of research. All burials that can be, with certainty, dated with the LgC have been found within settlement settings, most often in settlement pits, where they were interred in a ritual or non-ritual way (Čižmář et al. 2008, 77, 79–80).

Regular burial sites in the setting of the western branch of the Lengyel circle have not been known up to the present. Locations that can be considered as exceptions are Mauer near Vienna, where six skeleton graves were detected in a silex mining field (Ruttkay 1970), and Friebritz-Süd (Ruttkay 1970; Humpolová 1992, 61).

CREMATION BURIALS

A special phenomenon is cremation burials in the LgC. Cremation of the dead within the Neolithic period was long related nearly exclusively to the SPC, mainly due to the cremation burial site in Prague-Bubeneč and bi-ritual burial sites in Miskovice (Zápotocká 1981) and Plotiště nad Labem (Vokolek and Zápotocká 1997). Nevertheless, all three sites are found in Bohemia, and nowadays we know that the cremation rite occurred as early as the LPC period. This has been testified by Miroslav Šmíd at the site Kralice na Hané (2012).

Like in the case of skeleton graves, we have not recorded any regular cremation burial sites in the Western part of the Lengyel complex area. In the Lengyel circle, cremation graves are generally rare. The available information about this way of burial in Moravia was summarized by Alena Humpolová (1992). According to her information, only seven cremation graves can unquestionably be identified in Moravia, particularly in five locations: Jaroměřice nad Rokytnou, Křenovice, Vedrovice, Hluboké Mašůvky and Výrovice. The latter three showed two graves each, but one of the graves in Hluboké Mašůvky is sometimes classified in the literature as obscure (Humpolová 1992, 61). It is the find of a small tub of six handles, containing clay and burnt small human bones (?). An analogous case was reported from the site Eggenburg-Zogelsdorferstraße, where a similar small vessel was identified among grave gifts (Ruttkay and Teschler-Nicola 1985, 212). With a question mark, the find from Dobšice may be added to the LgC cremation burials as well. There the rescue excavations revealed fragments of vessels whose production technique and way of interment suggest a symbolic cremation burial (Geisler and Kovárník 1983, 75; Humpolová 1992, 62–64).

As for the dating of cremation burials, their placing in chronology is rather clear. The graves from Jaroměřice nad Rokytnou, Křenovice, and one of the graves from Vedrovice can be related to phase Ib considering the pottery finds. The same phase includes the potential cremation grave from Hluboké Mašůvky. Other graves belong to the later degree, specifically to phases IIa (the second grave from Vedrovice) and IIb (both graves from Výrovice), or possibly to the epi-Lengyel Jordanov group. Subsequently, hitherto we do not know a cremation grave belonging to the earliest phase Ia or the transitory phase Ic. A similar situation persists in Lower Austria (Humpolová 1992, 61; Hájek and Humpolová 2010, 63, 89). Particularly in connection with the earlier degree and in light of the new knowledge employing the data of absolute radiocarbon dating, one interesting question arises concerning the occurrence of cremation graves. Recently, the preliminary results of the correlation of the relative and absolute chronology of the Neolithic period in Moravia were published. On comparison of the data for the earlier degree, phases Ia and Ib showed a certain overlap in chronology. When the analysed locations were plotted on a map, they demonstrated some geographic exclusivity of the two phases. Therefore, at least for some time, they may have existed within the same time horizon. However, the people of the phase Ia traditionally inhabited lowland locations at the sides of the valley basins while the population of the phase Ib spread into higher altitudes. Another distinction between the two phases is the occurrence of rondel enclosures, which is virtually exclusively related to phase Ia, and the differences in materials used in the production of stone utensils (Kuča et al. 2012, 57). Therefore, the hypothesis that cremation burials, as well as some other social-economic aspects (mining and distribution of materials), may have been connected with affiliation to one of the co-existing culture entities cannot be ultimately excluded. Cremation graves in the later degree, in turn, may testify to the gradual development and merging of social models set in the earlier degree (Kuča et al. 2012, 59). Nevertheless, for definite confirmation of this hypothesis, more information about cremation burials will be needed, as we still have to work with a very limited and statistically hardly relevant set of conclusive data. The same problem persists in the issues of absolute chronology.

SKELETON BURIALS

Burial sites of the Eastern circle of the Lengyel complex (Hungary) comprise not only relatively standardized skeleton burials but also numerous anomalous ones.

As for skeleton burials, the information available is also rather fragmentary, and as in the case of cremation burials, we have not known any continuous burial fields in the Western branch of the Lengyel circle. From Moravia, we have recorded about fifty skeleton graves so far, all of them from settlement settings, where they are usually found in settlement pits. For example, as for the manner of interment of the remnants of the deceased, a considerable variability can be observed between particular burials. The dead bodies may be ritually buried or dumped, and in some cases, we can only find separate human bones. Multiple or mass graves are no exception, either. This phenomenon is sometimes explained as an absence of an established burial rite (Podborský and Vildomec 1972, 56; Kovárník 2002, 146; Podborský et al. 2005, 95; Podborský 2006, 172–173; Čižmář ed. 2008, 237).

Of the known funeral sites, a mass grave from the Džbánice location (district Znojmo) stands out in particular. In a rather small pit, twelve individuals of different ages were crammed with a dogs skull, 16 pottery vessels and artefacts located near the skulls. Another special case is the find of multiple burials in the southern part of Rajhrad (location "Sladovna"). In 1872, an LgC settlement was discovered there, and in one of the structures, five individuals were found, who had probably been violently thrown into the pit. Otherwise, most burials in which we can observe intentional, i.e. ritual interment of the deceased resemble the form of a funeral rite that was common throughout the Neolithic period. The dead body is interred in a crouched position on the left or right side and equipped with grave gifts, most often pottery vessels. To this type of grave we classify both finds from Těšetice-Kyjovice, location "Sutny," i.e. graves H3 and H14 (Košťuřík 1972; Košťuřík and Dočkalová 1992), of which grave H3 was dated according to the pottery present to phase IIa, and grave H14 to phase Ia. Prominent in the group of graves with the ritual interment of the dead person is the burial of a woman, aged 40–45 years, endowed with numerous grave gifts, and besides pottery vessels, chipped stone artefacts, remains of meaty food and pendants of deer. Of particular interest was the finding of a decoration consisting of a thin sheet of copper. Such a find is unique in the setting of Moravia (Schenk et al. 2007).

Non-ritual graves are terms used to describe situations where intentional and respectful interment of the individual in the pit cannot be presumed. Such a fact is proven, above all, by the position of the dead body indicating that it was thrown into the pit. This is manifested, e.g. in the find from Mašovice-Pšeničné (district Znojmo), where a male skeleton was not positioned in one level of the site. Moreover, the remains showed traces of unhealed injuries, which suggests a violent death (Dočkalová and Čižmář 2008a, 51). A special case of unintentionally interred human bodies was discovered at a mining area in the Krumlov forest in 2002. In one of the pits, a dish dating back to the earlier phase of LgC was found at a depth of two metres, with the skeleton of a hare underneath, which, however, may have fallen to the pit by accident. In a niche of the pit at a depth of 6 m, remains of a woman were found in non-anatomical position, with one arm dislocated. On the bottom of the niche, there was another woman buried lying on her back with her hand behind her head. The remains of the unborn foetus were also found there. Behind the woman's head was skeletal remains of a small dog (Dočkalová and Čižmář 2008a, 51).

In the survey of the skeleton burials known to the time, the theory mentioned above of different funeral rites employed in the older degree of LgC arises again. Among the skeleton burials found, none can be dated into phase Ib. Still, however, no definitive conclusion can be made on the nature of the burial rite during particular phases as the volume of relevant data available is very small. The said phenomenon, nevertheless, poses one of the most interesting questions to solve in the current research of the Neolithic period.

ON THE CHRONOLOGY

The original system of the relative chronology of the Moravian Painted Ware Culture was, like in other Neolithic cultures, based on the ornament of pottery vessels (see above). The basic division comprises two degrees—earlier (I) and later (II). Within these degrees, phases were also subdivided. J. Palliardi divided the earlier degree into two phases (a, b), while in the later degree he defined a third degree (c) as well. V. Vildomec extended his periodisation by distinguishing three phases in either degree. An attempt to make the periodisation more precise was made by V. Podborský, who first set out four degrees (I–IV), while he considered the fifth degree as Jordanov type pottery. The late degree was studied in detail by P. Koštuřík (1973) as well. Eventually, however, V. Podborský returned to the original periodisation coined by Palliardi and Vildomec. With a team of collaborators, he started the standardisation of the material of particular degrees: thus the Numeric Code of Moravian Painted Pottery was created (Podborský et al. 1977), which has been used by researchers till now. As early as in the mid-1980s, I. Rakovský separated the phase Ic (Rakovský 1985). Then continuously, more studies have been appearing, trying to refine or put more precisely the basic periodisation through the definition of sub-phases (Kazdová 1984; Čižmář et al. 2004).

In the past few years, with modern analyses available, new attempts appear of validation of the new data and matching of relative chronology to real calendar dating. In connection with these issues, several facts were revealed: In absolute dating, phases Ia, Ib and Ic are virtually contemporary.
- The differences between particular phases of the earlier degree pertain to settlement strategies.

- The differences between particular phases of the earlier degree are pronouncedly reflected by stone utensils and their production.
- The transition between the earlier and the later degree was very smooth and continuous.

The volume of the relevant data, however, is still rather small and in the future, it will be necessary to verify the said hypotheses through further research (Kuča et al. 2012). Another problem, which does not only involve the late Neolithic period, is the quantity of the data, or rather the quantity of archaeological material that has not yet been processed nor published. As the analysis of chipped stone utensils shows, the knowledge of material culture is vital for the reconstruction of the settlement strategy and way of life.

The material culture of LgC was last summarized in brief by a team of authors who dealt with the Neolithic life in general (Čižmář et al. 2008), and also through published manuscripts (Hájek 2014) and studies (Hájek, Humpolová, and Čerevková 2016). According to recent knowledge, however, it follows that the current state of research will require more complex updating, defining the prospective topics of the research for the years to come.

UPPER-SILESIAN LENGYEL GROUP

This term characterises one of the branches of the Lengyel complex, which in the Czech territory was spread in the region of North Moravia, particularly around Opava. The population of the Czech and later also Polish part of Silesia by the people of the Lengyel complex can reliably be dated to the later degree of the LgC. At that time, the Lengyel complex was at the apex of its spread, which was demonstrable in the areas of Central and South-East Moravia as well as in East Bohemia. The population of Upper Silesia as early as during the phase Ib has not been reliably proven, and for phase Ia, the evidence of population is absent. Within the Upper- Silesian Lengyel group, four phases of development were identified, the most prominent being phases I and III. Phase III corresponds to phase IIb of the LgC, and phase IV is contemporary with LgC IIc, i.e. early Eneolithic period (Pavelčík 1994; Janák 1990; 1991; 1998). The most important locations of the Upper Silesian Lengyel group include Velké Hoštice, with several sites within the cadastre (last Malík 2013, 162), Opava-Kylešovice (Stabrava 2008, 281–282; Stabrava and Kováčik 2009, 255; Hlubek 2011, 170–171; Hlas 2012b, 136; Langr and Hlas 2013, 150–151), Opava-Kateřinky, overlapping with the cadastre of Malé Hoštice (Juchelka 2009, 254) or Holasovice (Hlas 2012a, 129). All the said cases are settlement locations, and apart from Opava-Kylešovice, all show traces of funeral activities.

In the case of Opava-Kateřinky, the burial dated to the turn of phase III, and the grave gifts included a stemmed dish, a small vessel and a sharp axe (Juchelka 2009, 254). The Holasovice grave was dated to phase I, and the grave gifts consisted of a pottery vessel, a hammer axe, three lydite blades and two lydite chips (Hlas 2012a, 129). In Velké Hoštice, two graves were discovered, both containing grave gifts such as characteristic pottery, and grave 2, in addition, contained two-grain grinders of stone (Janák 2001, 326–327). With the anthropologic findings currently available, no details of the buried individuals could be communicated as their remains are very poorly preserved. In the area of the spread of the Upper Silesian Lengyel group, we have only had very few grave finds. All those graves without exception were skeletal ones (Janák 2001, 327, 330; Hlas 2012a, 129). Like in the other parts of Moravia, only sporadic burials within the settlements have been recorded. Proof of residential architecture, in turn, are missing altogether (Janák 2004, 76). One feature that is particularly characteristic of Silesia within the wider Moravian area is the finds of stone sinkers for fishing nets. These artefacts were present in the whole area virtually throughout the entire Neolithic as well as Eneolithic period, not excluding the Upper Silesian Lengyel group either. They have been known, for example, from Opava-Jaktař (Janák 2004, 78, 82) or Služovice/ Hněvošice (Janák 1989, 113, 198).

A particularly important role in the research of the Upper Silesian Lengyel group was played by Vratislav Janák, who explored the prominent site in Velké Hoštice (Janák 1984; 1985; 1987; 1990) and other locations, continuously summarizing the recent knowledge about the population of the Czech part of Silesia throughout the Neolithic as well as Eneolithic period (Janák 1989; 1998). Further, the assets of Lumír Jisl (1968) and Jiří Pavelčík (1974) must be mentioned. The state of research into the Upper Silesian Lengyel group in the said region, however, can still be judged as hardly satisfactory, which is, of course, a problem concerning some other periods too (Janák 1996, 202; 1998, 95).

OBTAINING NEW INFORMATION

The overview of the location used to be good thanks to synthetic studies dealing with specific regions, such as Znojmo (Podborský and Vildomec 1972), Třebíč (Košturík et al. 1986), and Brno-venkov (Belcredi et al. 1989). Although synthetic studies still do appear, they are usually focused on a wider scale rather than concentrating on particular sites. Nevertheless, the list of newly identified sites has been increasing since the 1990s mainly thanks to rescue explorations and prospection activity.

Prospection activity is predominantly connected with non-destructive methods. Aerial archaeology is widely used and in Moravia is connected with Radek Martin Pernička, Miroslav Bálek and Jaromír Kovárník. In relation to LgC, aerial photography was employed successfully in particular in photographic documentation of the rondel enclosure in Těšetice-Kyjovice at "Sutny" (Podborský 1988; Bálek and Podborský 2001, 73), and subsequently

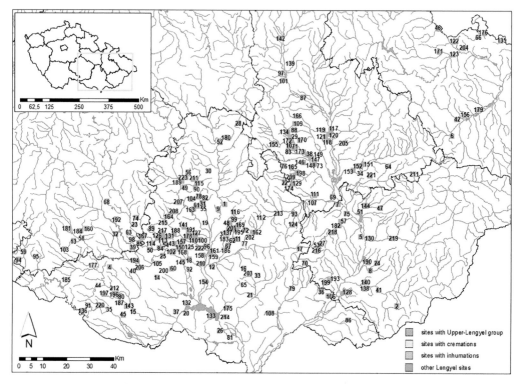

Fig. 17. The map of LgC sites in Moravia

1—Babice nad Svitavou 2—Bánov; 3—Bedřichovice; 4—Běhařovice; 5—Bělov; 6—Bernartice nad Odrou; 7—Bezměrov; 8—Bílovice u Uherského Hradiště; 9—Bílovice nad Svitavou; 10—Bílovice-Lutotín; 11—Blažovice; 12—Blučina; 13—Bohušice; 14—Bohutice; 15—Borotice; 16—Bošovice; 17—Brankovice; 18—Bratčice; 19—Brno; 20—Brod nad Dyjí; 21—Brumovice; 22—Březina; 23—Březník; 24—Březolupy; 25—Budkovice; 26—Bulhary; 27—Cetechovice; 28—Cetkovice; 29—Čechy pod Kosířem; 30—Černá Hora; 31—Česká; 32—Dalešice; 33—Dambořice; 34—Dluhonice; 35—Dobšice; 36—Domanín; 37—Drnholec; 38—Držovice; 39—Dukovany; 40—Džbánice; 41—Havřice; 42—Hladké Životice; 43—Hlína; 44—Hluboké Mašůvky; 45—Hodonice; 46—Holasovice; 47—Holešov; 48—Horákov; 49—Hradčany; 50—Hrubšice; 51—Hulín; 52—Chrudichromy; 53—Chvalnov—Lísky; 54—Ivančice; 55—Ivanovice u Brna; 56—Jamné; 57—Jarohnvěvice; 58—Jaroměřice nad Rokytnou; 59—Jemnice; 60—Jezeřany-Maršovice; 61—Jinačovice; 62—Jiříkovice; 63—Kladeruby nad Oslavou; 64—Kladmíky; 65—Klobouky u Brna; 66—Kobeřice; 67—Kobylnice; 68—Kojatín; 69—Kojetín; 70—Koryčany; 71—Kostelec na Hané; 72—Kovalovice; 73—Kralice na Hané; 74—Kralice nad Oslavou; 75—Kroměříž; 76—Krumsín; 77—Křenovice; 78—Kuřim; 79—Kyjov; 80—Kyjovice; 81—Lednice; 82—Lelekovice; 83—Lešany; 84—Letkovice; 85—Lhánice; 86—Lipov; 87—Litovel; 88—Luděřov; 89—Lukovany; 90—Malhostovice; 91—Mašovice; 92—Medlov; 93—Medlovice; 94—Menhartice; 95—Mladoňovice; 96—Modřice; 97—Mohelnice; 98—Mohelno; 99- Mokrá; 100—Moravany; 101—Moravičany; 102—Moravské Bránice; 103—Moravské Budějovice; 104—Moravské Knínice; 105—Moravský Krumlov; 106—Moravský Písek; 107—Mořice; 108—Mutěnice; 109—Náměšť na Hané; 110—Nebovidy; 111—Němčice na Hané; 112—Nemojany; 113—Neslovice; 114—Nová Ves u Oslavan; 115—Nuzířov; 116—Ochoz u Brna; 117—Olomouc-město; 118—Olomouc-Nemilany; 119—Olomouc-Neředín; 120—Olomouc-Povel; 121—Olomouc-Slavonín; 122—Opava-Kateřinky u Opavy; 123—Opava-Kylešovice; 124—Orlovice; 125—Ořechov; 126—Oslavany;

more round areas enclosed with ditches were identified using this method, e.g. Běhařovice etc. (Kovárník 1999, 25-40).

One of the most commonly used non-destructive methods of prospection is fieldwalking and sampling surveys. It is one of the least expensive while being very efficient as it provides information about the relative age of the site and its approximate area. Fieldwalking is also a form of archaeological activity that is available to the general public. Since time immemorial, people have gathered curious objects that attracted their attention in the landscape. Very often this happened during agricultural work, when people walked around more intensively, cultivating their fields, gardens and orchards. A considerable quantity of the artefacts found ended up being dumped as people did not know the real value of such finds. Some people, however, kept the items found in their homes as strange mementoes and curiosities—stone tools especially attracted such attention. With the origins of archaeology as a science, the interest in such objects increased, and people started searching the origin of their treasures. Some curious individuals succumbed to the keen interest in ancient curiosities and took up archaeological prospection as a hobby. Those were the first amateur explorers, who soon were no longer satisfied with bringing their finds to schools for consultation, but tried to obtain some level of education in archaeology themselves. Eventually, fieldwalking was also complemented with shovel-test pits as well as bigger explorations. The general public and amateur researchers were thus instrumental in the discovery of a large number of archaeological sites.

127—Ostopovice; 128—Ostrožská Nová Ves; 129—Otaslavice; 130—Otrokovice; 131—Padochov; 132—Pasohlávky; 133—Pavlov; 134—Pěnčín; 135—Píšť; 136—Podmolí; 137—Podolí u Brna; 138—Podolí u Uherského Hradiště; 139—Police; 140—Popovice; 142—Postřelmov; 143—Práče; 144—Pravčice; 145—Pravlov; 146—Prostějov; 147—Prostějov-Čechůvky; 148—Prostějov-Držovice; 149—Prostějov-Vrahovice; 150—Prštice; 151—Přerov-Lýsky; 152—Přerov-Předmostí; 153—Přerov-Dluhonice; 154—Přísnotice; 155—Ptení; 156—Pustějov; 157—Radostice; 158—Rajhrad; 159—Rajhradice; 160—Ratibořice; 161—Rebešovice; 162—Rousínov; 163—Rozdrojovice; 164—Říčany; 165—Seloutky; 166—Senička; 167—Senorady; 168—Silůvky; 169—Sivice; 170—Slatinky; 171—Slavkov; 172—Služín; 173—Smržice; 174—Sněhotice; 175—Starovičky; 176—Strahovice; 177—Střelice-Bukovina; 178—Střelice u Brna; 179—Studénka; 180—Sudice; 181—Šebkovice; 182—Šelešovice; 183—Šlapanice; 184—Štěpánovice; 185—Štítary; 186—Telnice; 187—Těšetice-Kyjovice; 188—Tetčice; 189—Tišnov; 190—Topolná; 191—Troubsko; 192—Třesov; 193—Tučapy; 194—Tulešice; 195—Tvarožná; 196—Tvořihráz; 197—Únanov; 198—Určice; 199—Vážany; 200—Vedrovice; 201—Velatice; 202—Velešovice; 203—Velké Hostěrádky; 204—Velké Hoštice; 205—Velký Týnec; 206—Vémyslice; 207—Veverská Bítýška; 208—Veverské Knínice; 209—Vincencov; 210—Vojkovice; 211—Všechovice; 212—Výrovice; 213—Vyškov; 214—Zaječí; 215—Zastávka u Brna; 216—Zástřizly; 217—Zbýšov; 218—Zdounky; 219—Zlín; 220—Znojmo; 221—Želatovice; 222—Želešice; 223—Železné

Amateur archaeologists mostly concentrated on the area of the place they were born or professionally active. One of the most prominent amateur archaeologists in Moravia was Vilém Gross (1894-1977). He explored many locations in the surroundings of Oslavany and along the Jihlava river, and his major assets include the research into the polycultural settlement in Nová Ves u Oslavan (Košťuřík 1994, 391-392). One of his friends was another prominent amateur archaeologist Jaroslav Mikulášek (1916-1996). The focus of his interest was the vicinity of his native village Neslovice. Gradually he widened the scope of his research and paid attention to the southern part of the Brno region as well, where he also explored several sites of the LgC (e.g. Popůvky, Radslavice, Střelice). Further, he played an important role in the research of Palaeolithic sites around Neslovice (Valoch 1997, 283). Another amateur archaeologist worth mentioning is Václav Růžička, who—together with Jiří Doležel of the Brno branch of the Archaeological Institute of the Czechoslovak Academy of Sciences—performed field surveys at the turn of the 1980s, particularly in the southern part of the Boskovice Furrow. Thereby he remarkably assisted in the extension of the list of Palaeolithic, Neolithic and Eneolithic sites in the area and gathered an extensive collection of archaeological material (Doležel 1985).

Field survey, naturally, also became a convenient tool for obtaining information by professional archaeologists, who are able to systematically spread sound knowledge of the prehistoric and medieval population. The prospecting activities of the archaeologist Martin Kuča (Museum and Gallery Prince House in Moravský Krumlov), mainly performed in cooperation with Milan Vokáč and Petr Škrdla (Archaeological Institute of the Academy of Sciences of the Czech Republic in Brno) were particularly important for the investigation of the LgC.

Recently, new sites have also been discovered due to the expanding construction activities, including the construction of both residences and the adjacent infrastructures. As required by national heritage legislation, the estate developers are required to report about their building plans in time and to allow the authorized archaeological institution to perform the rescue research or perhaps early prospection. These explorations often lead to the discovery of a new site. However, the main disadvantages of rescue research include the pressure of time, which is nearly invariably present, and also the limited size of the area under research, which rarely enables exploration of the whole site. Other pitfalls arise in connection with the subsequent processing of the data obtained, i.e. the material and documents, which may be too complicated and time-consuming. New information on the prehistoric population, therefore, naturally increases in amount rather than in quality, which may not be as good as that obtained through systematic exploration. Only a rather small percentage of the information obtained will then be brought into the attention of the general public as adequate publication output. In case of revision of the Lengyel population, one of the major problems is a more accurate chronological classification of the finds, especially where more attention has to be paid to the correlation of relative and absolute chronology (Kuča et al. 2012).

The number of LgC sites are continuously growing, mainly thanks to the intensive prospection and research activity in the past twenty years. Apart from discoveries of new, so far unknown sites, more accurate chronological classification of those already known is done, and the scope of archaeological material is extended (Bartík 2012; 2015, 167, 176, 190), which also applies to the region of Znojmo (Nejedlá 2012, 107–114).

The last study contributing to the topic of the development of the LgC dealt with its fixing within the absolute chronology. In recent years, suitable specimens for absolute dating through the radiocarbon method have been obtained. Some data collected from the sites in Moravia demonstrate that the phases Ia and Ib overlap in chronology and the differences between them consist in their geographic and geomorphologic spread. Geographically, the phases Ia, as well as Ib, take up the same regions of Moravia. While the sites of phase Ia are found at the edges of river valleys, the sites of Ib spread quite deep into the highlands. Another important difference is the connection of rondel enclosures to phase Ia. In this respect, a contentious location with possibly the presence of both phases is Bulhary. There are also some differences in the scope of materials used for processing. And a similar situation can be observed in the comparison of the phases Ic and IIa. In order to make more accurate definitive conclusions a substantially bigger bulk of data from reliable location-related finds will be needed, which at present is the main problem of a majority of Neolithic research activities (Kuča et al. 2012).

8. ANTHROPOLOGICAL ANALYSIS OF SKELETAL REMAINS OF PEOPLE OF THE LENGYEL CULTURE IN MORAVIA

MARTINA FOJTOVÁ, ZDENĚK TVRDÝ, IVANA JAROŠOVÁ

Unlike in the area of the Danube basin, no continuous skeleton burial sites of the Lengyel Culture (LgC) are known in the territory of Moravia. Therefore particular burials within the settlement areas are still the only source of information about anthropological characteristics of this population, which came to Moravia from the South-East. A few isolated cases of cremation were found (Čižmářová et al. 1996). Human remains dating back to the Late Neolithic period were also identified in the cave Jestřábí skála in the Moravian Karst. However, the situation is complicated by the absence of archaeological records and fragmentation of the discovered material due to secondary manipulation (Tvrdý 2016b). Ondroušková (2011) mentioned a child burial from the Lengyel Culture in the cave Slezákova díra as well, but these skeletal remains were probably lost some time in the past.

Anthropological analysis of skeletons from Moravian Neolithic settlements was performed earlier by M. Dočkalová (Čižmář and Dočkalová 2004; Dočkalová 2006; Dočkalová and Čižmář 2007, 2008a, b; Fojtová, Dočkalová and Jarošová 2008), and for the purpose of this publication the available data was revised, updated and completed with new finds.

Throughout the past century, skeletal remains of approximately 50 individuals of the Lengyel Culture have been discovered in Moravia, or of its local variety known as Moravian Painted Ware Culture. Of the found individuals, 34 were available for anthropological analysis (the map of the sites the individuals included in the research came from can be found in fig. 1). The study established the sex, basic anthropological measures of the skull and postcranial skeleton and estimated age at death. When possible, the approximate body height was also calculated. Further, traceological analysis of the surface of the teeth was performed and subsequently, using its results, the diet of the people of the Lengyel Culture was reconstructed. After, the data obtained were compared with identical analyses performed on skeletal remains of the people of the Linear Pottery Culture (LPC) and Stroked Pottery Culture (SPC), which preceded the Lengyel Culture population in the given area. The burials of these individuals can also be found within settlement structures (in case of LPC, even continuous burial fields are known, but individuals from these sites were not included in these comparisons). Unfortunately, the said analyses were considerably limited by the varying degrees of preservation of

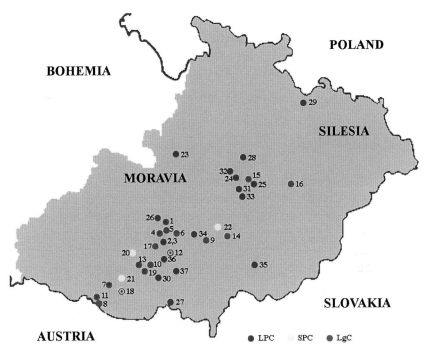

Fig. 1. Map of the Neolithic settlement burials in Moravia
1—Brno-Ivanovice, 2—Brno-Bohunice, 3—Brno-Starý Lískovec, 4—Brno-Komín, 5—Brno-Královo Pole, 6—Brno-Maloměřice, 7—Hluboké Mašůvky, 8—Hnanice, 9—Holubice, 10—Krumlovský les, 11—Mašovice, 12—Modřice, 13—Moravský Krumlov, 14—Orlovice-pískovna, 15—Prostějov-Čechůvky, 16—Předmostí-Dluhonice, 17—Střelice, 18—Těšetice-Kyjovice, 19—Vedrovice, 20—Nová Ves u Oslavan, 21—Trstěnice, 22—Vyškov, 23—Chornice, 24—Držovice, 25—Kralice na Hané, 26—Kuřim, 27—Mikulov-Jelení louka, 28—Olšany u Prostějova, 29—Opava, 30—Pohořelice-Šumice, 31—Seloutky, 32—Slatinky-Močílky, 33—Určice, 34—Velatice, 35—Žádovice, 36—Želešice, 37—Židlochovice.

the osteological material (ranging from virtually complete skeletons to small piles of nearly unidentifiable bone fragments).

METHODS OF ANTHROPOLOGICAL ANALYSIS

In order to identify the sex, methods employing intersexual differences in the pelvis morphology were used above all (Acsádi and Nemeskéri 1970; Novotný 1986; Brůžek 2002). In individuals whose pelvic bones had not been sufficiently preserved, morphology of bones of the skull was assessed (Acsádi and Nemeskéri 1970; Čihák 1987; Ferembach, Schwidetzky and Stloukal 1979), also considering the total robustness of the skeleton and degree of development of muscle insertions. In children and adolescents, the sex was not established because of insufficient development of sexually dimorph signs in immature skeletons, as in this case the methods of establishing the sex are unreliable.

In order to establish the biological age in immature individuals, methods that assess the degree of mineralization and dental eruption were used (Ubelaker 1978; Broadbent, Broadbent and Golden 1975), further methods were employed that assess the degree of epiphyseal union and general maturation of the skeleton (Brothwell 1972; Ferembach, Schwidetzky and Stloukal 1979; Schwartz 1995; Scheuer and Black 2004; Schaefer, Black and Scheuer 2009).

Opinions on accuracy and reliability of estimation of the age at death in adult individuals and appropriateness of the respective methods have passed through serious development in the past few years (see e.g. Bocquet-Appel 2008; Hoppa and Vaupel 2002; Falys and Lewis 2010; Garwin et al. 2012; Buckberry 2015). The set of skeletal remains from Neolithic settlement burials in Moravia had already been examined in this respect (Fojtová, Dočkalová and Jarošová 2008), however, on the basis of the latest knowledge the age estimation within the whole set was revised for the purposes of this research, and apart from the methods of age estimation used earlier (McKern and Stewart 1957; Gilbert and McKern 1973; Szilvássy 1980; Lovejoy 1985; Meindl and Lovejoy 1985; Meindl et al. 1985), the programme ADBOU (version 2.1), created on the basis of methodology described by Boldsen et al. (2002) was used in case of sufficiently preserved skeletons, even considering all its limitations and drawbacks (see Milner and Boldsen 2012). For each individual, the interval of the age at death was established using intersection of probable age intervals obtained through the said methods. Subsequently, all the individuals under research were divided into three basic age groups – younger adults (20–40 years), middle adults (40–60 years) and older adults (60–80 years). For those individuals whose probable age interval was on the border of two neighbouring groups, transient categories "younger to middle" and "middle to older" were created. Those individuals whose age interval was too wide (overlapping all three basic groups) or could not be established at all were not included in the subsequent analyses.

For the metric processing of the skeletal material of adult individuals, the system of measures according to Martin and Knussman as adopted by Drozdová (2004) was used. The body height was established through the method by Sjøvold (1990), always using the available measure with the highest correlation coefficient. In the situation when bones of the both sides could be measured, the average value was used to calculate the body height.

STRUCTURE OF THE EXAMINED SKELETAL SET IN TERMS OF SEX AND AGE

For anthropological analysis, skeletal remains of 34 individuals of the Lengyel Culture from as many as 18 sites were available. The data obtained were compared to those of 14 individuals of the Stroked Pottery Culture and

Tab. 1. List of localities with the number of skeletons

	LgC	SPC	LPC		LgC	SPC	LPC
Brno-Ivanovice	1		1	Nová Ves u Oslavan		2	
Brno-Bohunice	1			Trstěnice		1	
Brno-Starý Lískovec			12	Vyškov		1	
Brno-Komín	1		1	Chornice			1
Brno-Královo Pole	1			Držovice			1
Brno-Maloměřice	1			Kralice na Hané			2
Hluboké Mašůvky	1		3	Kuřim			1
Hnanice	1			Mikulov Jelení louka			1
Holubice	1			Olšany u Prostějova			2
Krumlovský les	3			Opava			1
Mašovice u Znojma	1		2	Pohořelice-Šumice			1
Modřice-Rybníky	3	2	3	Seloutky			1
Moravský Krumlov	1		1	Slatinky-Močílky			2
Orlovice-pískovna	2			Určice			1
Prostějov-Čechůvky	1			Velatice			2
Předmostí-Dluhonice	1			Žádovice			10
Střelice	6			Želešice			1
Těšetice-Kyjovice	7	8	10	Židlochovice			1
Vedrovice	1		24	Total	34	14	85

85 individuals of the Linear Pottery Culture. Therefore a total number of 133 skeletons from 37 sites (whose survey is given in tab. 1) were examined.

Out of the said 34 individuals buried in settlement structures of the Lengyel Culture, there were 6 men, 12 women, 11 children and adolescents,

Tab. 2. Basic population structure

	LPC		SPC		LgC	
Males	8	9.4%	3	21.4%	6	17.6%
Females	14	16.5%	3	21.4%	12	35.3%
Subadults	54	63.5%	4	28.6%	11	32.4%
?	9	10.6%	4	28.6%	5	14.7%
Total	85	100.0%	14	100.0%	34	100.0%

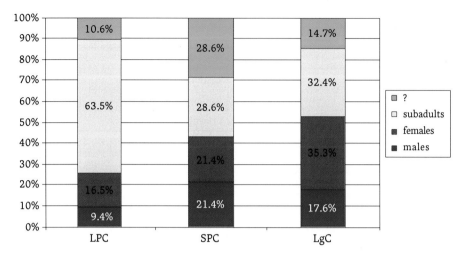

Graph 1. Basic population structure.

and another 5 were unidentifiable adult individuals. The Stroked Pottery Culture was represented by 3 men, 3 women, 4 children and/or adolescents and 4 unidentifiable individuals, while in settlement structures of the Linear Pottery Culture remains of 8 men, 14 women, 54 children and 9 anthropologically unclassifiable adults were found. (This data is summarized in surveys in tab. 2 and graph 1).

Considering a continuous transition of the Linear Pottery Culture to the Stroked Pottery Culture, as no population exchange of their creators is presumed (Zápotocká 2009; Končelová and Květina 2015; Link 2014, 2015), and

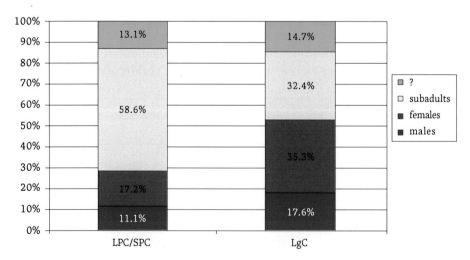

Graph 2. Basic population structure, LPC and SPC together.

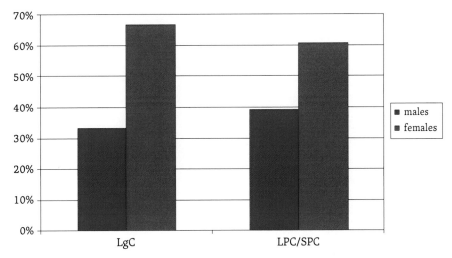

Graph 3. Sex ratio.

also keeping in mind the low number of adult skeletons available that can be ascribed to people of the Stroked Pottery Culture, then the data of the two cultures that preceded the Lengyel expansion in the territory of Moravia can be summarized, which provides the situation visualized in graph 2. There we can see that while in the period of the Linear and Stroked Pottery Cultures skeletal remains of children and adolescents prevailed in settlement burials, in the Lengyel Culture the number of children considerably decreased and the preponderance of female skeletons increased. The male-to-female ratio in Neolithic settlement burials is shown in more detail in graph 3. It is obvious that the Lengyel Culture buried twice as many women than men in this way, while in the earlier cultures women do prevail too but the number of men reaches about two-thirds of that number.

The basic distribution by age of the set under examination is summarized in tab. 3 (two skeletons of LPC could not be classified in the respective categories, so the number of individuals of this culture is different from the number given in tables 1 and 2 and visualized in graph 4). Here again, it is evident that the people from LPC and SPC used settlement pits for burials

Tab. 3. Age distribution

	LgC		SPC		LPC	
Adults	23	67.6%	10	71.4%	29	34.9%
Juveniles	3	8.8%	3	21.4%	8	9.6%
Children	8	23.5%	1	7.1%	46	55.4%
Total	34	100.0%	14	100.0%	83	100.0%

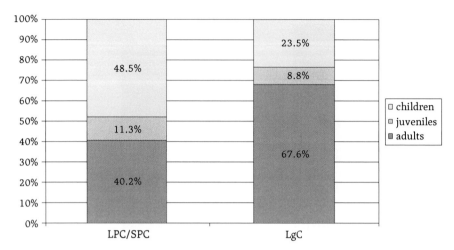

Graph 4. Basic age distribution.

mainly for children and adolescents under 20 years of age, and in the later Lengyel Culture most skeletons found belonged to adults individuals while the number of children and adolescents considerably decreased.

When inspecting the age structure of children in the examined set (tab. 4; again with only those skeletal remains included that could be classified within the respective age groups) and its visualization in Graph 5, it is obvious that—apart from the complete absence of children between the ages of 5 and 10 years in the set of LgC—the mortality curves in both groups follow the same pattern. The absence of the said age group may be due to the generally low number of child skeletons in LgC (i.e. remains of children of that age have yet to be unearthed). Ages 3–5 and 15–20 years are the most frequent age groups among the settlement burials of children in the Lengyel Culture,

Tab. 4. Age distribution of children

	LgC		SPC		LPC	
0–6m.	1	10.0%	0	0.0%	9	17.0%
6–12m.	0	0.0%	0	0.0%	4	7.5%
1–3	1	10.0%	0	0.0%	8	15.1%
3–5	3	30.0%	0	0.0%	7	13.2%
5–10	0	0.0%	1	25.0%	11	20.8%
10–15	2	20.0%	1	25.0%	6	11.3%
15–20	3	30.0%	2	50.0%	8	15.1%
total	10	100.0%	4	100.0%	53	100.0%

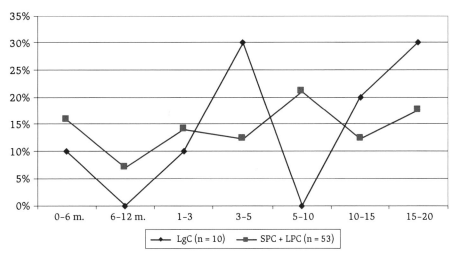

Graph 5. Age distribution of children (months and years).

while in earlier Moravian cultures (LPC/SPC) it is the category of children between 5 and 10 years that are most often found. The smallest group of children (apart from the absence, as mentioned above of the group 5-10 years in LgC) were in both cases the older infant age (6–12 months).

Tab. 5 displays the survey of approximate age structure of adults whose skeletal remains were found in settlement structures of the Moravian Neolithic (the total numbers in all three cultures being lower than in tables 1 and 2, as the state of preservation of some skeletal remains did not allow for a more accurate estimation of the age). From the data in the tables (and from graph 6) it follows that in the Lengyel Culture the highest number of adults buried in settlement structures were of the youngest age group (20–40 years) and the incidence of older individuals decreases with growing age. In the cultures of the early and middle Neolithic period (LPC/SPC) the maximum number of adult individuals also falls into the category of younger adults

Tab. 5. Age distribution of adults

	LgC		SPC		LPC		LPC+SPC	
younger adults (20–40)	14	70.0%	4	50.0%	10	41.7%	14	43.8%
younger to middle	4	20.0%	2	25.0%	3	12.5%	5	15.6%
middle adults (40–60)	0	0.0%	1	12.5%	1	4.2%	2	6.3%
middle to older	1	5.0%	1	12.5%	8	33.3%	9	28.1%
older adults (60+)	1	5.0%	0	0.0%	2	8.3%	2	6.3%
total	20	100.0%	8	100.0%	24	100.0%	32	100.0%

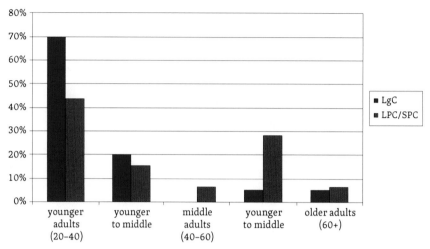

Graph 6. Cranial indices of LgC.

and the least numerous category is middle adults. However, the incidence of burials grows again as we observe the older age groups.

The general survey of the age composition of the two populations can be seen in graph 7. It shows that the individuals of the Lengyel Culture buried in settlement structures were predominantly children, adolescents and young adults below the age of 40, while the proportion of the older age categories was markedly lower. In earlier Moravian Neolithic cultures (LPC, SPC), children and adolescents prevail in settlement burials while towards the middle age there are fewer individuals buried that way, although some individuals of a higher age occur as well.

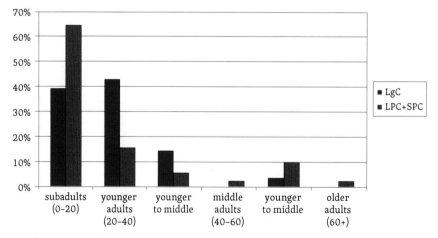

Graph 7. Age distribution by cathegories.

METRIC ASSESSMENT

In metric processing of human skeletal material from Moravian Neolithic settlements, we considered the values of the 15 main cranial indices, of dimensions of the postcranial skeleton we consider the most important dimensions correlating with the body height. Again, due to the insufficient state of preservation of the skeletons, we were not able to establish all the relevant measurements in all individuals, and some could not be taken at all.

Tables 6–8 display the survey of average values of these indices for men and women and all adult individuals of all the three Moravian Neolithic cultures. Table 9 shows the average values for individuals of LPC and SPC together. As it follows, intersexual differences within particular cultures as well as intercultural differences in adults are merely negligible. However, considering the low number of data, this conclusion cannot be generalized.

Tab. 6. Cranial indices of LgC

LgC		Males	Females			Adults
Cranial I. (I1)	78.31	mesocrany	73.36	dolichocrany	75.95	mesocrany
Length-Height I. (I2)	76.11	hypsicrany	80.27	hypsicrany	77.69	hypsicrany
Breadth-Height I. (I3)	100.23	acrocrany	101.48	acrocrany	99.20	acrocrany
Transversal Frontal I. (I12)	78.84		80.31	middle	79.51	middle
Fronto-Parietal I. (I13)	67.73	metriometopic	69.00	eurymetopic	68.42	metriometopic
Foramen Magnum I. (I33)	93.92	wide	85.29	middle	88.02	wide
Facial I. (I38)						
Upper Facial I. (I39)			48.74	euryeny	48.74	euryeny
Malar Upper Facial I. (I39(1))	68.56	chamae-prosopy	64.37	hyperchamae-prosopy	68.84	chamae-prosopy
Orbital I. (dx.) (I42)	85.00	mesoconchy	77.61	mesoconchy	82.99	mesoconchy
Orbital I. (sin.) (I42)	91.43	hypsiconchy	80.86	mesoconchy	85.08	hypsiconchy
Nasal I. (I48)	51.67	chamaerrhiny	57.29	chamaerrhiny	53.58	chamaerrhiny
Palatal I. (I58)	84.91	mesostaphyline	81.48	mesostaphyline	83.20	mesostaphyline
Jaw I. (I60)	92.17	orthognathy	86.87	orthognathy	90.37	orthognathy
Mandibular I. (I62)	54.20	dolichosteno-mandibular	62.75	dolichosteno-mandibular	58.47	dolichosteno-mandibular

I. = Index

Tab. 7. Cranial indices of LPC

LPC	Males		Females		Adults	
Cranial I. (I1)	71.85	dolichocrany	75.46	mesocrany	74.32	dolichocrany
Length-Height I. (I2)	76.19	hypsicrany	73.11	orthocrany	74.27	orthocrany
Breadth-Height I. (I3)	108.36	acrocrany	97.30	metriocrany	100.98	acrocrany
Transversal Frontal I. (I12)	82.48		83.79		83.30	
Fronto-Parietal I. (I13)	73.11	eurymetopic	70.50	eurymetopic	71.41	eurymetopic
Foramen Magnum I. (I33)	82.21	middle	84.42	middle	83.68	middle
Facial I. (I38)	94.70	leptoprosopy	90.98	leptoprosopy	92.84	leptoprosopy
Upper Facial I. (I39)	59.99	lepteny	48.95	euryeny	55.57	lepteny
Malar Upper Facial I. (I39(1))	79.43	leptoprosopy	71.80	chamaeprosopy	75.19	leptoprosopy
Orbital I. (dx.) (I42)	89.10	hypsiconchy	73.38	chamaeconchy	82.36	mesoconchy
Orbital I. (sin.) (I42)	83.83	mesoconchy	78.34	mesoconchy	80.54	mesoconchy
Nasal I. (I48)	45.55	leptorrhiny	50.93	mesorrhiny	48.91	mesorrhiny
Palatal I. (I58)	70.40	leptostaphyline	76.12	leptostaphyline	73.26	leptostaphyline
Jaw I. (I60)	104.62	prognathy	94.61	orthognathy	99.61	mesognathy
Mandibular I. (I62)	66.67	dolichosteno-mandibular	75.09	dolichosteno-mandibular	73.40	dolichosteno-mandibular

I. = Index

Tab. 8. Cranial indices of SPC

SPC	Males		Females		Adults	
Cranial I. (I1)	70.97	dolichocrany	75.95	mesocrany	73.96	mesocrany
Length-Height I. (I2)			71.67	orthocrany	71.67	orthocrany
Breadth-Height I. (I3)			96.27	metriocrany	96.27	metriocrany
Transversal Frontal I. (I12)	87.61		80.05		81.94	
Fronto-Parietal I. (I13)	67.93	metriometopic	68.81	metriometopic	68.46	metriometopic
Foramen Magnum I. (I33)						
Facial I. (I38)						
Upper Facial I. (I39)						
Malar Upper Facial I. (I39(1))			71.11	chamaeprosopy	71.11	chamae-prosopy
Orbital I. (dx.) (I42)			80.56	mesoconchy	80.56	mesoconchy
Orbital I. (sin.) (I42)			80.56	mesoconchy	80.56	mesoconchy

Nasal I. (I48)						
Palatal I. (I58)			72.12	leptostaphyline	72.12	leptostaphyline
Jaw I. (I60)			94.95	orthognathy	94.95	orthognathy
Mandibular I. (I62)			62.16	dolichosteno-mandibular	62.16	dolichosteno-mandibular

I. = Index

Tab. 9. Cranial indices of LPC+SPC

LPC/SPC	Males		Females		Adults	
Cranial I. (I1)	71.41	dolichocrany	75.71	mesocrany	74.14	dolichocrany
Length-Height I. (I2)	76.19	hypsicrany	72.39	orthocrany	72.97	orthocrany
Breadth-Height I. (I3)	108.36	acrocrany	96.79	metriocrany	98.63	acrocrany
Transversal Frontal I. (I12)	85.05		81.92		82.62	
Fronto-Parietal I. (I13)	70.52	eurymetopic	69.66	eurymetopic	69.94	eurymetopic
Foramen Magnum I. (I33)	82.21	middle	84.42	middle	83.68	middle
Facial index (I38)	94.70	leptoprosopy	90.98	leptoprosopy	92.84	leptoprosopy
Upper Facial I. (I39)	59.99	lepteny	48.95	euryeny	55.57	lepteny
Malar Upper Facial I. (I39(1))	79.43	leptoprosopy	71.46	chamae-prosopy	73.15	chamae-prosopy
Orbital I. (dx.) (I42)	89.10	hypsiconchy	76.97	mesoconchy	81.46	mesoconchy
Orbital I. (sin.) (I42)	83.83	mesoconchy	79.45	mesoconchy	80.55	mesoconchy
Nasal I. (I48)	45.55	leptorrhiny	50.93	mesorrhiny	48.91	mesorrhiny
Palatal I. (I58)	70.40	leptostaphyline	74.12	leptostaphyline	72.69	leptostaphyline
Jaw I. (I60)	104.62	prognathy	94.78	orthognath	97.28	orthognath
Mandibular index (I62)	66.67	dolichosteno-mandibular	68.63	dolichosteno-mandibular	67.78	dolichosteno-mandibular

I. = Index

From the measurements of the skulls we can conclude that a typical woman of the Lengyel Culture had a long high head with a wide forehead, low face, medium height orbits, wide nose, medium width palate, orthognathic jaws, long narrow mandible and a rather circular foramen magnum. The average man of LgC had a medium length tall skull with a medium width forehead and unequally shaped orbits. The nose was broad, palate of medium width, jaws orthognathic, and the mandible long and narrow. The male foramen magnum was wider and shorter than that of the female.

The men of LPC and SPC, vice versa, had longer skulls than their female counterparts, and women of LPC and SPC had lower skulls compared to women of LgC. Men and women of both earlier Neolithic cultures, compared to those of LgC, had narrower and longer faces, narrower noses and palates and the typical man had prognathic jaws. The foramen magnum of the skull was somewhat circular in both sexes.

Tab. 10. Body height

	n	Mean	Median	Maximum	Minimum
LgC females	8	152.7	152.9	163.5	146.1
LgC males	4	159.8	157.6	170.2	154.0
SPC females	0				
SPC males	3	163.3	167.0	169.6	153.4
LPC females	9	154.8	152.6	168.3	145.4
LPC males	6	165.5	165.7	169.3	158.5
LPC/SPC females	9	154.8	152.6	168.3	145.4
LPC/SPC males	9	164.8	165.9	170.2	153.4
LgC	12	155.3	154.0	170.2	146.1
SPC	3	164.4	165.5	169.6	153.4
LPC	15	159.1	162.4	169.3	145.4
SPC/LPC	18	157.7	163.0	169.6	145.4

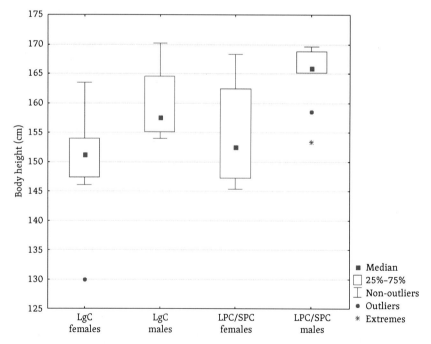

Graph 8. Body height

Estimation of body height was performed in 30 skeletons, 12 of which belonged to the people of the Lengyel Culture (4 men and 8 women), 15 to the Linear Pottery Culture (6 men, 9 women) and 3 to men of the Stroked Pottery Culture. The mean, median, maximum and minimum values found are summarized in tab. 10. Regretfully, due to the complete absence of suitable skeletal material, the body height of women of the Stroked Pottery Culture could not be done. Therefore, the set of individuals from the early and middle Neolithic (LPC/SPC), who are presumed to be of common origin, was again used for comparison. Further, the pathologic skeleton of the adult woman of the Lengyel Culture that was found in Brno-Ivanovice (H803/2010), whose body height was estimated at 130 cm (Jiří Kala, pers. comm., June 13, 2018), was excluded from the calculation. It follows from the given data that the average body height of the people of the Lengyel Culture, who had come to Moravia ca 4500 B.C., was lower than the body height of the earlier local Neolithic population. The difference is, above all, evident in men (see also graph 9).

DENTAL PATHOLOGY

Analysis of dental pathologies in individuals buried in Moravian Neolithic settlement structures has been done in the past (see Jarošová and Dočkalová 2008; Jarošová, Dočkalová and Fojtová 2008). In particular, the authors focused on dental caries and enamel hypoplasia. The methodology of the research is described in detail in the above publications, which we refer to here. In total, 27 people of the Lengyel Culture (11 children, 9 women, 4 men and 3 unidentifiable adults) were assessed. The obtained results were compared to the findings on the teeth of 82 members of the Linear Pottery Culture and 13 of the Stroked Pottery Culture. The total number was 1,540 permanent and 436 deciduous teeth.

Caries (tooth decay) is defined as a multifactorial, multibacterial disease of calcified tooth tissues. It is characterized by demineralisation of the inorganic portion and destruction of the organic component (Langsjoen 1998, 402). From the published results it follows that the caries intensity I-CE (ratio of decayed teeth in the total number of the teeth examined in all individuals, increased by the percentage of intravital loss) was the highest in individuals belonging to the Linear Pottery Culture (total 13.3%, or 19.4% in men and 12.6% in women) and the lowest in the Stroked Pottery Culture (total 1.7%, or 3,5% in women and 0.0% in men). However, these results could be considerably altered due to the low number of teeth examined. The caries intensity in individuals of the Lengyel Culture was 9.8% (4.0% in men and 14.5% in women) (see tab. 11). The most frequently decayed tooth both in LgC and LPC was the second molar, while in SPC it was the first molar. In individuals of all three

Moravian Neolithic cultures alike, the teeth of the lower jaw got generally decayed more often than the upper teeth.

In case of *caries frequency* (F-CE, percentage of individuals suffering from decayed teeth and/or intravital tooth loss; tab. 11), the results of comparison of various Neolithic cultures were similar—most decayed teeth per person was recorded in LPC (F-CE = 42.9%), least in SPC (25.0%), while in the LgC people 38.5% individuals suffered from dental caries. However, considering the relatively low number of individuals available for establishing of the F-CE value (28 adults of LPC, 8 of SPC and 13 of LgC), these results should be taken with a pinch of salt.

Tab. 11. *Caries intensity* (I-CE) and *frequency* (F-CE) in adults (adapted after Jarošová and Dočkalová 2008)

		I-CE	F-CE
LPC	males	19.4	50.0
	females	12.6	53.3
	M+F+?	13.3	42.9
SPC	males	0.0	0.0
	females	3.5	66.7
	M+F+?	1.7	25.0
LgC	males	4.0	50.0
	females	14.5	42.9
	M+F+?	9.8	38.5

One common sign of all the cultures was the complete absence of dental caries in adolescents between the ages of 15 to 20 years (I-CE as well as F-CE = 0). In children under 15 years of age, the only case of dental caries was found on the second right upper deciduous molar in an eleven-year-old child of the Linear Pottery Culture.

Dental enamel hypoplasia (DEH) is a structural defect of the enamel of the tooth resulting from a non-specific metabolic stress disrupting ameloblastic physiology (Langsjoen 1998, 405). At the macroscopic level, it can be seen as transverse grooves or row of pits on the labial side of the crown of the tooth. As after eruption of the tooth the enamel loses the ability of regeneration (Klepáček and Mazánek 2001), hypoplasias provide a unique record of distress undergone in childhood, which persists on the teeth of adult individuals as well. These defects can be interpreted as manifestations of nutritional and/or infectious diseases (El-Najjar, DeSanti and Ozebek 1978; Hodges and Wilkinson 1990; Lukacs 1992; Goodman 1993; Malville 1997; Wright 1997).

Tab. 12. Distribution of individuals displaying *dental enamel hypoplasia* (acute and chronic type). (adapted after Jarošová and Dočkalová 2008)

		DEH absence	DEH presence	DEH %	Individuals analyzed	Acute DEH (lines/pits)	Chronic DEH	Both acute and chronic DEH
LPC	subadults	28	4	12.5	32	3/0	1	0
	M	6	0	0.0	6	0/0	0	0
	F	10	2	16.7	12	0/1	1	0
	?	1	1	50.0	2	1/0	1	1
	total	45	7	13.5	52	4/1	3	1
SPC	subadults	1	1	50.0	2	1/0	0	0
	M	1	0	0.0	1	0/0	0	0
	F	4	0	0.0	4	0/0	0	0
	?	1	0	0.0	1	0/0	0	0
	total	7	1	12.5	8	1/0	0	0
LgC	subadults	4	2	33.3	6	1/0	1	0
	M	3	0	0.0	3	0/0	0	0
	F	5	1	16.7	6	1/0	0	0
	?	1	0	0.0	1	0/0	0	0
	total	13	3	18.8	16	2/0	1	0

Incidence of DEH was examined on a total of 346 teeth (specifically, 243 permanent and 103 deciduous incisors and canines) belonging to 76 individuals with front teeth present. The criteria included the presence/absence of DEH, its form (acute or chronic) and the type of the hypoplastic defect (grooves and/or pits). A survey summarising all the above facts is given in tab. 12.

The problem, once more, is the low number of individuals whose dentitions could be studied for hypoplasia (particularly in LgC and SPC). There is some uncertainty, but perhaps the incidence of dental hypoplasia in people of the Lengyel Culture was somewhat higher than in those of the two earlier cultures who were buried in settlement structures. But the non-parametric Kruskal-Wallis ANOVA test did not prove statistical relevance of this difference. Moreover, as isolated finds rather than continuous populations were studied, it would be precarious to conclude the degree of nonspecific distress from the obtained data or even the degree of general fitness of individuals of the particular archaeological cultures.

The teeth most frequently affected by hypoplastic defects in the Lengyel Culture were the lower permanent canines (27.3%). The same is true about the

Linear Pottery Culture (15%), while in individuals from the Stroked Pottery Culture, medial incisors in both jaws were most often affected (hypoplasia was observable in 20%). None of the 103 deciduous teeth of individuals of all the three cultures in the study bore any signs of hypoplasia.

RECONSTRUCTION OF THE DIET BASED ON DENTAL MICROWEAR

Very interesting findings has also been provided by analysis of dental microwear, which adds important characteristics to the picture of the nutritional strategy of the population of Moravia in the Neolithic period, relating to climate changes throughout the era. The results of the research done by Jarošová et al. (2008) confirm considerable differences in strategies of obtaining food between the people of the Lengyel Culture and those of the earlier Moravian Neolithic cultures. In the Lengyel culture, the state of microwear of the enamel shows a high percentage of meat in the diet (up to 50%), while in the earlier Linear Pottery Culture the vegetable component prevails (meat only represents ca 25%). Further differences were revealed when comparing the dental microwear of adults and children. Unlike the adult individuals of LgC, the children of this culture were nourished differently, probably a diet with a high proportion of plants. In the earlier periods (LPC and SPC), no statistically relevant nutritional difference between children and adults was proven (Jarošová et al. 2008, 113). The conclusions match the results of osteological analyses, where at the sites populated by the Lengyel Culture, a higher proportion of bones of young cattle and sheep/goats (i.e. animals killed for food sooner than they could be used for production of milk) is found, compared to the situation in the era of the Linear Pottery Culture. At the same time, there was a higher proportion of pig bones, kept exclusively for meat (Jarošová et al. 2008, 119). Another shift in food strategies of the people of the Lengyel Culture was a significant increase in the consumption of wild animals (from the original 5% in the early Neolithic period up to 50–60% in the period of LgC) (Pavúk 1991).

The cause of these dramatic changes in food strategies throughout the Moravian Neolithic era should be looked for in climatic fluctuations. During the period corresponding to the presence of the Lengyel Culture in Moravia, a mild decrease in temperatures and precipitations in comparison to the previous Neolithic stage occurred, which led to a relative decrease in the yields of cereal crops and concurrently to an extension of the forest area (Ložek 1980; Pavúk 1991, 1994). This fact was reflected in the increase of hunting (Ambros 1986). The change in nutrition strategies in the late Neolithic period in Moravia is, therefore, an example of human adaptation to changes in the environment.

CONCLUSION

For contemporary researchers, human skeletal remains are an essential source of information about the appearance, health state, population structure and lifestyle of ancient cultures. People of the Lengyel Culture, coming to Moravia before the middle of the 5th millennium B.C. and rapidly assimilating the previous middle Neolithic cultures, regretfully, did not leave much information of this kind. No continuous burial fields are known (and it is unlikely that they have not been discovered if they had existed). So, it is possible that the burial rite used did not leave any archaeological traces. Dumped skeletons, as well as ritual burials in settlement structures, should be held as proof of a burial rite that has not been codified yet (Podborský 1993, 132). Therefore the data of representation of sexes and particular age groups in individuals so buried naturally cannot reflect the actual structure of the given population but rather some kind of selection, whose ritual background and other reasons we can only speculate about. Really limiting is the degree of preservation (or rather decay) of the skeletal material as well.

Considering the anthropological analysis of skeletal remains of the people of the Lengyel Culture in Moravia we can conclude that, unlike the earlier Neolithic cultures (LPC and SPC) which left mainly children's skeletons in their settlements, the Lengyel Culture buried adults rather than children, and the number of women buried in this manner is twice as high as that of the men. The estimated age of these children is most often between 3 and 5 years, and equally frequent are finds of adolescent individuals (15–20 years). Among the adults, the age group of young adults (20–40 years) prevails, and with the growing estimated age the number of skeletons found decreases (while in LPC and SPC the minimum matches the middle age, and the number of older individuals buried in settlement structures is again higher).

People of the Lengyel Culture buried in settlement structures in Moravia had, on average, shorter and taller skulls than their predecessors from LPC and SPC, and their faces were wider, with wider noses as well as jaws. Their body height reached, on average, 152.7 cm in women and 159.8 cm in men, which was somewhat lower than the body height of people of LPC and SPC (men 164.8 cm tall on average and women 10 cm smaller than male).

As for the diet, it was found through analysis of dental microwear and animal osteological material that in the earlier Moravian cultures, meat only constituted about a quarter of the consumed food. This percentage was not significantly different in adults and children. However, the adult individuals of the Lengyel Culture consumed meat much more often than their children and their predecessors from the earlier stages of the Neolithic era (as meat constituted more than 50% of their diet). The cause of these changes was most probably a climatic fluctuation and the ensuing decrease in the yields of field crops and expansion of the forest area, which the expanding Neolithic population flexibly adapted. One of the outcomes of the shortage of saccharides in the diet of the people of the Lengyel Culture, compared to earlier Neolithic cultures, may have been the decrease of incidence of tooth decay in adults as well. On the other hand, the incidence of dental hypoplasia was obviously not very changeable during the Neolithic period, so the influence of nonspecific distress throughout this period was probably relatively constant, and therefore the Lengyel Culture was not very different from its predecessors in Moravian sites in terms of nutrition and general fitness.

9. SURVEY OF BONE DISEASES IN MORAVIAN NEOLITHIC CULTURES

VÁCLAV SMRČKA, ZDENĚK TVRDÝ

The objective of this study is to characterize the state of health in population of the Moravian Painted Ware Culture (also Lengyel Culture, "LgC,"
4700–4500/4000 B.C.), dated into the later Neolithic period, with its latest
phase falling into the Eneolithic (Chalcolithic) period, and to compare this
culture to earlier Neolithic cultures, such as the Linear Pottery Culture (hereinafter "LPC," 5700–4900 B.C.) and the Stroked Pottery Culture (hereinafter
"SPC," 4900–4700 B.C.), in terms of morbidity.

The skeletal material employed in the comparison includes 121 individuals
and comes from Neolithic settlements in the area of Moravia, Czech Republic
(fig. 1).

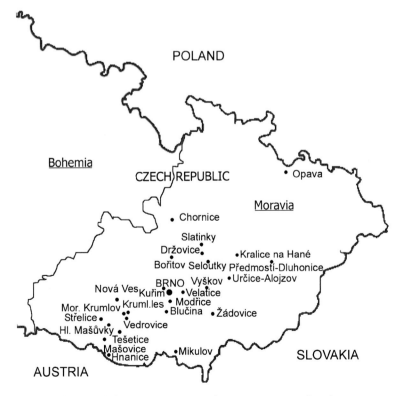

Fig. 1. Location of the Neolithic sites in Moravia that were mentioned in chapter 9.

Its previous anthropological analysis was performed by Dočkalová et al. (Dočkalová and Čižmář 2007, 2008a; Fojtová, Dočkalová and Jarošová 2008). The palaeopathological assessment was done by Smrčka and Tvrdý (2009), and for the purposes of this study, the material was revised, re-assessed and completed with new items. The unique feature of this study consists in judging the morbidity in Neolithic cultures in a unified way, and we also tried to match the material assessed to morbidity in other Neolithic cultures in Moravia for the practical purposes of archaeological interpretation.

In total, 26 skeletons from the LgC settlements were assessed, including 5 men, 9 women, 9 children and 3 unidentifiable adults. The scope of the palaeopathological investigation was limited due to the poor state of preservation of many skeletons. The bones were examined macroscopically, and in case of traumatic lesions, an x-ray investigation was performed. Together with the description of the pathology, the state of preservation of the bones was recorded as well, which enabled the establishment of the frequency of occurrence of particular pathologies in the population. For comparison, a set of skeletons from settlement burials was used, dated to the LPC period, i.e. 83 individuals—13 men, 19 women, 42 children and 9 unidentifiable adults, and into the SPC period, i.e. 12 individuals—3 men, 3 women, 3 children, 3 unidentifiable adult individuals (Smrčka and Tvrdý 2009) (tab. 1).

Tab. 1. List of individuals from the Neolithic Period analyzed in chapter 9

Locality	Grave/Inventory number	Culture	Sex	Age Category	Age (years and months)
Brno-Ivanovice	H 802	LPC	N	child	2
Brno-Komín	IČ 9 (Pa44/38)	LgC	M	adult	25–40
Brno-Komín (Nivy)	800/2006	LPC	N	child	12
Brno-Královo Pole	IČ 18	LgC	F	adult	20–30
Brno-Maloměřice	IČ 11	LgC	N	adult	ADULT
Brno-Starý Lískovec	obj. 658/K410/2005	LPC	N	child	4–5M
	obj. 2601/K801/2006	LPC	N	adult	45–55
	obj. 534/K800/2006	LPC	N	child	6M
	K803/2007	LPC	M	adult	20–21
	obj. 2565/K800/2007	LPC	M?	adult	ADULT
	obj. 4689/K801/2007	LPC	N	child	9
	obj. 6605/K804/2007	LPC	N	child	4–10M
	obj. 5575/K802/2007	LPC	N	child	1–6M
	K805/obj.7714/2008	LPC	M	juvenile	15–20
	K806/obj.7727/2008	LPC	M	adult	65–90
Držovice	2/1998	LPC	F	adult	20–30

Locality	Grave/Inventory number	Culture	Sex	Age Category	Age (years and months)
Hluboké Mašůvky	IČ 17/1897	LgC	N	adult	30–60
Hluboké Mašůvky	654/1/2003	LPC	F	adult	20–30
	654/2/2003	LPC	N	child	13–15
	654/3/2003	LPC	N	child	5
Hnanice I	obj. 3/1992	LgC	F	adult	20–25
Holubice 9	IČ 10/1897	LgC	N	juvenile	19–20
Chornice	1/1939	LPC	N	adult	35–80
Kralice na Hané	548/2003	LPC	N	child	1
	1683/2003	LPC	N	juvenile	18–20
Krumlovský les	2a/2002	LgC II	F	adult	35–40
	2b/2002	LgC II	N	child	0–1M
	1/2002	LgC II	F	adult	25–35
Kuřim	obj. 243	LPC	N	N	N
Mašovice u Znojma	1–1066/1/2003	LgC	M	adult	20–30
Mašovice u Znojma	H1/2003 (jáma 613)	LPC	F	juvenile	15–17
Mašovice u Znojma-Pšeničné	J821/K1308	LPC	N	child	0–1M
Mikulov-Jelení louka	1/1970	LPC	N	adult	ADULT
Modřice-Rybníky	IČ 35/1939	SPC	F	adult	30–70
Modřice	obj. 551/K800/2004	LPC	F	adult	50–90
	obj. 796/K802/2004	LPC	N	child	0–1M
	obj. 734/K801/2004	LPC	F	adult	50–85
Moravský Krumlov	1/1980	LgC	F	adult	25–35
Moravský Krumlov	obj. 513/2002	LPC	N	child	9
Nová Ves u Oslavan	IČ 37/1950	SPC	N	adult	ADULT
	1/16/1950	SPC	M	adult	25–30
Olšany u Prostějova	K506/H1/2001	LPC	N	adult	30–40
	K507/H1/2016	LPC	N	child	9–10
Opava	IČ IV-1612/1959	LPC	F	adult	20–40
Pohořelice-Šumice	IČ IV-1611/1959	LPC	N	adult	20–25
Prostějov-Čechůvky	K1535/2004	LgC	F	child	15
Předmostí-Dluhonice	126/1/2006	LgC	F	adult	20–40
Seloutky	527/1/1999	LPC	N	child	3
Slatinky-Močílky	576/1/2002	LPC	N	child	11
	576/2/2002	LPC	N	child	6–9M
Střelice	H I (IČ 12)	LgC	M	adult	50–90
	IČ 13	LgC	N	child	7–15
	9 (IČ 15)	LgC	N	adult	25–50

Locality	Grave/Inventory number	Culture	Sex	Age Category	Age (years and months)
	IČ 16	LgC	N	child	5
	IČ 14 (H2)	LgC	F	adult	25–50
	obj.523/K800/2005	LgC	N	juvenile	16
Těšetice-Kyjovice	1/1967	LgC	N	child	2
	3/1972	LgC	M	adult	25–40
	4/1974	LgC	M	adult	25–50
	6/1967	LgC	N	child	5
	8/1976	LgC	F	adult	20–35
	14/1988	LgC	F	adult	25–40
Těšetice-Kyjovice	2_1/1968	SPC	M	adult	35–50
	2_2/1968	SPC	N	adult	35–45
	7/1976	SPC	N	juvenile	15–18
	10/3/1981	SPC	N	child	7
	10/2/1981	SPC	F	adult	50–90
	10/1/1981	SPC	M	adult	30–35
	12/1987	SPC	N	adult	ADULT
Těšetice Kyjovice	11/1986	LPC	F	adult	40–50
	15/1991	LPC	N	child	11
	17/1991	LPC	N	child	9–10
	18/1992	LPC	F	juvenile	15–20
	19/1992	LPC	M	juvenile	18–20
	20/1992	LPC	M	juvenile	17–19
	21/1992	LPC	M	adult	20–30
	22/1993	LPC	N	child	1–6
	23/1993	LPC	N	child	4
	26/2005	LPC	N	child	0–1M
Trstěnice	IČ 36	SPC	F	adult	25–40
Určice	K529/1999	LPC	N	adult	ADULT
Vedrovice, Široká u lesa-sídliště	109/1984	LgC	N	child	4–5
Vedrovice, Široká u lesa-sídliště	1/1963	LPC	N	child	6–9M
	2/1963	LPC	N	child	6–7
	3/1966	LPC	N	child	9
	4/1969	LPC	N	child	8
	5/1971	LPC	N	child	6–7
	6/1972	LPC	N	child	3
	7/1972	LPC	N	child	0–1M

Locality	Grave/Inventory number	Culture	Sex	Age Category	Age (years and months)
	8/1974	LPC	N	child	0–1M
	9/1974	LPC	F	adult	70–90
	10/1974	LPC	M	adult	40–70
	11/1974	LPC	M	adult	40–80
Vedrovice, Za dvorem (obj. 37)	H1/1985	LPC	F	adult	20–30
Vedrovice, Za dvorem (pohřebiště)	H2/1985	LPC	M	adult	25–40
Vedrovice, Za dvorem (obj. 56)	H3/1986	LPC	N	child	1.5–2
Vedrovice, Za dvorem (pohřebiště)	H5/1988	LPC	N	child	3
	H6/1988	LPC	F	adult	50–80
	H7/1988	LPC	F	adult	40–80
	H8/1988	LPC	N	child	14
	H9/1988	LPC	F	juvenile	18
	H10/1989	LPC	F	adult	25–40
Vedrovice, Za dvorem (sídliště)	H11/1997	LPC	F	adult	50–90
	H12/1996	LPC	N	child	4
	H13/1997	LPC	N	child	2
Vedrovice, Za dvorem (příkop rondelu)	H14/1997	LPC	M	juvenile	18–20
Velatice	IČ 278	LPC	F	adult	ADULT
	obj. 725/K800	LPC	N	child	2
Vyškov	37/1960	SPC	N	juvenile	15–17
Žádovice	82/1/1986	LPC	N	child	6–7
	82/2/1986	LPC	N	child	2
	H237	LPC	N	child	7
	obj. 95	LPC	N	child	0–1M
	obj. 109/1986	LPC	N	adult	35–45
	obj. 142/H1/1986	LPC	N	child	3–4
	obj. 142/H2/1986	LPC	N	child	5
	obj. 52/H1/1986	LPC	N	child	5
	obj. 52/H2/1986	LPC	N	child	8
	obj. 52/H3/1986	LPC	N	child	5
Želešice	I/79	LPC	F	adult	30–50
Židlochovice	IČ 1617	LPC	M	adult	ADULT

PALAEOPATHOLOGICAL CHARACTERISTICS

WORKLOAD

Traces of workload were found in bones and even teeth of both men and women of all three Neolithic cultures in Moravia. There were some cases recorded of a pronounced muscle relief on the bones of the upper and lower extremities, more obvious in middle-aged and older individuals. On the phalanges of fingers of 6 women from the LPC period, one from the LgC and also two men (LgC, Těšetice-Kyjovice, grave 3; LPC Vedrovice, grave 10), longitudinal bone rims with pronounced insertion sites for short flexors (m. interossei et lumbricales) were found at the edges of the palmar surface of the proximal phalanges of three-phalanx fingers, and also on middle phalanges for the flexor digitorum superficialis, "phalanx flexor hypertrophy" (Lai and Lowell 1992), which occurred as a result of long-term workload (fig. 2).

The said bone rims on the phalanges of fingers were due to long-term work, probably on processing textile fibres, and they also have been interpreted so (Dočkalová and Čižmář 2008a).

In a man (age 25–40 years, grave 3/1972 from Těšetice-Kyjovice) from the LgC period and a woman (age 50–90 years, grave 10/2/1981 from Těšetice-Kyjovice) from the SPC period, bone rims on the phalanges were just indistinct.

In a woman (age 50–85 years; 734/H801/2004) from the LPC period in Modřice, apart from the above mentioned bone rims on three-phalanx fin-

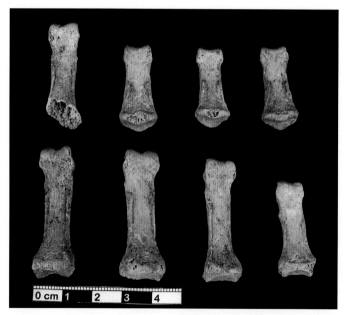

Fig. 2. Pronounced bone rims on phalanges of the hand in a woman (age 50–85 years) from Modřice (734 H801/2004).

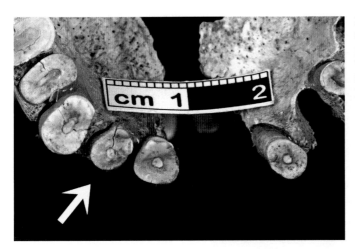

Fig. 3. *Grooves on the canine* and first premolar due to their use as a working tool in a woman (age 50–85 years) from Modřice (734/H801/2004).

gers, we found rounded grooves on the canine and first premolar in the left half of the upper jaw (fig. 3), which were probably connected with the use of the teeth as working tools.

On the lumbar vertebrae of a woman, aged 35–40 years, found in a mining pit in Krumlov forest (LgC, 2a/2002), Schmorl's nodes were detected.

CONGENITAL DEFECTS

On the skull of a man of the LPC, age 40–70 years (Vedrovice, grave 10/1974), a widened canalis incisivus was found, with 14% frequency (N7 individuals examined).

In the region of the cervical spine of a five-year-old child (Žádovice, grave 52/H11986), a *congenital deformity of the atlas* (fig. 4a) and fusion of the axis with C3 were found, with 15% prevalence (N13 children's cervical spines examined) (fig. 4b).

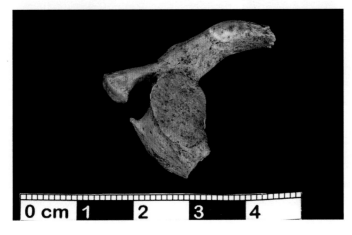

Fig. 4a. *Congenital deformity of the atlas,* Žádovice H52/1/1986. LPC, a 5-year-old child.

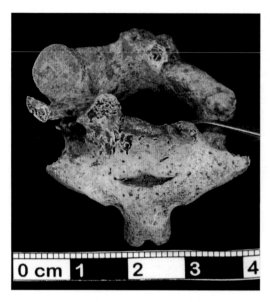

Fig. 4b. *Klippel-Fail syndrome,* fusion of the axis with the 3rd cervical vertebra, Žádovice H52/1/1986, LPC, a 5-year-old child.

In a man at the age of 65–90 years (LPC, Brno-Starý Lískovec, K 806/obj. 7727/2008), the congenital fusion of the anterior parts of cervical vertebrae C3–C5 occurred, with 16.7% frequency (N6 well-preserved male cervical spines examined) (fig. 5a, b).

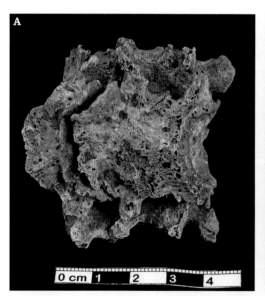

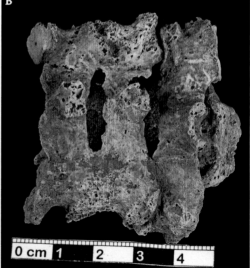

Fig. 5a–b. Fusion of the front bodies of cervical vertebrae C3–C5, Brno-Starý Lískovec LPC, K 806/feature 7727/2008, a man, age 50–59 years, A: ventral view, B: dorsal view.

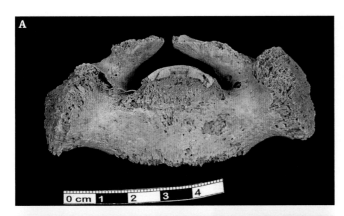

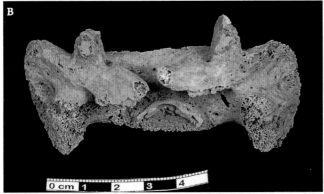

Fig. 6a–b. *Spina bifida,* woman, age 15–17 years (LPC, Mašovice-Pšeničné, H1/feature 613/2003), A: ventral view, B: dorsal view.

Bone fusions in the region of the cervical spine are usually classified within *Klippel-Feil syndrome,* described in 1912 (Dungl 2005; Helmi and Pruzansky 1980).

In the upper part of the sacral bone, spina bifida was found in a young woman, age 15–17 years, from Mašovice (grave 1/feature 613/2003, LPC), with 20% frequency (N5 female sacral bones examined) (fig. 6a, b).

In the region of the lower part of the sacral spine, a totally cleft sacral bone (*canalis sacralis apertus*) was found in a 20-to-25-year-old woman of the LgC population from the site Hnanice I u Znojma, with 33% frequency (N3 sacral bones examined) (fig. 7).

The population that was most severely affected by congenital defects was the LPC, with the most often inflicted part of the skeleton being the vertebral column.

TRAUMAS

Multiple injuries were found on the skeleton of a man, aged 20–29 years, from the burial 2/feature 705/2003 (LgC) at the site Mašovice-Pšeničné. On

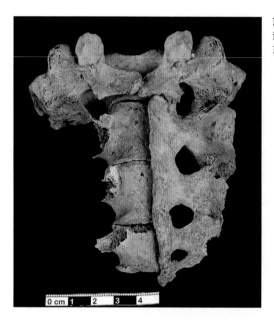

Fig. 7. *Canalis sacralis apertus* in a woman, age 20–25 years, Hnanice, feature 3/1992, LgC.

his skull, at the border of the left temporal and parietal regions, there was an oval opening (22 × 18 mm), with a perpendicular edge cranially and sloping inwards caudally. The edges did not show any signs of healing. In the occipital direction, there is a loose part, 10 × 5 mm large, at the edge of the opening. It may have been pushed inside by violent force. Diverging from the opening, three fracture lines exit, the lower two into the fossa temporalis, which is broken into six fragments, while the third is directed towards the frontal region (fig. 8a).

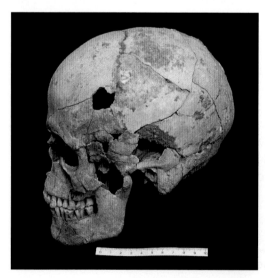

Fig. 8a. *Perimortal defect* of the calvaria vault in the parietal region with a star-shaped break line and a *splintered fracture* in the left temporal region in a man, age 20–29 years, Mašovice H1/ K 1066/41/2003, LgC.

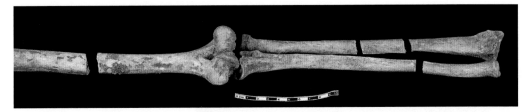

Fig. 8b. *Complex comminuted fracture* of the forearm and humerus of a man from Mašovice
(age 20–29 years, H1/K1066/41/2003,LgC).

In the middle part of the right clavicle, a fracture line is found, running
mediolaterally and with edges covered with calcareous crust. The left clavicle
is intact. On the right humerus, a *supratrochlear fracture* with the fracture line
being found near the fossa olecranii, running sideways craniocaudally. There
is a triangular fragment, around 7 × 3 mm, in the fossa olecrani, and is partially pushed inwards. This might be proof of a violent assault from behind.
On the border of the medial and distal third of the left humerus, a transverse
fracture is found, with fracture lines being covered with calcareous crust.
Fractures were also found on the bones of the left forearm. In the middle part
of the radius, there was a 4-centimetre fragment with a horizontal fracture
line running about 8 cm from the distal edge of the bone. The left ulna shows
a transverse fracture in the distal third, about 7 cm from the distal end of the
bone. Distal break lines on both bones are approximately at the same level
(fig. 8b).

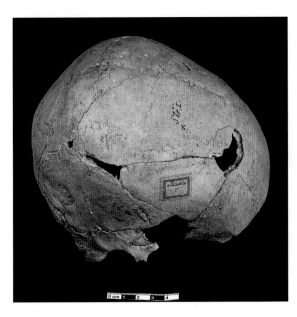

Fig. 9. *Perimortal fracture*
with a star shaped break line,
Střelice H1/12, grave no. 12, LgC,
a woman over 50 years of age.

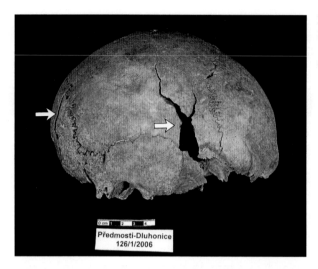

Fig. 10. *Perimortal fractures,* Předmostí-Dluhonice (126/H1/2006, LgC, woman aged 20–40 years).

Bones of the right forearm are intact. On the ribs, there are fracture lines at the angles of 4 left and 5 right ribs. This may suggest a *serial fracture of ribs* due to pressure on the thorax from the sides.

Another trauma of the skull in the LgC was found in a 50-to-90-year-old woman from Střelice (H 1/12), who had a *perimortal fracture* with a star-shaped break line and a central round fragment, 30 mm in diameter, on the right parietal bone adjacent to the frontal bone (fig. 9).

On the right parietal bone of a woman from Předmostí-Dluhonice (LgC, 126/1/2006), aged 20–40 years (Schenk et al. 2007), a depression is found, sized 30 × 20 mm, with rounded edges, with a prominence on the inner surface of the skull and slight trabecular reaction at the base of the skull. Anterior to this lesion, a Y-shaped fracture line is found in the parietal region, with its front branch reaching the temporal region via the coronal suture.

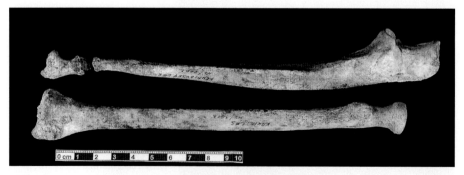

Fig. 11a. *Fracture of the left ulna with a pseudoarthrosis* in a woman (age 35–40 years), LgC, in Krumlov forest (2a/2002).

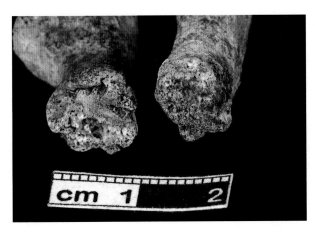

Fig. 11b. *Fracture* of the left ulna with a *pseudoarthrosis* in a woman (age 35–40 years), LgC, in Krumlov forest (2a/2002), detail with beginning arthrotic signs.

Another fracture line can be seen in the occipital region. Both fractures have sharp edges and are not healed (fig. 10).

On the postcranial skeleton of the 35-to-40-year-old woman from a mining pit in the Krumlov forest (LgC, 2a/2002), a poorly healed fracture of the cervix of the left ulna was found, where the two bone ends did not unite and a *pseudoarthrosis* occurred (fig. 11a, b).

VERTEBRAL OSTEOPHYTES

In total, vertebrae were examined in 39 individuals of the LPC (fig. 12), 16 of the LgC and 3 of the SPC. Osteophytes were examined separately for each portion of the vertebral column. The cervical spine was examined in 27 individuals of the LPC, 12 individuals of the LgC and 2 individuals of the SPC; thoracic spine in 18 individuals of the LPC, 9 individuals of the LgC and 2 individuals

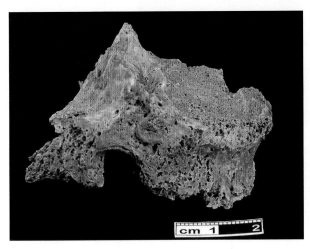

Fig. 12. *Deformation spondylosis*, adult, age 40–50 years (LPC, Určice-Alojzov, 1/K,529/199).

of the SPC; lumbar spine in 20 individuals of the LBK, 9 individuals of the LgC and 2 individuals of the SPC. Osteophytes occurred most often in the LPC women on the thoracic spine (25% with 2 osteophytes) and on the lumbar spine (25% with 3 osteophytes).

PERIOSTITIS

In an LgC woman from Hnanice I (feature 3/1992), aged 20–25 years, *periostitis of a rib* near the tuberculum costae (7 × 5 mm) was found—*tuberculosis* cannot be excluded. Other periostitic changes were identified in three cases in the LPC, in a neonate (0–1 month) from Těšetice-Kyjovice (KH 26/2005), where periostitis is found supraglabellarly to the extent of 30 × 20 mm in the horizontal direction. Further, in an LPC neonate from Vedrovice (7/1972) parietal periostitis was identified, with radial arrangement of the grooves in facies interna ossis parietalis, suggesting suspected *meningitis* (fig. 13), and a 4-year-old child (Vedrovice H12/1996 from the settlement Za Dvorem, LPC), where we identified osteoplastic periostitis changes on the inner surface of the cranium along the sulcus sagittalis superior, to the extent of 90 × 40 mm.

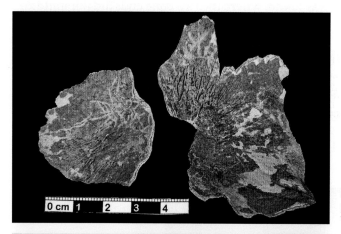

Fig. 13. *Intracranial periostitis*, neonate from Vedrovice, LPC (7, 1972).

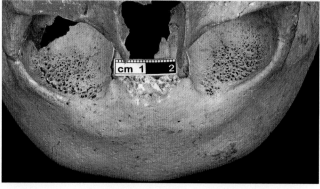

Fig. 14. Bilateral *cribra orbitalia*, trabecular form, Prostějov-Čechůvky K15/35/2004, LgC, age 14–15 years.

CRIBRA ORBITALIA

Cribra manifest themselves macroscopically as delimitated areas of holes and porosities in the internal part of the roof of the orbit (fig. 14). In the LPC, some of the types of orbital cribra were found in 8 out of 26 right orbits (30.7%) and in 14 out of 28 left orbits (50%). In the LgC, cribra orbitalia were found in 4 out of 14 right orbits (25%) and in 5 out of 12 left orbits (41%). In the SPC, cribra orbitalia were found in 1 out of 6 right orbits (16.7%) and 1 out of 5 left orbits (14.3%).

The frequency of these pathologic lesions decreases from the LPC and the LgC to the SPC in the right orbit (LPC 30.7%, LgC 25%, SPC 16.7%) as well as in the left orbit (LPC 77.8%, LgC 41%, SPC 14.3%). On the other hand, the frequency of the most serious type 3 increases from 7% in the LPC (2 out of 28 left orbits) up to 25% in the LgC (3 out of 12 left orbits).

POROTIC HYPEROSTOSIS

Occurred on parietal and occipital bones (fig. 15) and on ribs.

PARIETAL BONES

The set examined included 41 left and 42 right parietal bones of adults as well as children of the LPC, 18 left and 20 right parietal bones of the LgC and 6 left and 7 right parietal bones of the SPC.

In the LPC, porotic hyperostosis was found on one unidentified left parietal bone and two unidentified right parietal bones. In the LgC, porotic hyperostosis was found in the woman 2a/2002 from the mining pit in Krumlov forest.

OCCIPITAL BONES

In the LPC, the condition was found in eight women (12.5%) and in one unidentified individual (50%). In the LgC, there was a finding in the woman 2a/2002 from the mining pit in Krumlov forest.

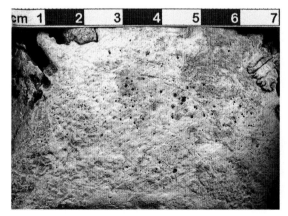

Fig. 15. *Porotic hyperostosis* on the occipital bone in a woman (age 25–35 years, LPC, Držovice 2/1989).

RIBS
In the LPC, the condition was found in 1 out of 8 men (12.5%) and 1 out of 8 women (12.5%). Traces of porosity were only found in the LPC but none in the LgC or SPC.

HARRIS LINES
Periods of distress (illness, famine) within the period of growth of the individual manifest as Harris lines (*growth arrest lines*), horizontal lines of dense bone tissue formed due to retardation of growth, which are visible on x-rays of the tibias. In the set from the Neolithic settlements in Moravia, Harris lines were identified in 11 women and 4 men (Dočkalová and Čižmář 2008a). At the LPC burial site in Vedrovice, Harris lines were found in 15 men, 4 women and 8 children (Dočkalová 2008).

TUMOURS
Of tumours we only found incipient meningioma in a woman, aged 40–50 years (LPC, Těšetice-Kyjovice, grave 11/ 1986), who showed increased vascularization around the left, deepened middle meningeal artery, entering a 5 mm pacchionian granulation adjacent the sagittal sinus, i.e. the signs that were described by Campillo (1977, 143–156) for *parasagittal meningioma* (fig. 16).

PAGET'S DISEASE OF BONE
Osteitis deformans, known as Paget's disease, is bone dysplasia of unknown aetiology, affecting individuals over 40 years of age. In the morphological aspect, excessive bone remodelling is characteristic (Adler 2000). In an individual of unidentified sex from Střelice 9/15, aged 25–50 years (fig. 17a, b), this disease was diagnosed on the basis of thickening of the wall of the cranium

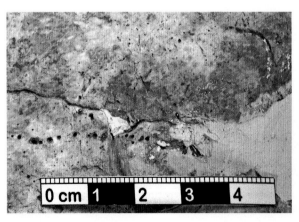

Fig. 16. Incipient *meningioma* with increased vascularization around the left middle meningeal artery in woman (age 40–50 years, Těšetice-Kyjovice H11/1986), LPC.

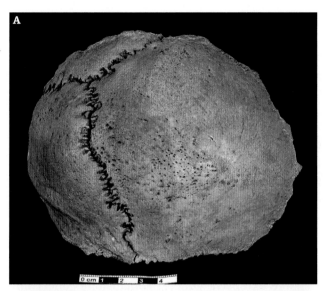

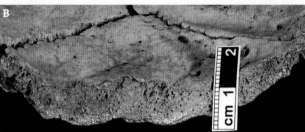

Fig. 17a–b. *Paget's disease*, Střelice, grave no. 9/15, LgC, unidentified individual, age 30 to 40 years, A: porous lamina of the outer wall, B: detail of the cranial wall.

by 1–2 cm and the x-ray findings of an enlarged, sclerotic lamina interna and a thickened, porous lamina externa as well as the cluster of osteosclerosis.

DISCUSSION

The transition from the hunting and gathering way of life to agriculture had an extensive impact on the health state of the population of the first farmers. Changes occurred, apart from other things, in the development, growth and robustness of the skeleton. It was an individual's body height that indirectly indicated their state of health. In the populations from the upper Palaeolithic to Neolithic period, a considerable decrease of body height can be observed (Meiklejohn et al. 1984; Cohen 2009, 592). Fojtová et al. (2008) discovered that the process of body height decrease had continued in the Neolithic period as well. In the set from Moravia (N21), during the Neolithic period (from the LPC to LgC) the body height decreased by 10 cm in men and by 5 cm in women, eventually reaching the lowest values in women of the Moravian Painted Ware Culture (LgC) with the minimum of 145 cm in some women (chapter 8).

Genomically, it has been proven that the mixing of the LPC with hunter-gatherers in Central Europe was still ongoing even in 5545 ± 65 B.C. From Germany, 29 individuals from the early Neolithic LPC and 11 individuals of the middle Neolithic period were analysed, four of them from the site Blätterhöhle were the result of the mixing of Neolithic peasants and hunters-gatherers relatively late in the Neolithic period (Bollongino et al. 2013).

In Blätterhöhle, evidence was found for asymmetrical gene transfer between Neolithic farmers and hunter-gatherers. Three farmers identified by stable isotopes were found to be of hunter descent in 40–50%, while the individual Bla 8, who presented with findings depicting their fisher way of life was genetically close to hunters-gatherers and showed 27% farmer descent on mixing (Lipson et al. 2017).

The state of dentition and epidemiologic conditions worsened as well (Cohen and Armelagos 1984; Larsen 1995; Eshed et al. 2010; Macintosh et al. 2016). However, the lack of skeletal material, from the late Neolithic period, in particular, does not enable extensive general conclusions concerning the differences in the state of health between the populations in particular phases of the Neolithic period in the territory of Moravia.

PHYSICAL ACTIVITIES IN THE FARMING WAY OF LIFE

Physical activities in the farming way of life manifested themselves with specific changes on bones that were caused by the exertion of work (Eshed et al. 2004). Men and often also women had a pronounced muscle relief on the skull and upper as well as lower extremities. In women and some men, longitudinal rims on phalanges of the fingers were found, as proof of long-term and hard manual work.

As an example, we can mention two women (aged 50–90 years; feature 551/K800/2004 and feature 734K801/2004) from the LPC in Modřice, who showed pronounced longitudinal rims on proximal and medial phalanges of the fingers (fig. 2). These rims occurred at the same time as mutilation of the teeth, groove-like impressions on upper incisors. The teeth were used as a working tool.

Rims on medial phalanges of fingers, "phalanx flexor hypertrophy," were caused by excessive activity of the superficial flexor of the hand (m. flexor digitorum superficialis), which bends the middle phalanx in the 2nd to 5th finger. Similar changes were described, for example, in an Egyptian scribe from Thebes, who had them on his right hand (Kennedy et al. 1986), but also in Canadian fur traders, who had to hold the paddle in a firm grip for several days in line when travelling (Lai and Lowell 1992).

Rims on the proximal phalanges were created by excessive activity of the interosseous muscles (mm. interossei) and the lumbricals of the hand, which flex the proximal phalanges but also extend the medial and distal phalanges at the same time. From the above-mentioned changes, the pattern of motion is obvious, with precise excessive muscle activity of the superficial long flexors at the beginning of the motion with the maximum in metacarpophalangeal joints, and with subsequent stabilization of short flexors and minor motion in the interphalangeal joint on extension of the distal two phalanges. All that was done in opposition of the thumb, which was not involved in the muscle activities in any way that could cause the rims. Such a pattern of motion could correspond to weaving, which also suggests the use of incisors in the two women as a third hand. Nor can the use of the teeth as a tool be excluded, either, in production of baskets of wicker, held in the mouth, or in the production of strings by pulling them between the teeth. Grooves connected with such activity were identified in one man and three women from Nitra as well as in 14 individuals from Vedrovice, predominantly women (Frayer 2004; Tvrdý 2016a).

Considering the fact that the *grooves in the canine and the premolar* in the woman from Modřice (Feature 734 / H801/2004) are parallel (fig. 3) and over 2 mm wide, we would rather incline to believe in holding firmly suspended fibres on weaving the fishing nets, as we know from ethnologic sources (Larsen 1985), and in men, in turn, on processing of tendons prepared for bow production, as described by Hansen (1984) in case of the Eskimo from Greenland.

In the LPC population from the burial site in Vedrovice, the percentage of adult individuals with bone rims on phalanges of the fingers even exceeded 80% (Dočkalová 2008).

In individuals of the LgC and SPC from Těšetice-Kyjovice, however, the rims observed on the phalanges of three-phalanx fingers were less conspicuous and often just as mere traces.

The vertebral column is another part of the skeleton that is often affected by a heavy workload. *Osteophytes* may occur, as well as reduction of the height of the vertebral bodies, reduction of intervertebral discs and the *Schmorl's nodes* (intraspongious vertebral herniations), which originate due to prolapse of the tissue of intervertebral discs into the vertebral bodies, most often on the lower thoracic and lumbar spine. Many changes on the vertebral column are due to the process of ageing, and not always they can be discriminated from the changes due to excessive workload, as the cause of the damage to the vertebral column often involves more factors. In our set, the damage to the vertebral column, particularly in the form of osteophytes, mainly occurred in women from the period of the LPC. In the LgC, conspicuous traces were found on the skeletons of two women buried in the mining pit in the Krumlov forest. These women ranked among the shortest within the Neolithic period in Moravia and their skeletons showed osteophytes, Schmorl's nodes, porotic hyperostosis, Harris lines, pronounced muscle relief as evidence of long-term physical exertion and periods of distress. One factor that cannot be excluded is their involvement in the chert mining in the Krumlov forest (Tvrdý 2010), as the stress factors involved are flexion and lateral motion of the spine on lifting heavy weights, which can be expected in prehistoric hunters and farmers as well as stone cutters.

Capasso et al. (1998, 38) distinguished the types of bone changes on a herniated nucleus pulposus in various directions: (A) intraspongious herniation, without crossing the anulus fibrosus (Schmorl's node properly); (B) herniated nucleus pulposus with a posterior crossing of anulus fibrosus ("intracanal herniation"), particularly connected with physical exertion when the vertebral column is in flexion; (C) herniated nucleus pulposus with anterior crossing of the anulus fibrosus; (D) herniated nucleus pulposus with posterolateral crossing of the anulus fibrosus (only this type of herniation can compress the nerve roots so that pain will occur in the lower extremities).

On the material from Herculaneum, Capasso also identified various degrees of development of *Schmorl's node*: *type A*—in progress, where microscopic porosity and erosion are present at the base; *type B*—recent, when the herniation affected the nucleus pulposus just a short time before the death and the base shows microscopic porosity with bone reaction; *type C*—old herniation, in which the base is microscopically created by the cortical bone, a "finished aspect"; *type D*—very old herniation, with the same microscopic appearance.

CONGENITAL DEFECTS

The vertebral column was the most affected part of the skeleton, too, as for congenital defects. The most common ones were, in particular, fusions of vertebrae and spina bifida, mainly in the region of the cervical spine, first described by Klippel together with Feil in 1912. The incidence is reported between 1:30,000 and 1:50,000.

Klippel-Feil syndrome is congenital synostosis of two or more cervical vertebrae which clinically manifests in shortening of the neck with a low scalp margin and considerable limitation in motion of the cervical spine. It is due to a disorder of segmentation of mesodermal somites during the 3rd to 8th week of pregnancy, fusion of C2 and C3 is inherited in the autosomal dominant way.

Three morphologic types are distinguished: *Type I*, with massive fusion of several cervical and upper thoracic vertebrae; *type II* is fusion of one to two intervertebral spaces with occurrence of abnormally shaped "half-vertebrae"; and in *type III* the cervical fusions are accompanied with fusion in the lower thoracic or upper lumbar spine (Dungl 2005, 671–676; Helmi and Pruzansky 1980, 65–88).

CRIBRA ORBITALIA

Cribra orbitalia are commonly seen on skeletal material of all periods and their aetiology is believed to be connected with disturbances in haematopoiesis and with anaemia due to malnutrition, distress and infectious diseases (Rivera and Mirazon Lahr 2017). In our set, the frequency of these pathologic lesions decreases from the LPC to the LgC and eventually the SPC in the right as well as left orbits. On the other hand, the frequency of the most serious type 3 increases from 7% in the LPC (2 out of 28 left orbits) to 25% in the LgC (3 out of 12 left orbits). In the LPC population within the whole region of Central Europe, children and women were more often affected (Hedges et al. 2013, 371). In children, the worse state of health is observed, probably due to premature weaning, which is rather common is settler communities, unlike in those of hunters-gatherers (Ash et al. 2016).

Porotic hyperostosis usually has similar signs and causes like cribra orbitalia and often accompanies them but its accurate aetiology may be different (Rivera and Mirazon Lahr 2017). In Neolithic settings in Moravia, it was most often found in individuals of the LPC.

Harris lines in some cases occur together with cribra orbitalia, which may suggest poor nutrition, infectious diseases or other factors influencing the incidence of these signs.

PERIOSTITIS

Inflammation of the periosteum can occur for various causes, such as infectious disease, injury or tumour (Adler 2000). The bone with the periosteum similarly responds to various influences—in infectious diseases by lines, in tumours—as a rule—by projections and tubercles, either generalized with more bones affected, or to a limited extent with only one bone affected (Gladykowska-Rzeczycka 1998).

In a woman of the LgC from Hnanice I (feature 3/ 1992), aged 20-25 years, periostitis of a rib was found near the tubercle of the rib (7 × 5 mm), and tuberculosis could not be excluded. TB did occur in Neolithic cultures, e.g. in the man of the LPC (grave 34/1965, Nitra-Horné Krškany), aged 35-40 years, periostitis not only occurred on the ribs but even the bodies of two thoracic vertebrae collapsed, which contributed to the development of a deformity of the vertebral column (Whittle et al. 2013; Tvrdý 2016a).

The cause of periostitis may or may not be just specific inflammation as TB in the above cases. In a neonate of the LPC (in grave 7/1972 from Vedrovice) it was a nonspecific bacterial inflammation, which manifested in the radial pattern of the grooves on the inner side of the parietal bone, and inflammation of the meninges. It was meningitis that killed the baby. The infection was probably contracted from the birth canal.

TUMOURS

In the set described, we only found a stigma of a benign tumour, incipient *meningioma*, in a woman of the LPC (Těšetice-Kyjovice, grave 11/1986), aged 40–50 years, who showed increased vascularization around the left deep middle meningeal artery, entering a large pacchionian granulation. Similar stigmata were found by the neurosurgeon Domingo Campillo (1977, 145) at the Neolithic burial site of Bóvila Madurel.

In our set, we only found benign tumours. The incidence of malignant tumours indisputably begins in the Neolithic period, which was undoubtedly connected with the existence or rather the rise of risk factors in the environment. Only in the case of European prehistoric cultures, can they be described as relatively rare (Strouhal and Němečková 2008, 165).

In the view of differential diagnosis, the finding from Střelice must be judged as well, where Paget's disease of bone (osteitis deformans) was suspected. The view may be taken that there were bone changes due to blood disease, especially some type of haemolytic anaemia. Vyhnánek (1976, 144) also took thalassemia major, sickle cell anaemia and familial haemolytic icterus into consideration as possible causes of the brush-shaped skulls that he had found in Mikulčice. As an important diagnostic sign, he pinpointed the fact that the thickening of the skull wall completely disappears adjacent to the sutures, where the thickness of flat bones of the skull is adequate in anaemias. In our case, i.e. the finding from Střelice, the thickness of the skull wall seems to be even, which does not match a skull in anaemia or a rachitic skull, which Vyhnánek also considered for differential diagnosis and which would, vice versa, show some thickening at the edges of the flat bones.

EVIDENCE OF VIOLENCE

Evidence of violence is no exception in the Neolithic period (Schulting and Fibiger 2012), which is testified by sets of skeletons with traces of violence from the German LPC (5600–4900 B.C.) sites Talheim (Wahl and Trautmann 2012) or Schöneck-Kilianstädten (Meyer et al. 2015). Some sites that had been considered as possible locations of war conflicts, however, according to some interpretations served as places of a specific funeral rite, e.g. the well-known Herxheim (Orschiedt and Haidle 2006). In the early Neolithic period, execution of adult males (non-local) was newly proven in Halberstadt in Germany. Individuals number 5 to 8 had one *cranial trauma* each, the ninth two, and another five-six traumas each. The injuries were found on the dorsal side of the skull (12.92%), affecting the posterior part of the parietal area (7.54%) and the upper part of the occipital area (1.8%). Only one perimortal trauma was found on the frontal bone (1.8%). This injury was found in the individual number 4 (Meyer et al. 2018).

TRAUMAS

Traumas are sometimes identified even on children's skeletons, for example in the two 4-to-5-year-old children buried together with a young woman in the triple grave H48-49-50/65 at the LPC burial site Nitra-Horné Krškany in Slovakia. Both children had perimortal traumas on their skulls (Whittle et al. 2013; Tvrdý 2016a). From the late Neolithic (LgC) period in Moravia, multiple injuries were found on the skeleton of a young man from Mašovice-Pšeničné (fig. 8), suggesting the idea of stoning a lying person to death, or burying him with rocks within the six weeks following the death, when bones can still be broken in this specific way.

Traumas on the skulls of the women from Střelice or Předmostí-Dluhonice match hits from the side with blunt instruments, probably shoe-adze or stone, which subsequently leave a star-shaped fracture, like in Střelice (fig. 9), or break lines at the sides of the impact area, as in Předmostí-Dluhonice (fig. 10).

Fracture of the cervix of the *left ulna with a pseudoarthrosis* in an LgC woman from the mining pit in the Krumlov forest, aged 35 to 40 years, most probably happened after a fall onto the ulnar edge of an abducted hand, but direct violence cannot be excluded either. The fragment did not heal to unite, and a pseudoarthrosis developed. Considering the early arthrotic changes, the accident happened 4-7 years prior to death. The woman suffered from painful clicking and skipping on pronation and supination movement. The lower end of the ulna protruded on the dorsal or volar side of the ulnar region (figs. 11a, b).

We can only speculate whether the said cases were about intra- or interpopulation violence, directed rather against adult individuals or whether they were, for example, executed or sacrificed.

Also mentioned must be the evidence of therapeutic interventions in Neolithic populations in Moravia, which can be traced at the site of Vedrovice.

A mature man (grave 82/79 Vedrovice) had an *amputated left forearm*, 10 cm above the wrist. The forearm was healed well, which proves the success of the therapeutic intervention, whether it was done by the affected person alone or with assistance, or by a person from the Vedrovice Neolithic community who was skilled in healing. A previous serious injury or fracture accompanied by infection (Lillie 2008, 143; Crubézy 1996) does not seem very likely, as some signs of inflammation would be inevitably present. The treatment must have followed immediately after the amputation, which may have been a form of punishment too. Even with a missing left hand, the man may have been handicapped socially.

In an adult man, aged 35-40 years (grave 15/75; Vedrovice), two artificial openings in the skull were found, with signs of healing at the edges. According to Crubézy (1996) and Lillie (2008, 144), it seems that the trepanation was performed in response to an injury which the individual survived.

In both these cases, we can see elements of primitive surgical therapeutic intervention.

CONCLUSION

In the survey of pathologic findings on the skeletons of 122 individuals buried in Neolithic settlements in Moravia in the period of the Linear Pottery Culture, LPC, 5000–4700 B.C. (N 82), Stroked Pottery Culture, SPC, 4900–4700 B.C. (N13), and Moravian Painted Ware Culture (also Lengyel Culture, LgC), 4700–4000 B.C., *congenital defects, signs of anaemias* and *traumas* were detected. The incidence of infections was sporadic.

In the population of Neolithic settlements, congenital defects were usually found in the area of the vertebral column, predominantly in the LPC. The frequency of orbital cribra in Neolithic populations showed a descending tendency from the LPC to the LgC and eventually the SPC, in both the right and left orbits.

Vice versa, an ascending frequency of the more complicated type 3 of orbital cribra was found in 7% cases in the LPC but in 25% in the LgC. Porotic hyperostosis occurred on parietal and occipital bones and on the ribs. Signs of porosity, however, were only found in the LPC.

A special group of traumas was injuries to the cranial wall with impression fractures and penetrating injuries. In long bones, fractures of particular bones occurred as well as multiple injuries. In two cases, both at the site of Vedrovice, evidence of primitive surgical treatment was found.

10. COMPARISON OF THE DIET OF THE LENGYEL CULTURE WITH THOSE OF EARLIER NEOLITHIC CULTURES OF MORAVIA: STABLE CARBON AND NITROGEN ISOTOPE ANALYSIS

VÁCLAV SMRČKA, FRANTIŠEK BŮZEK, JARMILA ZOCOVÁ, IVAN ZOC, MARTA DOČKALOVÁ

The possibilities of reconstruction by means of stable isotopes were described by Jiří Šantrůček and his colleagues: "Different places on our planet are specific due to the stable isotopes of biogenic elements contained in them (their concentration can be measured, denoted by the Greek letter delta, δ) and this specificity of the location is transferred into the bodies of all living things through their food. We, as well as all living things, become isotope representatives of the locations where we stay.

If the isotope content was exhibited in colours, then our bodies would change colour according to the places as we would move house. If a body contains a "recording medium" (hair, fingernails...) which constantly grows, it is possible to reconstruct the time and place of one's stay based on the changing isotope "colour" (Šantrůček, Šantrůčková, et al. 2018, 13).

The goal of this research was to compare the diet reconstruction using carbon and nitrogen isotopes of the Lengyel Culture (LgC) in Moravia with preceding Neolithic cultures—the Linear Pottery Culture (LPC) and Stroked Pottery Culture (SPC). In diet reconstruction, it has proved useful to supplement isotope analyses with multi-elemental trace element analysis.

The comparison was conducted in several stages: The 1st stage (10.1) was conducted at the multicultural burial site in Těšetice-Kyjovice using 21 individuals of all the Neolithic Cultures (LgC, LPC, and SPC). Dietary trends were compared between children and adults in terms of plant ($\delta^{13}C$) and animal ($\delta^{15}N$) components of the diet. Preliminary results from the pilot research were published in 2008 (Smrčka et al. 2008; Smrčka, Bůzek, and Zocová 2008) including a summary of archaeological and anthropological research at the site.

In the 2nd stage (10.2), 59 individuals from the whole region of Moravia were tested in the same manner. This allowed for further division into age groups—infants (up to 1 year of age), children (up to age 14), adolescents (juvenis, up to age 20), adults (up to age 40) and maturus (up to age 60), whereas adults were also separated into groups of males and females.

Tab. 1. Stable C, N isotopes in the Neolithic population (N = 21) at the multicultural site of Těšetice-Kyjovice for the LPC (N = 9), LgC (N = 5), SPC (N = 7) Neolithic cultures in age groups (children up to age 14, juvenis up to age 20, adults up to age 40, maturus up to age 60)

TES	$\delta^{13}C$(‰) N	$\delta^{13}C$(‰) Mean	$\delta^{13}C$(‰) SD	$\delta^{13}C$(‰) Min	$\delta^{13}C$(‰) Max	$\delta^{15}N$(‰) N	$\delta^{15}N$(‰) Mean	$\delta^{15}N$(‰) SD	$\delta^{15}N$(‰) Min	$\delta^{15}N$(‰) Max
LPC	9	-20.59	1.09	-22.77	-19.26	9	9.54	0.69	8.85	11.18
Child	4	-21.59	0.83	-22.77	-20.89	4	9.64	1.05	8.85	11.18
Juv	3	-19.74	0.42	-20.00	-19.26	3	9.51	0.43	9.05	9.91
Adult	1	-19.97	0.00	-19.97	-19.97	1	9.50	0.00	9.50	9.50
Matur	1	-19.77	0.00	-19.77	-19.77	1	9.29	0.00	9.29	9.29
LgC	5	-21.84	2.94	-27.02	-19.65	5	10.07	1.54	8.71	12.46
Child	2	-20.29	0.90	-20.92	-19.65	2	11.60	1.22	10.74	12.46
Juv	0					0				
Adult	3	-22.88	3.59	-27.02	-20.64	3	9.04	0.29	8.71	9.22
Matur	0					0				
SPC	7	-20.14	0.38	-20.63	-19.43	7	9.95	1.01	8.42	11.47
Child	1	-20.24	0.00	-20.24	-20.24	1	10.13	0.00	10.13	10.13
Juv	1	-20.18	0.00	-20.18	-20.18	1	8.88	0.00	8.88	8.88
Adult	2	-20.13	0.26	-20.32	-19.95	2	10.86	0.87	10.24	11.47
Matur	3	-20.10	0.62	-20.63	-19.43	3	9.64	1.06	8.42	10.27
Total	21	-20.74	1.64	-27.02	-19.26	21	9.80	1.01	8.42	12.46

LPC — Linear Pottery Culture; LgC — Lengyel, Moravian Painted Ware Culture; SPC — Stroked Pottery Culture

Tab. 2. Stable C, N isotopes in the Neolithic population (N = 21) at the multicultural site of Těšetice-Kyjovice in the LPC (N = 9), LgC (N = 5), and SPC (N = 7) cultures separated according to sex into groups of children, males and females

TES	$\delta^{13}C(‰)$ N	$\delta^{13}C(‰)$ Mean N	$\delta^{13}C(‰)$ SD	$\delta^{13}C(‰)$ Min	$\delta^{13}C(‰)$ Max	$\delta^{15}N(‰)$ N	$\delta^{15}N(‰)$ Mean	$\delta^{15}N(‰)$ SD	$\delta^{15}N(‰)$ Min	$\delta^{15}N(‰)$ Max
LPC	9	-20.59	1.09	-22.77	-19.26	9	9.54	0.69	8.85	11.18
Child	4	-21.59	0.83	-22.77	-20.89	4	9.64	1.05	8.85	11.18
Male	3	-19.74	0.42	-20.00	-19.26	3	9.38	0.29	9.05	9.58
Female	2	-19.87	0.14	-19.97	-19.77	2	9.60	0.44	9.29	9.91
LgC	5	-21.84	2.94	-27.02	-19.65	5	10.07	1.54	8.71	12.46
Child	2	-20.29	0.90	-20.92	-19.65	2	11.60	1.22	10.74	12.46
Male	1	-27.02	0.00	-27.02	-27.02	1	9.22	0.00	9.22	9.22
Female	2	-20.81	0.24	-20.98	-20.64	2	8.96	0.35	8.71	9.20
SPC	7	-20.14	0.38	-20.63	-19.43	7	9.95	1.01	8.42	11.47
Child	1	-20.24	0.00	-20.24	-20.24	1	10.13	0.00	10.13	10.13
Male	3	-20.15	0.19	-20.32	-19.95	3	10.20	1.29	8.88	11.47
Female	3	-20.10	0.62	-20.63	-19.43	3	9.64	1.06	8.42	10.27
Total	21	-20.74	1.64	-27.02	-19.26	21	9.80	1.01	8.42	12.46

10.1 TĚŠETICE-KYJOVICE: STABLE CARBON AND NITROGEN ISOTOPE ANALYSIS

In the **Linear Pottery Culture (LPC)** of Těšetice-Kyjovice, 9 individuals were tested in age groups (children 4, juvenis 3, adult 1, maturus 1) (tab. 1) and according to their sex (children 4, males 3, females 2) (tab. 2).

In the *plant component ($\delta^{13}C$) of the diet*, changes in dietary trends relative to age were discovered. Significant differences at 5% level of significance were found on testing according to age between the 4 children ($\delta^{13}C$ –21.59 ± 0.83‰) and 3 juvenis ($\delta^{13}C$ –19.74 ± 0.42‰), and at 10% level of significance between the children and one adult as well as the one maturus individual (tab. 3 age—analysis of variance; Figure 1 tesage 13LPC).

Tab. 3. Analysis of Variance: Analysis of stable C, N isotope variance in Těšetice-Kyjovice according to age groups in the LPC, LgC and SPC Neolithic cultures. The samples are very small, so statistical results need to be viewed with reservations.

Analysis if variance						
Cult	Isot	F	df	p	Different groups	Graph (.jpg)
All	$\delta^{13}C$	1.147	3;17	0.359		tesage13
	$\delta^{15}N$	0.890	3;17	0.501		tesage15
LPC	$\delta^{13}C$	4.999	3;5	0.058	ChildxJuv p = 0.05; ChildxAdult p = 0.10; ChildxMatur p = 0.10	tesage13LPC
	$\delta^{15}N$	0.046	3;5	0.985		tesage15LPC
LgC	$\delta^{13}C$	0.907	1;3	0.411		tesage13LgC
	$\delta^{15}N$	14.297	1;3	0.032	ChildxAdult p = 0.05	tesage15LgC
SPC	$\delta^{13}C$	0.019	3;3	0.996		tesage13SPC
	$\delta^{15}N$	1.030	3;3	0.490		tesage15SPC
Kruskal–Wallis						
Cult	Isot	χ^2	df	p	Different groups	Graph (.jpg)
All	$\delta^{13}C$	5.918	3	0.116		tesage13
	$\delta^{15}N$	0.764	3	0.858		tesage15
LPC	$\delta^{13}C$	6.300	3	0.098	ChildxAdult p = 0.10	tesage13LPC
	$\delta^{15}N$	3.263	3	0.353		tesage15LPC
LgC	$\delta^{13}C$	0.139	1	0.709		tesage13LgC
	$\delta^{15}N$	5.000	1	0.025	ChildxAdult p = 0.10	tesage15LgC
SPC	$\delta^{13}C$	2.236	3	0.525		tesage13SPC
	$\delta^{15}N$	2.236	3	0.525		tesage15SPC

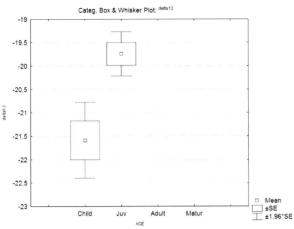

Fig. 1. Significant differences in the plant component of the diet ($\delta^{13}C$) in LPC of Těšetice between children and juvenis; children and adults, at a significance level of 10%. Note: If only one individual is contained in the group, than it is not displayed in the boxplot.

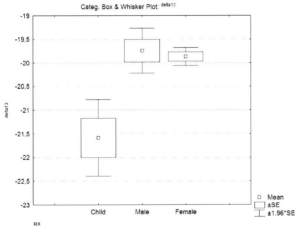

Fig. 2. Differences in the plant component of the diet ($\delta^{13}C$) in LPC of Těšetice between children and males at 1% level of significance, and between children and females at 5% level of significance.

On testing according to sex and separating the group into males (N = 3) and females (N = 2) (tab. 4) there were significant differences between children and females ($\delta^{13}C$ –19.87 ± 0.14‰) at 5% level of significance, and also between children and males ($\delta^{13}C$ –19.74 ± 0.42‰) at 1% level of significance (fig. 2).

In the *animal component ($\delta^{15}N$) of the diet*, in the LPC of Těšetice, on testing according to sex and age, no significant differences were found between children and adults (tab. 3), not even upon differentiation between males and females (tab. 4).

In the **Lengyel Culture (Moravian Painted Ware Culture) (LgC)**, of Těšetice, 5 individuals—2 children and 3 adults (1 male, 2 females)—were tested with respect to sex.

In the *plant component of the diet* on testing according to sexes and on comparison of the children (N = 2) ($\delta^{13}C$ –20.29 ± 0.90‰) and the separated

Tab. 4. Analysis of stable C, N isotope variance in Těšetice-Kyjovice with respect to sex for the groups of children, males, and females, in the LPC, LgC and SPC Neolithic cultures

Cult	Isot	F	df	p	Different groups (LSD)	Graph (.jpg)
				Analysis if variance		
All	$\delta^{13}C$	0.467	2;18	0.634		tessex13
	$\delta^{15}N$	1.263	2;18	0.306		tessex15
LPC	$\delta^{13}C$	8.893	2;6	0.016	ChildxMale p = 0.01; ChildxFemale p = 0.05	tessex13LPC
	$\delta^{15}N$	0.099	2;6	0.907		tessex15LPC
LgC	$\delta^{13}C$	39.286	2;2	0.025	ChildxFemale p = 0.05; ChildxMale p = 0.05	tessex13LgC
	$\delta^{15}N$	4.927	2;2	0.169	ChildxFemale p = 0.10	tessex15LgC
SPC	$\delta^{13}C$	0.034	2;4	0.967		tessex13SPC
	$\delta^{15}N$	0.177	2;4	0.844		tessex15SPC

Cult	Isot	χ^2	df	p	Different groups	Graph (.jpg)
				Kruskal–Wallis		
All	$\delta^{13}C$	2.673	2	0.263		tessex13
	$\delta^{15}N$	0.382	2	0.826		tessex15
LPC	$\delta^{13}C$	6.300	2	0.043	ChildxFemale p = 0.10	tessex13LPC
	$\delta^{15}N$	1.238	2	0.539		tessex15LPC
LgC	$\delta^{13}C$	0.833	2	0.659		tessex13LgC
	$\delta^{15}N$	5.000	2	0.082	ChildxFemale p = 0.10	tessex15LgC
SPC	$\delta^{13}C$	1.556	2	0.459		tessex13SPC
	$\delta^{15}N$	1.556	2	0.459		tessex15SPC

adult group, males (N = 1) and females (N = 2) (tab. 2), significant differences were found between children and females ($\delta^{13}C$ –20.81 ± 0.24‰) as well as between children and the male ($\delta^{13}C$ –27.02 ± 0.00‰) at a significance level of 5% (tab. 4, fig. 3).

In the *animal component of the diet* represented by values of stable nitrogen isotope ($\delta^{15}N$), on testing according to sexes of the 5 LgC individuals, significantly different $\delta^{15}N$ values were found between the children (N = 2) (11.60 ± 1.22‰) and females (N = 2) (8.96 ± 0.35‰) at a significance level of 10% (tab. 4; fig. 4).

It was possible to separate the 5 LgC individuals from Těšetice into age groups (2 children and 3 adults) (tab. 1).

In the *plant component of the diet* represented by the carbon isotope ($\delta^{13}C$), no significant differences were determined for the age groups of LgC (Lengyel, Moravian Painted Ware Culture) of Těšetice.

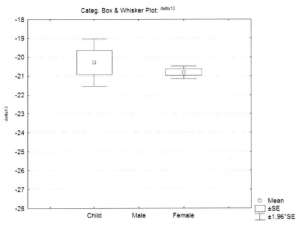

Fig. 3. Differences in the plant component of the diet (δ^{13}C) in LgC of Těšetice between children and females at a significance level of 5%.

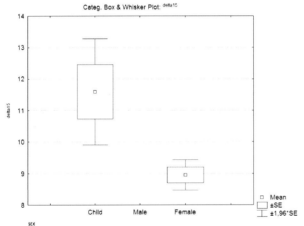

Fig. 4. Differences in the animal component of the diet (δ^{15}N) in LgC of Těšetice, relative to sex, between groups of children and females at 10% level of significance.

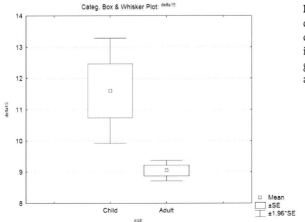

Fig. 5. Illustration of the differences in the animal component of the diet (δ^{15}N) in LgC of Těšetice, in the age groups of children and adults at 5% level of significance.

In the *animal component of the diet ($\delta^{15}N$)*, there were different values for the children (N = 2) (11.60 ± 1.22‰) and the 3 adults, at a significance level of 5% (tab. 3; fig. 5).

In the comparison of $\delta^{15}N$ in the 2 children (11.6 ± 1.22‰) and the adults (N = 3) (9.04 ± 0.29‰) there is an evident decrease in $\delta^{15}N$ values with age within LgC, while the adult diet in both LPC and LgC cultures was similar.

In Těšetice, the highest amounts of protein were found in children, who would apparently catch fish as indicated by the nitrogen isotope analysis (however, in Těšetice, there is only archaeozoological evidence of a catfish) (Smrčka et al. 2008). Archaeological evidence of fishing in this time period is represented by a bone harpoon found in Jezeřany-Maršovice (Rakovský 1985).

In Těšetice, archaeozoological analysis was conducted on 11,025 bones of which approx. 1000 were identified in the 24 LPC objects and 2000 in the 21 LgC objects (Dreslerová 2006).

The proportion of hunted animals grew to 50–60% in LgC in contrast with the 5% of LPC. Domestic animals of the LPC were slaughtered at the age of 4, and so the number of older animals producing milk was higher in LPC than in LgC where animals were slaughtered at the age of 3 already.

The most frequently hunted animals in LgC were beaver, red deer, wild boar and horse (*Equus hydruntinus* and *Equus ferus*). From domestic animals, sheep and goat's bones prevailed.

Trace element analyses showed that in the two LgC males, the concentration of nickel in bones (13.40 μg Ni/g of bone) was significantly higher than that of the 4 LPC males (10.56 μg Ni/g of bone). The increased nickel concentrations of the LgC period could have been caused by consumption of river mussels (Smrčka et al. 2008).

In the **Stroked Pottery Culture** (SPC) in Moravia, no significant differences were determined on testing the animal and plant components of the diet with respect to sex and age.

The conclusion of the pilot research into the diet at the multicultural site in Těšetice demonstrated that in the Lower Neolithic, there was a difference in the diet of children and adults, particularly between children and males, at 1% level of significance.

The LPC population consumed more milk than that of LgC. This was proved by archaeozoological research. In LPC, the older beasts were let to live up to 4 years of age while in LgC, which focused on meat production, cattle would be slaughtered at age 3 already.

10.2 MORAVIAN NEOLITHIC SETTLEMENTS: STABLE CARBON AND NITROGEN ISOTOPE ANALYSIS AND TRACE ELEMENT ANALYSIS

In the **Linear Pottery Culture (LPC)** of Moravia, 34 individuals were tested in age groups (tab. 1) and 30 individuals were tested relative to their sex (tab. 2).

On expanding the Moravian LPC set to 34 individuals, it became possible to separate it into age groups (infants 2, children 17, juvenis 6, adults 8, maturus 1).

In the *plant component of the diet ($\delta^{13}C$)*, changes in dietary trends with respect to age were discovered. There were significant differences at 1% level of significance between the 17 children (**$\delta^{13}C$** –22.27 ± 1.87‰) and 8 adults (**$\delta^{13}C$** –20.23 ± 0.33‰) on testing in relation to age (tab. 1; fig. 1). The information that the diet of children and adults of the LPC differed previously discovered in Těšetice was confirmed for the whole Neolithic region of Moravia.

On testing according to sexes and on splitting the adult group into males (N = 6) and females (N = 7) (tab. 2), significant differences were found between the 17 children and females (**$\delta^{13}C$** –20.22 ± 0.36‰) as well as between children and males (**$\delta^{13}C$** –20.34 ± 1.23‰) at a significance level of 1% (tab. 2; fig. 2).

Trace element analysis at the Vedrovice settlement revealed the reason for the difference in diets of LPC children and adults.

The children's plant-based diet was mostly obtained through forest fruit picking and was similar to that of wild animals, contrarily, the diet of adults was obtained from sources outside the forest.

In comparison with the other members of the LPC population of Vedrovice, children had high concentrations of lead and cadmium. The concentrations of lead, cadmium, as well as rare-earth elements (Yb and Lu) in bones

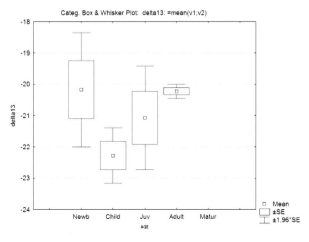

Fig. 1. Differences in the plant component of the diet ($\delta^{13}C$), in the region of Neolithic Moravia in LPC (N = 34), separated into the age groups of children (N = 17) and adults (N = 8), at a significance level of 1%.

Tab. 1. Stable C, N isotopes in the Neolithic population (N = 59) in the region of Moravia in the LPC (N = 34), LgC (N = 13), SPC (N = 12) Neolithic cultures according to age groups (infants up to age 1; children up to age 14; juvenis up to age 20; adults up to age 40; maturus up to age 60)

	$\delta^{13}C(‰)$ N	$\delta^{13}C(‰)$ Mean	$\delta^{13}C(‰)$ SD	$\delta^{13}C(‰)$ Min	$\delta^{13}C(‰)$ Max	$\delta^{15}N(‰)$ N	$\delta^{15}N(‰)$ Mean	$\delta^{15}N(‰)$ SD	$\delta^{15}N(‰)$ Min	$\delta^{15}N(‰)$ Max
LPC	34	−21.38	1.83	−25.03	−19.25	34	10.63	1.59	7.62	14.59
Newb	2	−20.17	1.31	−21.10	−19.25	2	13.32	1.80	12.05	14.59
Child	17	−22.27	1.87	−25.03	−19.91	17	10.61	1.43	8.70	13.20
Juv	6	−21.07	2.07	−24.48	−19.26	6	9.49	1.06	7.62	10.63
Adult	8	−20.23	0.33	−20.75	−19.80	8	11.03	1.56	9.50	14.54
Matur	1	−19.77	0.00	−19.77	−19.77	1	9.29	0.00	9.29	9.29
LgC	13	−20.96	1.89	−27.02	−19.65	13	10.28	1.23	8.71	12.46
Newb	1	−20.61	0.00	−20.61	−20.61	1	8.85	0.00	8.85	8.85
Child	2	−20.29	0.90	−20.92	−19.65	2	11.60	1.22	10.74	12.46
Juv	1	−20.78	0.00	−20.78	−20.78	1	12.02	0.00	12.02	12.02
Adult	7	−21.26	2.59	−27.02	−19.66	7	9.94	1.08	8.71	11.72
Matur	2	−20.85	0.19	−20.99	−20.71	2	9.99	0.07	9.94	10.04
SPC	12	−20.03	1.33	−23.05	−17.71	12	9.97	0.95	8.42	11.47
Newb	0					0				
Child	1	−20.24	0.00	−20.24	−20.24	1	10.13	0.00	10.13	10.13
Juv	2	−20.01	0.25	−20.18	−19.83	2	10.13	1.76	8.88	11.37
Adult	6	−19.97	1.92	−23.05	−17.71	6	10.06	0.90	9.17	11.47
Matur	3	−20.10	0.62	−20.63	−19.43	3	9.64	1.06	8.42	10.27
Total	59	−21.01	1.80	−27.02	−17.71	59	10.42	1.41	7.62	14.59

LPC — Linear Pottery Culture; LgC — Lengyel, Moravian Painted Ware Culture; SPC — Stroked Pottery Culture

Tab. 2. Stable C, N isotopes in the Neolithic population of Moravia (N=50) separated according to sex into groups of children, males and females for the LPC, LgC and SPC Neolithic cultures

	δ¹³C(‰) N	δ¹³C(‰) Mean	δ¹³C(‰) SD	δ¹³C(‰) Min	δ¹³C(‰) Max	δ¹⁵N(‰) N	δ¹⁵N(‰) Mean	δ¹⁵N(‰) SD	δ¹⁵N(‰) Min	δ¹⁵N(‰) Max
LPC	30	−21.41	1.80	−25.03	−19.26	30	10.48	1.24	8.70	13.20
Child	17	−22.27	1.87	−25.03	−19.91	17	10.61	1.43	8.70	13.20
Male	6	−20.34	1.23	−22.78	−19.26	6	10.25	1.27	9.05	12.58
Female	7	−20.22	0.36	−20.75	−19.77	7	10.36	0.76	9.29	11.34
LgC	10	−21.04	2.17	−27.02	−19.65	10	10.28	1.19	8.71	12.46
Child	2	−20.29	0.90	−20.92	−19.65	2	11.60	1.22	10.74	12.46
Male	3	−22.56	3.92	−27.02	−19.66	3	10.32	1.28	9.22	11.72
Female	5	−20.43	0.48	−20.98	−19.81	5	9.73	0.88	8.71	11.06
SPC	10	−19.99	1.45	−23.05	−17.71	10	9.77	0.88	8.42	11.47
Child	1	−20.24	0.00	−20.24	−20.24	1	10.13	0.00	10.13	10.13
Male	5	−19.26	1.23	−20.32	−17.71	5	9.89	1.02	8.88	11.47
Female	4	−20.84	1.55	−23.05	−19.43	4	9.53	0.90	8.42	10.27
Total	50	−21.05	1.86	−27.02	−17.71	50	10.30	1.18	8.42	13.20

LPC — Linear Pottery Culture; LgC — Lengyel, Moravian Painted Ware Culture; SPC — Stroked Pottery Cultur

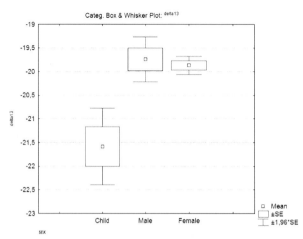

Fig. 2. Differences in the plant component of the diet (δ^{13}C) in the region of Neolithic Moravia for LPC (N = 30) separated according to sex into groups of children (N = 17) and males (N = 6), and children and females (N = 7) at 1% level of significance. (LPC—Linear Pottery Culture).

were also higher in wild animals (roe deer, stag) than in domestic ones (Smrčka et al. 2006).

The Pb concentration in the bones of five children (4.91 ± 5.20 µg/g) was higher than that of the two infants (3.78 ± 1.91 µg/g), two males (1.09 ± 0.87 µg/g) and one female (0.35 µg/g); the mean concentration of lead in bones of the population being 3.5 ± 4 µg Pb/g of bone. The lead content in the soil at the settlement was 16.62 µg/g. When related to calcium, the Pb/Ca ratio was also higher in the five children than in the adults, males and the female.

The Pb concentration in the bones of wild animals, roe deer and stag, (1.82 ± 0.01 µg/g) was higher than that of ten small herbivores (1.02 ± 0.6 µg/g), eight omnivores (0.9 ± 1.0 µg/g) and eleven large herbivores (0.81 ± 0.46 µg/g); the mean Pb concentration in bones of the animal population being 1.0 ± 0.7 µg/g.

The concentration of Cd in the bones of five children (0.23 ± 0.07 µg/g) was higher than in the two infants (0.22 ± 0.10 µg/g), two males (0.11 ± 0.03 µg/g) and one female (0.06 µg); the average concentration for the human population being 0.2 µg/g. The cadmium content in the soil of the settlement was 0.35 µg/g.

The Cd concentration in the bones of wild animals, roe deer and stag, (0.46 ± 0.27 µg/g) was higher than that of ten small herbivores (0.21 ± 0.11 µg/g), eleven large herbivores (0.16 ± 0.05 µg/g), eight omnivores (0.08 ± 0.04 µg/g) and one carnivore (0.08 µg/g)(p < 0,009); the mean Cd concentration in the animal population being 0.2 ± 0.1 µg/g. The differences between the groups were significant reaching the level p = 0.009 (Smrčka et al. 2006).

The most probable source of the aforementioned elements was accumulation of fallout on forest fruits, mushrooms, but also acorns, beechnuts, and conkers (Vencl 1985), which are popular foods of deer. The concentration of heavy elements in forests in contrast to the open fields and meadows was proved even in today's landscapes (Ettler et al. 2005).

It is presumed that children collected forest fruits to a higher extent. The diet of mothers of the infants during pregnancy must have also been supplemented with forest products (Smrčka 2005). Infants would obtain some of the Cd and Pb through the placenta. The degree depended on placental perfusion (Kelman and Walter 1977).

In times of crop failure, flour would be mixed half-and-half (Beranová 2015, 100) with substitutes of grains, among other things: ground rootstocks of bracken, also known as eagle fern, Iceland moss (*Cetraria islandika*)—lichen which had to be debittered, roots of couch grass (*Elytrigia repens*) as well as acorns and conkers.

Yet, what was the essential component of the Neolithic diet of the C3 photosynthetic cycle identified through carbon isotopes in Neolithic Denmark (Tauber 1981), as well as in Central Europe at the Neolithic LPC settlement in Vedrovice (Smrčka et al. 2005) and the burial site in Vedrovice (Smrčka, Bůzek, and Zocová 2008)?

In the Neolithic, the most frequently grown crop in Central Europe was emmer wheat, often in combination with einkorn, in 2:1 ratio. Contrarily, in the Balkans, einkorn wheat was more common. C4, millet, was not common and there was not much of it (Miller et al. 2016; Motuzaite-Matuzeviciute et

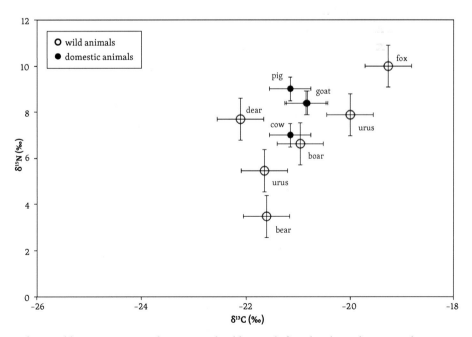

Tab. 3. Stable C,N isotopes in domestic and wild animals found at the Vedrovice settlement.

al. 2013). The most widespread prehistoric cereal had one peculiarity—it was hulled. Both the wheat types—einkorn and emmer, as well as ancient barley varieties, were hulled. Beranová (2015) stated, that dehulling was possible by heating the grains quickly. The husks would then largely fall off by themselves or could be easily removed with fingers.

Prehistoric farmers preferred hulled cereals, because they were less challenging to grow and guaranteed good yields. They would grow even in badly cultivated soil, without the need for fertilisers, it resisted diseases and weather conditions and not a large amount of seeds was needing for sowing.

Tab. 4. Analysis of stable C, N isotope variance in the region of Neolithic Moravia with respect to age groups (infants up to age 1; children up to age 14; juvenis up to age 20; adults up to age 40; maturus up to age 60) in the LPC, LgC and SPC Neolithic cultures

Analysis if variance						
Cult	**Isot**	**F**	**df**	**p**	**Different groups (LSD)**	**Graph (.jpg)**
All	$\delta^{13}C$	2.452	4;54	0.057	ChildxAdult p = 0.01; ChildxMatur p = 0.05; ChildxJuv p = 0.10	allage13
	$\delta^{15}N$	1.679	4;54	0.168	NewbxJuv p =0.05; NewbxMatur p = 0.05	allage15
LPC	$\delta^{13}C$	2.757	4;29	0.047	ChildxAdult p = 0.01	allage13LPC
	$\delta^{15}N$	3.149	4;29	0.029	NewbxJuv p = 0.01; NewbxChild p = 0.05; NewbxAdult p = 0.05	allage15LPC
LgC	$\delta^{13}C$	0.084	4;8	0.985		allage13LgC
	$\delta^{15}N$	2.237	4;8	0.155	NewbxChild p = 0.10; NewbxAdult p = 0.10	allage15LgC
SPC	$\delta^{13}C$	0.011	3;8	0.998		allage13SPC
	$\delta^{15}N$	0.121	3;8	0.942		allage15SPC
Kruskal-Wallis						
Cult	**Isot**	**χ2**	**df**	**p**	**Different groups**	**Graph (.jpg)**
All	$\delta^{13}C$	7.390	4	0.117	ChildxAdult p = 0.10	allage13
	$\delta^{15}N$	2.231	4	0.693		allage15
LPC	$\delta^{13}C$	10.931	4	0.027	ChildxAdult p=0.10	allage13LPC
	$\delta^{15}N$	6.225	4	0.183		allage15LPC
LgC	$\delta^{13}C$	4.090	4	0.394		allage13LgC
	$\delta^{15}N$	5.240	4	0.264		allage15LgC
SPC	$\delta^{13}C$	3.343	4	0.343		allage13SPC
	$\delta^{15}N$	1.333	4	0.721		allage15SPC

LPC—Linear Pottery Culture; LgC—Lengyel, Moravian Painted Ware Culture; SPC—Stroked Pottery Culture

In favourable conditions, 1 ha could yield 25q, but even 10q would be enough in prehistoric conditions.

Ancient food from grains would be made quite easily (Beranová 2015, 63). Coarsely ground wheat would be mixed with water, small flatbreads would be formed and baked in the fireplace or on a hot stone. In ancient Greece, and possibly before that, flatbreads would be eaten unbaked, kneaded from barley flour and dried. These were called maza. It was the food of common men and would be made for storage. It would be moistened with water before consumption.

Tab. 5. Analysis of stable C, N isotope variance in the region of Neolithic Moravia with respect to sex in the groups of children, males and females in the LPC, LgC and SPC Neolithic cultures

Analysis if variance						
Cult	**Isot**	**F**	**df**	**p**	**Different groups (LSD)**	**Graph (.jpg)**
All	$\delta^{13}C$	4.709	2;47	0.014	ChildxFemale p = 0.01; ChildxMale p = 0.01	allsex13
	$\delta^{15}N$	1.943	2;47	0.155	ChildxFemale p = 0.10	allsex15
LPC	$\delta^{13}C$	6.193	2;47	0.006	ChildxFemale p = 0.01; ChildxMale p = 0.01	allsex13LPC
	$\delta^{15}N$	0.216	2;47	0.807		allsex15LPC
LgC	$\delta^{13}C$	1.066	2;47	0.007	ChildxFemale p = 0.01; ChildxMale p = 0.05	allsex13LgC
	$\delta^{15}N$	2.215	2;47	0.698		allsex15LgC
SPC	$\delta^{13}C$	1.471	2;47	0.325		allsex13SPC
	$\delta^{15}N$	0.234	2;47	0.345		allsex15SPC
Kruskal-Wallis						
Cult	**Isot**	**χ2**	**df**	**p**	**Different groups**	**Graph (.jpg)**
All	$\delta^{13}C$	9.820	2	0.007	ChildxMale p = 0.01; ChildxFemale p = 0.05	allsex13
	$\delta^{15}N$	1.336	2	0.513		allsex15
LPC	$\delta^{13}C$	11.002	2	0.004	ChildxFemale p = 0.05; ChildxMale p = 0.05	allsex13LPC
	$\delta^{15}N$	0.868	2	0.648		allsex15LPC
LgC	$\delta^{13}C$	0.533	2	0.766		allsex13LgC
	$\delta^{15}N$	4.133	2	0.127	ChildxFemale p > 0.10	allsex15LgC
SPC	$\delta^{13}C$	3.800	2	0.150		allsex13SPC
	$\delta^{15}N$	1.200	2	0.549		allsex15SPC

LPC—Linear Pottery Culture; LgC—Lengyel, Moravian Painted Ware Culture;
SPC—Stroked Pottery Culture

Flatbreads were made ever since the origins of agriculture, however, there are not many pieces of archaeological evidence.

The best conditions for preservation existed in Switzerland in pile dwellings, where in the wet, muddy layers many remains of plants and products made of these were preserved.

In the Twann settlement dated to 5000–6000 years ago (3700 B.C., according to C14 calibrated dating almost 1000 years earlier) from the late to final Stone Age, patty-like lumps of moistened cereal mixed with flour and baked either directly in the fireplace or in ashes, were discovered.

Dough-like lumps of grains mixed with flour from the Twann settlement we "pre-baked" and then stored in a pot as a reserve. Before consumption they were likely to be heated or prepared otherwise.

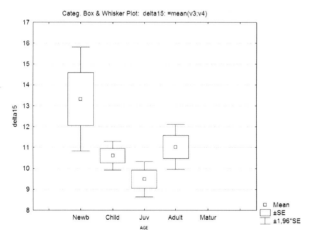

Fig. 3. Illustration of the differences in the animal component of the diet (δ^{15}N) in the region of Neolithic Moravia for the age groups of infants (N = 2) and children (N = 17), and infants and adults (N = 8) at 5% level of significance; infants and juvenis (N = 6) at 1% level of significance.

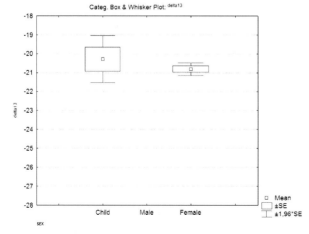

Fig. 4. Differences in the plant component of the diet (δ^{13}C) for LgC in the region of Neolithic Moravia between children (N = 2) and females (N = 5) at 10% level of significance (LgC—Lengyel, Moravian Painted Ware Culture).

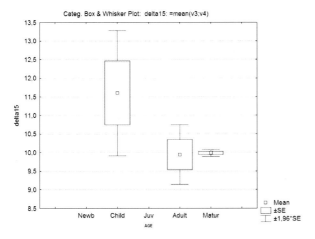

Fig. 5. Illustration of the differences in the animal component of the diet ($\delta^{15}N$) for LgC in the region of Neolithic Moravia, according to age groups—1 infant, children (N = 2) and adults (N = 7) at 10% level of significance (LgC—Lengyel, Moravian Painted Ware Culture).

At the site in Twann, a settlement of the Cortaillod Culture in Switzerland, the oldest preserved leavened bread was also discovered (around 3500 B.C., that is, about 200 years later than the flatbreads from the same site).

It was found in 1976 and weighed 25.20 g. It was subjected to detailed examination by Max Währen (1984), who proved that it was a leavened bread and not an unleavened flatbread. He presumed that the first leavening agent was fermented milk. At the Twann settlement, he found fermented cereal porridge and remains of baked porridge in the shape of flatbreads. Technologically, these items would be the precursors of bread. The same porridge was also found at the Portalban settlement. The samples belonged to the lower layer of Cortaillod Culture, dated to 3830–3700 B.C. through C14 dating.

In the *animal component* ($\delta^{15}N$) *of the diet,* in LPC, testing according to sexes did not reveal any significant differences between children and adults (tab. 4) not even on separating males and females (tab. 5).

An animal food source for both children and adults was milk. In terms of ^{13}C values, children and women were more likely to have consumed cow's milk ($\delta^{13}C$ –21.15‰; $\delta^{15}N$ 7‰), while males were more likely to have consumed that of goats ($\delta^{13}C$ –20‰; $\delta^{15}N$ 8.4‰) (tab. 3). No comparison was found for children's diet as Richards (2008) did not analyse the diet of children.

In testing for *the animal component* ($\delta^{15}N$) of the diet with respect to age, there was a decline in the ^{15}N values from infants, through childhood to the juvenis age group (tab. 4; fig. 3).

Significant differences in the content of animal proteins at 5% level of significance were noted in the diet of 2 infants and 17 children; and at 1% level of significance between infants and the 6 juvenile individuals (juvenis). Juvenis (N = 6) (^{15}N 9.49 ± 1.06‰) exhibited lower levels than adults (N = 8) ($\delta^{15}N$ 11.03 ± 1.56‰). It follows that the dietary trends among juvenile individuals and adults as discovered by Richards (2008) in Vedrovice also hold for

LPC at the Neolithic settlements in Moravia. Juvenis/adolescents had a different diet than the adults. Significant differences at 5% level of significance were also found between infants and adults (tab. 4; fig. 3).

In the **Lengyel Culture (Moravian Painted Ware Culture) LgC**, in the whole Moravian region, 10 individuals were tested with respect to their sex: 2 children and 8 adults (3 males and 5 females).

In the *plant component of the diet*, on testing with respect to sexes in children and the adult group separated into males (N = 3) and females (N = 5) (tab. 2), significant differences were detected between children and females ($\delta^{13}C$ −20.22 ± 0.36‰), as well as between children and males ($\delta^{13}C$ −20.43 ± 0.48‰) at a significance level of 10% (tab. 5; fig. 4).

In the *animal component of the diet*, represented by stable nitrogen isotope ($\delta^{15}N$) values, on testing according to sexes, no significant difference in $\delta^{15}N$ was found between the groups of LgC individuals.

On increasing the set to 13 LgC individuals, age groups could be formed (1 infant; 2 children; 1 juvenis—in our notation an adolescent; 7 adults and 2 individuals of the maturus group) (tab. 1).

In the animal component of the diet, $\delta^{15}N$, the isotope values differed between the infant (8.85 ± 0.00‰) and the children (N = 2)(11.66 ± 1.22‰) at a significance level of 10%, and the 7 adults, also at a 10% level of significance (tab. 4).

It can be said, that in the *animal component* of the diet, $\delta^{15}N$, the values of the nitrogen isotope increase with age from the infant (8.55‰) to the children (N = 3) and the juvenile individual (12,02‰). Then there is a breakpoint, because the juvenis individual has a higher $\delta^{15}N$ value than the 7 adult individuals (9.94 ± 1.08‰)(fig. 5).

On comparing $\delta^{15}N$ in the two children (11.6 ± 1.22‰) and adults (N = 7) (9.94 ± 1.08‰) and the maturus group (N = 2) (9.99 ± 0.07‰), an apparent decrease in $\delta^{15}N$ values relative to age can be observed in the LgC; whereas the diet of adults in both the LPC and LgC cultures is similar.

In the animal component ($\delta^{15}N$) of the LgC infants' diet, a substantial role could have been played by goat's milk, in the groups of children and juvenis by fish, and in adults the meat of domestic and hunted animals (Smrčka et al. 2008).

In the **Stroked Pottery Culture (SPC)** of Moravia, on testing with respect to sex and age, no significant differences were found for the vegetal and animal components of the diet.

The comparison of results from the pilot research at the multicultural site in Těšetice into early Neolithic cultures of LPC, SPC and the late Neolithic LgC with the results of the subsequent research in Neolithic settlements across Moravia proved that the same as was discovered for diet reconstruction in Těšetice also holds for the rest of Moravia.

The diet of children and adults was different in the LPC. The main source of food of children and pregnant women was similar to that of wild animals, roe deer and red deer.

The LPC population consumed more milk than the LgC population. Women and children would probably consume milk of cows while men that of goats. The diet of adolescents (juvenis) was different from that of adults. The nutrition of children was not sufficient as children suffered from anaemias as is apparent from the incidence of cribra orbitalia (Dočkalová and Čižmář 2007).

METHODS

After mechanically removing the adhering dirt, bone samples were ultrasonically cleaned in demineralised water. Collagen extracts were prepared using the Longin (1971) method modified by Bocherens (1992). Powdered samples were demineralised in 1 M HCl for 20 minutes, followed by removal of humic acids with 0,125 M NaOH (for 18–20 hours), and gelatinisation in 0,01 M HCl at 100°C for 17 hours. Then, the samples were freeze-dried for approximately 72 hours.

11. NEOLITHIC HUMAN MIGRATION OF MORAVIA IN STRONTIUM ISOTOPES

VOJTĚCH ERBAN, VÁCLAV SMRČKA, MARTA DOČKALOVÁ

Human skeletal remains from Neolithic settlements of Southern Moravia (Czech Republic) were analyzed for strontium isotopic composition. The aim was to determine migration mobility of Neolithic cultures in Moravia and to compare the Lengyel Culture (Moravian Painted Ware Culture) with other Neolithic cultures.

The method is based on the observation that the $^{87}Sr/^{86}Sr$ isotopic ratio in the tissues reflects the composition of the diet. The dental enamel is formed in early childhood and it is not renewed later on, while the bone tissue is gradually renewed until the very end. The dental enamel thus preserves the isotopic fingerprint of the childhood region. The bone tissue, on the other hand, reflects the diet of last few years of the individual's life. Contrasting composition of these two tissues suggests that the examined person spent his/her childhood and the years before his/her death in different geochemical ambient (Hillson 1997; Price, Burton, and Bentley 2002).

To distinguish local and migrant individuals, background $^{87}Sr/^{86}Sr$ signal should be identified. The $^{87}Sr/^{86}Sr$ isotopic ratio in the food chain reflects the composition of the local water sources. The primary source of strontium in the water is the bedrock, either sedimentary or crystalline. Unfortunately, most rocks are composed of various minerals of differing isotopic compositions, each mineral weathering and releasing strontium into the water at various rates. That is why in most cases the information about local geology (usually well known) provides only indirect evidence of local bioavailable $^{87}Sr/^{86}Sr$. Due to the variability of hydrological and hydrogeological conditions also direct measuring of water sources is problematic. Skeletons of minor rodents or domestic animals, especially those of pigs, which are very near to humans in the trophic chain (Price, Burton, and Bentley 2002; Bentley and Knipper 2005; Bentley et al. 2002), prove to be the best indicator of the local $^{87}Sr/^{86}Sr$ signal. Another approach is statistical, when the average $^{87}Sr/^{86}Sr$ composition of the population (with obvious outliers being rejected) is considered to be representative for non-migrant individuals (Bickle et al. 2014; Scheeres et al. 2014).

MATERIAL AND METHODS

1. SAMPLING
Samples of 41 skeletons from the graves of Neolithic settlements kept at the Anthropos institute in Brno were sampled to determine the mobility. Pair samples of the enamel from the first molars in the lower jaw right and from the right femur were taken.

2. SAMPLE PROCESSING
Bone and tooth enamel samples were mechanically abraded to obtain pure and clean, compact tissue. Samples were further cleaned using dilute ultra-pure acetic acid, sonicated in deionized water and incinerated in a muffle furnace. Ashed samples were dissolved in double distilled nitric acid. Strontium fraction was isolated using cation-exchange chromatography columns filled with Eichrom's Sr-spec resin.

Isotopic analyses were performed using a Finnigan MAT 262 Thermal Ionization Mass Spectrometer in dynamic mode with a double Re filament assembly. The $^{87}Sr/^{86}Sr$ ratios were corrected for mass fractionation assuming $^{88}Sr/^{86}Sr = 0.1194$. External reproducibility is given by the results of repeat analyses of the NBS 987 ($^{87}Sr/^{86}Sr = 0.710250 \pm 0.000024$ (2δ), n = 21) isotopic standards.

RESULTS

1. MOBILITY AT THE TĚŠETICE POLYCULTURAL SETTLEMENT
The largest dataset represents the population in the polycultural Neolithic settlement at Těšetice. Fourteen skeletons were sampled in the course of the first stage of the excavations. Domestic pig tooth was taken to represent local background.

The whole $^{87}Sr/^{86}Sr$ dataset ranges between 0.7087 and 0.7137. This large spread is a consequence of high variability of the enamel samples. The range of the femur samples is significantly narrower (0.7110–0.7121). Data of both types of material (enamel and femur) have very close mean value (0.7115). The Sus Scrofa sample, which presumably represents a proxy of local bioavailable Sr (e.g. Price, Burton, and Bentley 2002), has the value $^{87}Sr/^{86}Sr = 0.7117$, which is close to the averages of both datasets.

Regarding the overall variability, there are two possible explanations of $^{87}Sr/^{86}Sr$ data scatter in case of the prehistoric skeletal sample sets. As mentioned above, the primary variability is a result of contrasting composition of bioavailable Sr in the environment, e.g. it is caused by migration. This information may be obscured by secondary variability, caused by sample diagenesis and post-mortem changes. The latter affects more often the bone tissue samples than the enamel bioapatite. The secondary $^{87}Sr/^{86}Sr$ alteration should, therefore, lead to significantly larger scatter (or drift towards contaminating agent composition) in femur samples compared to enamel data. However, this is not the case of the situation we observe in case of the available Těšetice data. There is no overall shift between the enamel and femur data. On top of it, we see significantly lower scatter for the femur data compared to enamel results. We thereby consider the larger scatter of the enamel data (compared to femur numbers) to be a strong evidence that the $^{87}Sr/^{86}Sr$ variability is primary rather than diagenetic.

As mentioned above, the $^{87}Sr/^{86}Sr$ range of femur data is very narrow (0.7110–0.7121). Statistically, all the femur data are within 2 standard deviation range from the dataset mean. Therefore we consider all studied individuals as locals during their adult age.

If we look at the enamel composition to explore lifetime mobility, the range is significantly larger than in case of the femur data. The two standard deviation range (±2SD) for all the enamel and femur analyses defines a range between 0.7096 and 0.7133. All the data beyond this range are statistical outliers and we interpret these individuals as the non-locals (migrants). In this way we have identified three non-locals, one in each cultural group (fig. 1): grave 11/1986 in the Linear Pottery Culture (LPC); grave 8/1976 in the Moravian Painted Ware Culture (LgC); and grave 2-2 in the Stroke Ornamented Pottery Culture (SPC).

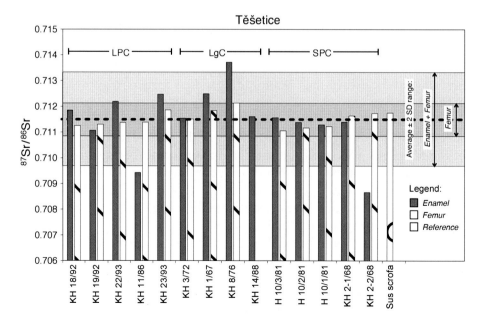

Fig. 1. Migration at the multicultural settlement at Těšetice-Kyjovice.

Tab. 1. Migration at the Moravian Neolithic settlements.

Grave	Culture	Locality	Sex	Age	Enamel	Femur	Migrant	Comment
H2/1998	LPC	Držovice	F	20-30	0.710216 (15)	0.710389 (18)	No	
654/H3/2003	LPC	Hluboké Mašůvky	N	5	0.712364 (14)	0.712094 (12)	No	
654/H2/2003	LPC	Hluboké Mašůvky	N	13-15	0.711559 (08)	0.712127 (12)	No	
654/H1/2003	LPC	Hluboké Mašůvky	F	20-30	0.711644 (11)	0.712415 (13)	No	
17/1897	LgC	Hluboké Mašůvky	N	30-60	0.713184 (13)	0.712270 (12)	No	
10/1897	LgC	Holubice	N	19-20	0.709640 (17)	0.709953 (16)	No	Mandibula
K1683/2003	LPC	Kralice na Hané	N	18-21	0.711075 (17)	0.710184 (18)	Yes	
548/2003	LPC	Kralice na Hané	N	1	0.710258 (12)	0.710337 (09)	No	Pars petrosa ossis temporalis
H2a/2002	LgC	Krumlovský les	F	35-40	0.710823 (19)	0.710957 (14)	No	
1-K-1066/H1	LgC	Mašovice u Znojma	M	20-30	0.715171 (17)	0.713057 (10)	Yes	
1/16/1950	SPC	Nová Ves u Oslavan	M	25-30	0.711370 (16)	0.711137 (10)	No	
IV/1612	LPC	Opava	F	20-40	0.711758 (16)	0.711583 (13)	No	
IV/1611	LPC	Pohořelice-Šumice	N	20-25	0.710492 (11)	0.710756 (15)	No	
126-H1/2006	LgC	Předmostí-Dluhonice	F	20-40	0.710336 (12)	0.710302 (14)	No	
35/1939	SPC	Rybníky	F	30-70	0.712045 (17)	0.713119 (13)	No	Ramus mandibulae
K527-H1/1999	LPC	Seloutky	N	3	0.710429 (17)	0.710592 (14)	No	
H1/2002	LPC	Slatinky, Močílky	N	11	0.710653 (11)	0.711233 (09)	No	
HI,12	LgC	Střelice	M	50-90	0.710733 (14)	0.711519 (20)	No	
KH6/1967	LgC	Těšetice – Kyjovice	N	5		0.711153 (14)	No	
36,1957	SPC	Trstěnice	F	25-40	0.712453 (19)	0.712815 (14)	Yes	
H37/1960	SPC	Vyškov	N	15-17	0.713423 (19)	0.711228 (14)	Yes	
82-H1/1986	LPC	Žádovice	N	6-7	0.709631 (11)	0.709826 (16)	No	
95-H237	LPC	Žádovice	N	7	0.709680 (17)	0.709886 (19)	No	
82-H2/1986	LPC	Žádovice	N	2	0.709590 (13)	0.709941 (18)	No	Humerus
52-H1/1986	LPC	Žádovice	N	5	0.709711 (08)	0.709978 (13)	No	
52-H2/1986	LPC	Žádovice	N	8	0.709652 (08)	0.710020 (12)	No	
I/1979	LPC	Želešice u Brna	F	30-50	0.710382 (13)	0.710489 (15)	No	
6397 Sus A		Krumlovský les			0.711120 (15)			Reference
6397 Sus B		Krumlovský les			0.711123 (17)			Reference
95-H237/1986 Cep		Žádovice			0.710073 (15)			Reference

If we consider the $^{87}Sr/^{86}Sr$ 2SD of the femur data only as a better proxy of local population variance (e.g. more strict approach), three more individuals emerge as suspect migrants: In the LPC these are graves 23/1993 and 22/1993, of the LgC the individual with different birthplace was buried in the grave 1/1967. However, as the 22/1993 is a child not older than 2.5 years and the enamel value is very close to the statistical boundary, we do not consider this one to be a migrant.

Although the small number of analyzed skeletons is hardly representative for the whole population, we can estimate that between 20 and 40% of population were mobile in Těšetice during the period of LPC (n = 5). On the contrary, only 20% of population migrated from their birth place in the period of the SPC (n = 5), and 25 to 50% of population were mobile in the period of the LgC (n = 4, fig. 1). It should be also stressed that the numbers above represent only lower estimate of the migrating population, as the method is not able to identify migrants from areas with same $^{87}Sr/^{86}Sr$ background.

2. DETERMINATION OF MOBILITY AT OTHER MORAVIAN NEOLITHIC SETTLEMENTS

Pairs of samples of enamel of M1 and of middle part of the thigh bone were analyzed for 27 skeletons from 19 Moravian Neolithic settlements in addition to the Těšetice dataset (tab. 1, fig. 2). As the number of skeletons available

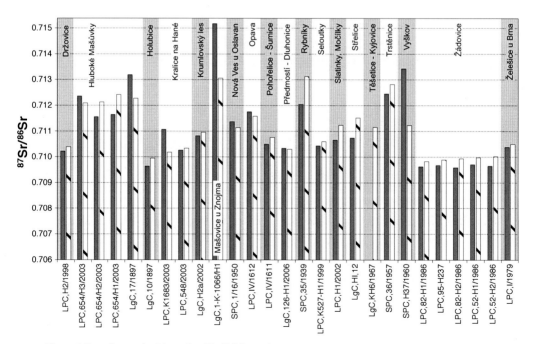

Fig. 2. Migration at the Moravian Neolithic settlements.

for isotopic research was limited, most localities are represented by one or two individuals only. Also suitable proxies of bioavailable Sr were lacking for most locations. The situation is further obscured by complicated geology of the Moravian region (e.g. Cháb et al. 2010). It is situated at the border between Bohemian Massif (pre-Mesozoic igneous and metamorphic rocks, mostly elevated $^{87}Sr/^{86}Sr$) and Pannonian basin (Neogene marine sediments, generally lower $^{87}Sr/^{86}Sr$), covered by abundant quaternary loess and fluvial sedimentary cover (intermediate $^{87}Sr/^{86}Sr$). Such situation does not allow unequivocal deduction of background Sr or sound distinction between localities. This limits considerably the interpretation. The only reliable parameter indicating possible migration is in most cases the contrast between enamel and femur $^{87}Sr/^{86}Sr$ composition. As a general rule, difference larger than the 2SD of the Těšetice femur data (0.0006) is considered to indicate the migration, if no other hints are available.

Individual from only 1 of 16 investigated graves of the LPC have contrasting ratio of $^{87}Sr/^{86}Sr$ in the femur compared to the enamel of M1. In Kralice na Hané the enamel of H1683/2003 is 0.0009 higher than femur, which suggest migration origin. In the Hluboké Mašůvky locality, the high overall $^{87}Sr/^{86}Sr$ variability in this locality is attributed to combination of loess and more radiogenic (high $^{87}Sr/^{86}Sr$) orthogneiss in the background, rather than to the mobility (Czech Geological Survey, 2018).

Apart from the migration considerations, it should be noted that the $^{87}Sr/^{86}Sr$ of the skeletons from five children graves of the settlement at Žádovice are remarkably homogeneous (0.7096–0.7100, 2SD ~0.0003). Even within this narrow range, the results for enamel are systematically lower than for the femur. All the enamel and femur numbers are slightly lower than the value determined for the local reference sample of the Cepaea Vindobonensis (0.7101). The data are in good agreement with the overall low age of the tested individuals, which also suggest low probability of migration.

This also points towards geographical differences in the period of the Linear Pottery Culture. All individuals of the settlement at Žádovice (n = 5) are local; on the contrary, the mobility is between 20% and 40% at Těšetice in this period, as we have already mentioned.

In the set of four SPC individuals outside the Těšetice locality the data indicate that one or two individuals resettled during their lifetime. In the grave H 37/1960 at Vyškov there is extreme difference (0.0022) between $^{87}Sr/^{86}Sr$ in femur and enamel; the difference in 35/1939 at Rybníky is somewhat lower (0.0011), which also suggests migratory background. Together with the Těšetice results the SPC era migration rate is estimated between 22% and 33%.

Apart from four individuals at Těšetice seven LgC individuals from seven distinct localities were investigated. The data indicate that only one individual was non-local. At Mašovice u Znojma the grave 1-K-1066/H1 reveals the highest $^{87}Sr/^{86}Sr$ value (0.7152) together with high contrast between femur and enamel values. It must be admitted that also variable geology at this locality may play also rule (loess vs. presumably more radiogenic granites of the Thaya massif). If all LgC data are counted, the overall migration for this cultural period would be 27%.

3. REGIONAL CONSIDERATIONS

With regard to the fact that almost all the measured isotopic ratios are higher than ~0.7097, it can be supposed that the individuals did not come from the region of the Viennese basin stretching to the south-east. The sea basin sediments of the Neogene age have considerably lower isotopic ratio of bioavailable Sr (below 0.709; DePaolo and Ingram 1985). The only one exception is the grave H 2-2/1968 (SPC at Těšetice) with enamel $^{87}Sr/^{86}Sr$ = 0.7087. On the contrary, in the region of the Bohemian Massif (roughly to the north-west of the Brno–Znojmo line; Czech Geological Survey 2018) the igneous and metamorphic rocks are sources of considerably higher $^{87}Sr/^{86}Sr$ isotopic ratio. We see increased $^{87}Sr/^{86}Sr$ values at the localities situated near the contact of sedimentary and crystalline rocks: Mašovice u Znojma, Huboké Mašůvky, Rybníky, Trstěnice and Těšetice. This implies that the suspected migration may be only short distance resettlement. On contrary, there is no high-$^{87}Sr/^{86}Sr$ source near the Vyškov site, pointing to longer-distance migration for the H37/1960.

CONCLUSIONS

Human skeletal remains (n = 41) from Neolithic settlements in southern Moravia, the Czech Republic, were analyzed for $^{87}Sr/^{86}Sr$ composition of femur and enamel to investigate human migration.

In Těšetice we performed a pilot study of the population mobility on 14 skeletons. We identified 3 to 5 migrants (non-locals): two in the Linear Pottery Culture (LPC) in graves 22/93 and 11/86; two in the Moravian Painted Ware Culture (LgC), grave 8/76 and possibly also H 1/1967; and one in the Stroke Ornamented Pottery Culture (SPC) in grave 2-2/68. The Stroke Ornamented Pottery Culture population seems to be less mobile compared with the Linear and Painted Pottery Cultures. Between 20 and 40% of the Těšetice population were mobile during the period of LPC, while only 20% during SPC and 40% in the time of LgC.

Taken together, results of analysis of 21 LPC (Linear Pottery Culture) individuals, 9 SPC (Stroke Ornamented Pottery Culture) individuals and 11 LgC (Moravian Painted Ware Culture) from the whole region of the South Moravia indicates that 9 individuals had moved during their lifetime.

It should be also pointed out that all children aged 8 or younger have very alike strontium values in the enamel and bone tissue. This juvenile $^{87}Sr/^{86}Sr$ homogeneity justifies the original methodological assumptions and also provides an independent control of the samples quality and of laboratory protocol relevance.

Comparison of the mobility of Neolithic cultures in Moravia shows that the mobility of the LgC was similar to that of LPC (40%). The mobility of the SPC, the successor of the LPC in Moravia, was lower than in both the LgC and LPC.

This finding would agree with the view of archaeologists that the SPC was passively pushed by the LgC to today's Bohemia, and northern Moravia (Pavlů and Zápotocká 2007).

12. TRACE ELEMENTS IN BONES OF THE NEOLITHIC CULTURES OF MORAVIA

VÁCLAV SMRČKA, MARTIN MIHALJEVIČ, JARMILA ZOCOVÁ, IVAN ZOC, IVO NĚMEC

The aim of this research was to determine at which life stages trace elements exhibit the highest metabolic activity, represented by their highest concentration in bones. Samples were taken from the standard compartment of the upper femur (Smrčka 2005) in 46 individuals belonging to Neolithic cultures—Linear Pottery Culture (LPC), Lengyel Moravian Painted Ware Culture (LgC) and Stroked Pottery Culture (SPC). Individuals were categorised by age (from infants aged 0–1, to adults aged 60) and gender (children, females and males).

Concurrently, environmental factors of the Neolithic Age that could lead to trace element deficiencies were also determined.

The following trace elements affecting bone metabolism were selected: arsenic (As), barium (Ba), cobalt (Co), magnesium (Mg), chromium (Cr), copper (Cu), lead (Pb), sodium (Na), strontium (Sr), calcium (Ca), zinc (Zn), and iron (Fe).

The bone collection comprised of 27 individuals (13 children, 6 females, 4 males, and 4 unidentified individuals) of the Linear Pottery Culture (LPC), 12 individuals (3 children, 5 females, 2 males, and 2 unidentified individuals) of the Lengyel Culture (LgC—Moravian Painted Ware), and 7 individuals (1 child, 2 females, 2 males, and 2 unidentified individuals) of the Stroked Pottery Culture (SPC).

METHOD

Bone samples were weighed and placed into 25 ml volumetric flasks. 5 ml concentrated HNO_3 (p.a. Merck Germany) was added and the flask was heated on a hot plate until the sample had completely dissolved. The volumetric flask was filled with deionised water and the sample was then diluted 10 times before analysis at a final concentration of HNO_3 2% v/v. The concentrations of Ca, Na, Mg, Fe and Al were determined by inductively coupled plasma emission spectrometry (ICP OES—Agilent 5110, Agilent Australia) under standard analytical conditions. The concentrations of As, Ba, Co, Ce, Cr, La, Mn, Cu, Pb, Pr, Sr and Y were determined by inductively coupled plasma mass spectrometry (ICP MS, X Series II- Thermoscientific Germany) with Ge, Rh and Re internal standardisation and instrument optimization. The method accuracy

Tab. 1. An overview of average concentrations of elements (µg/g of bone) in the 46 individuals belonging to the Neolithic populations of Moravia

	dx					sin			
	n	Mean	Min	Max	SD	n	Mean	Min	Max	SD
Ca	45	315297.26	268105.26	356401.71	22385.14	38	312209.13	199050.95	355302.28	31137.80
Sr	45	302.75	194.56	528.18	81.86	38	297.94	167.03	525.47	85.29
Zn	46	312952.96	261562.05	342146.42	22003.20	38	106.71	52.42	286.30	50.95
Pb	45	1.18	0.00	14.18	2.40	38	0.77	0.00	6.61	1.35
Mn	45	157.70	2.18	1935.87	393.44	38	122.51	0.72	1726.30	293.14
Mn*	43	76.21	2.18	373.45	95.86	37	79.16	0.72	465.66	122.26
Fe	45	1520.26	54.98	22810.11	4232.47	38	1041.40	20.02	21436.92	3444.92
Fe*	43	639.97	54.98	4119.94	806.20	37	490.17	20.02	2390.89	574.38
Mg	45	1367.66	650.79	3782.13	624.72	38	1343.93	712.40	3649.30	645.92
K	45	173.35	40.36	753.75	172.79	38	134.75	36.26	670.65	121.50
Na	45	2178.71	1188.52	4526.93	673.79	38	2204.20	1105.95	4645.15	722.78
Cu	45	6.65	1.88	19.47	3.53	38	6.21	1.51	21.97	3.79
V	45	11.48	3.30	43.90	8.02	38	10.64	3.43	38.25	8.13
Cr	45	9.41	0.95	30.93	5.55	38	8.72	1.02	25.18	5.08
Co	45	1.96	0.89	7.68	1.46	38	1.63	0.73	4.31	0.81
Ni	45	14.68	9.62	27.23	4.51	38	14.11	8.99	27.02	4.17
As	45	2.58	0.49	16.13	3.07	38	2.22	0.44	16.70	2.67
Y	45	2.88	0.00	19.33	4.21	38	2.07	0.00	10.58	2.88
Cd	45	0.05	0.00	0.55	0.13	38	0.01	0.00	0.32	0.06
Ba	45	172.46	46.65	452.39	98.26	38	161.63	58.10	422.65	88.44
La	45	2.26	0.00	13.89	3.47	38	1.57	0.00	6.95	2.16
Ce	45	2.13	0.00	24.53	3.80	38	1.50	0.00	7.06	1.80
Pr	45	0.41	0.00	3.04	0.72	38	0.28	0.00	1.32	0.41
Nd	45	1.47	0.00	12.04	2.91	38	0.94	0.00	5.07	1.60
Sm	45	0.13	0.00	2.25	0.47	38	0.03	0.00	0.37	0.09
Eu	45	0.03	0.00	0.59	0.11	38	0.01	0.00	0.15	0.03
Gd	45	0.11	0.00	1.74	0.36	38	0.04	0.00	0.40	0.12
Tb	45	0.02	0.00	0.38	0.07	38	0.01	0.00	0.09	0.03
Dy	45	0.12	0.00	1.96	0.40	38	0.05	0.00	0.54	0.14
Ho	45	0.02	0.00	0.39	0.07	38	0.00	0.00	0.04	0.01
Er	45	0.05	0.00	1.14	0.20	38	0.01	0.00	0.15	0.03
Tm	45	0.00	0.00	0.11	0.02	38	0.00	0.00	0.00	0.00
Yb	45	0.02	0.00	0.87	0.13	38	0.00	0.00	0.00	0.00
Lu	45	0.00	0.00	0.09	0.01	38	0.00	0.00	0.00	0.00
U	45	6.16	0.37	38.10	6.32	38	5.19	0.85	21.41	4.30

dx = dexter, right; sin = sinister, left

was controlled by CRM 1400 (Bone Ash, NIST USA) certified reference material, and was generally better than 10% relative standard deviations (RSD) for
all elements.

ARSENIC (As)

As has a positive and negative role in terms of bone metabolism; it is both
essential and toxic. It has an essential role related to the metabolism of
methionine and phosphorylation.

Excess levels of As lead to pathological effects on bone metabolism through
inhibition of endochondral ossification, reducing bone mineral density and
trabecular bone structure in femoral bones, leading to osteomalacia. It affects
mineralisation by lowering alkaline phosphatase, stimulating osteoclasts and
inducing bone resorption (Hu et al. 2012).

Research in humans involving exposure to arsenic in osteomalacia shows
a higher prevalence of Paget's disease (Lever 2002) and disrupted foetal development (Kippler et al. 2012).

The acute toxicity of arsenic is well known (Dermience et al. 2015). The
study of Neolithic material may help clarify the influence of this element's
dual role in bone metabolism. The average concentration of As in femoral
bones of the 46 individuals was 0–5,6 µg/g (tab. 1, 2).

The arsenic concentrations in bones of the 6 females of the Neolithic
Linear Pottery Culture were higher (5.2 µg/g) than in the two females of the
succeeding Stroked Pottery Culture (1.03 µg/g). The children (N = 3) of
the Moravian Painted Ware Culture (LgC) had higher bone As concentration
(2.8 ± 1.08 µg/g) than the children of LPC and SPC. The arsenic concentrations
were approximately the same for the male individuals across all examined
cultures (tab. As, sex).

With respect to age, infants under 1 year of age (N = 2) and children
under 10 years of age (N = 13) exhibited the highest bone concentrations of As. Similar values were also found in the LPC females aged 20–40
(N = 6). This increase was also relative to Ca (p 0.542) (tab. As, age; fig. Ascaage;
fig. Ascult).

In femoral bones of the Neolithic cultures, As can be said to have been
metabolically active in infants under 1 year of age, children under 10 years of
age, and in females 30 years old.

The recommended daily intake of arsenic for our contemporary population is derived from experiments on animals and is very low, between
12–25 µg/day. No deficiency in humans has been described (Ulthus and
Nielsen 1993).

Tab. 2. Analysis of variance of dual classification with the influence of culture and sex

Element	Factor	Without interactions				With interactions				graph
		F (2,37)	signif	p	different groups	F (2,37)	p	signif	different groups	
Ca	cult	3.321	5.00%	0.049	SPCxLgC,LPCxLgC	3.169	0.057	10%	SPCxLgC	cacult
Sr/Ca	sex	2.615	10.00%	0.088	ChxM					srcasex
	cult	2.368	>10.00%	0.109	SPCxLgC,LPCxLgC	2.540	0.096	10%	LgCxSPC	srcacult
Pb	sex	6.865	0.01%	0.003	ChxF,ChxM	2.763	0.080	10%	ChxF,ChxM	pbsex
Pb/Ca	sex	6.290	0.01%	0.005	ChxM,ChxF	2.575	0.093	10%	ChxM,ChxF	pbcasex
Mg	cult	3.146	10.00%	0.056	LgCxLPC,LgCxSPC	2.487	0.101	>10%	LgCxLPC,SPCxLPC	mgcult
Mg/Ca	cult	4.261	5.00%	0.023	LgCxLPC,LgCxSPC	3.481	0.044	5%	LgCxLPC,	mgcacult
Na	cult	3.597	5.00%	0.039	LgCxLPC,LgCxSPC					nacult
Na/Ca	cult	4.663	5.00%	0.016	MMxLPC	2.746	0.081	10%	LgCxLPC,	nacacult
Cu	sex	3.273	10%	0.051	ChxM,FxM,ChxF					cusex
Cu/Ca	sex	3.385	5.00%	0.046	ChxM,ChxF					cucasex
Co	sex	3.974	5.00%	0.028	ChxM,ChxF	2.133	0.137	>10%	ChxM,ChxF	cosex
Co/Ca	sex	4.064	5.00%	0.026	ChxM,ChxF	2.245	0.124	>10%	ChxM,ChxF	cocasex
Ni	sex	2.106	>10.00%	0.138	ChxF					nisex
Ni/Ca	sex	2.287	>10.00%	0.117	ChxM					nicasex
Y	sex	2.504	10.00%	0.097	ChxM					ysex
Y/Ca	sex	2.693	10.00%	0.083	ChxM					ycasex
La	sex	2.287	>10.00%	0.117	ChxM					lasex
La/Ca	sex	2.416	>10.00%	0.105	ChxM					lacasex
Ce	sex	5.580	0.01%	0.008	ChxM,ChxF	3.587	0.041	5%	ChxM,ChxF	cesex
Ce/Ca	sex	5.548	0.01%	0.008	ChxM,ChxF	3.684	0.038	5%	ChxM,ChxF	cecasex
Pr	sex	2.309	>10.00%	0.115	ChxM					prsex
Pr/Ca	sex	2.413	>10.00%	0.105	ChxM					prcasex

Tab. As, sex. Arsenic concentration in bone with regard to sex of the Neolithic populations

	As									As/Ca		
	dx µg/g Mean	dx N	dx µg/g SD	sin µg/g Mean	sin N	sin µg/g SD	aver.µg/g Mean	N	aver.µg/g SD	Mean	N	SD
LPC	2.994	26	3.793	2.737	21	3.439	2.984	27	3.730	9.67E-06	27	1.23E-05
Children	1.828	13	0.825	2.033	10	0.964	1.867	13	0.866	5.99E-06	13	2.84E-06
Females	5.215	6	5.960	5.190	5	6.773	5.172	6	5.999	1.67E-05	6	1.94E-05
Males	1.588	4	0.331	2.074	4	1.240	1.831	4	0.764	5.62E-06	4	2.10E-06
Undef	5.481	3	7.069	1.450	2	0.120	4.481	4	6.108	1.51E-05	4	2.08E-05
LgC	2.465	12	1.855	1.887	10	1.163	2.417	12	1.903	7.97E-06	12	5.95E-06
Children	2.700	3	0.881	2.919	3	1.323	2.809	3	1.080	9.65E-06	3	4.77E-06
Females	2.485	5	2.945	0.873	4	0.402	2.362	5	2.995	7.46E-06	5	9.04E-06
Males	1.978	2	0.015	1.923	2	0.317	1.950	2	0.151	6.77E-06	2	3.95E-07
Undef	2.551	2	0.975	2.773	1	0.000	2.434	2	0.810	7.91E-06	2	2.18E-06
SPC	1.224	7	0.284	1.149	7	0.386	1.186	7	0.184	3.69E-06	7	6.09E-07
Children	1.342	1	0.000	1.375	1	0.000	1.359	1	0.000	4.35E-06	1	0.00E+00
Females	0.952	2	0.017	1.117	2	0.019	1.034	2	0.018	3.18E-06	2	5.49E-08
Males	1.258	2	0.178	1.174	2	0.854	1.216	2	0.338	3.61E-06	2	1.07E-06
Undef	1.403	2	0.472	1.041	2	0.293	1.222	2	0.089	3.94E-06	2	9.68E-08

LPC — Linear Pottery Culture; LgC — Lengyel Culture; SPC — Stroked Pottery Culture; dx = dexter, right; sin = sinister, left

Tab. As, age. Arsenic concentration in bone in age groups of the Neolithic populations

	As									As/Ca		
	dx µg/g Mean	dx N	dx µg/g SD	sin µg/g Mean	sin N	sin µg/g SD	aver.µg/g Mean	N	aver.µg/g SD	Mean	N	SD
LPC	2.994	26	3.793	2.737	21	3.439	2.984	27	3.730	0.0000097	27	1.23E-05
Newborn	2.924	1	0.000	2.722	1	0.000	2.823	1	0.000	0.0000100	1	0.00E+00
1–10 years	1.729	10	0.862	1.937	7	1.138	1.766	10	0.941	0.0000057	10	2.97E-06
10–20 years	3.268	7	4.584	1.661	6	0.333	3.320	7	4.559	0.0000108	7	1.56E-05
20–40 years	5.269	6	5.921	5.607	5	6.576	5.373	6	5.879	0.0000173	6	1.90E-05
40–60 years	1.567	2	0.094	1.831	1	0.000	1.616	2	0.164	0.0000050	2	1.33E-07
Undef		0		1.365	1	0.000	1.365	1	0.000	0.0000049	1	0.00E+00
LgC	2.465	12	1.855	1.887	10	1.163	2.417	12	1.903	0.0000080	12	5.95E-06
Newborn	2.080	1	0.000	2.546	1	0.000	2.313	1	0.000	0.0000076	1	0.00E+00
1–10 years	3.011	2	0.987	3.105	2	1.814	3.058	2	1.400	0.0000107	2	6.28E-06
10–20 years		0			0			0			0	
20–40 years	2.542	8	2.215	1.611	6	0.767	2.473	8	2.216	0.0000080	8	6.62E-06
40–60 years	1.143	1	0.000	0.443	1	0.000	0.793	1	0.000	0.0000026	1	0.00E+00
Undef		0			0			0			0	
SPC	1.224	7	0.284	1.149	7	0.386	1.186	7	0.184	0.0000037	7	6.09E-07
Newborn		0			0			0			0	
1–10 years	1.342	1	0.000	1.375	1	0.000	1.359	1	0.000	0.0000043	1	0.00E+00
10–20 years	1.069	1	0.000	1.248	1	0.000	1.159	1	0.000	0.0000040	1	0.00E+00
20–40 years	1.277	3	0.406	1.248	3	0.483	1.262	3	0.205	0.0000038	3	5.73E-07
40–60 years	1.162	2	0.314	0.837	2	0.377	1.000	2	0.031	0.0000030	2	2.04E-07
Undef		0			0			0			0	

LPC — Linear Pottery Culture; LgC — Lengyel Culture; SPC — Stroked Pottery Culture; dx = dexter, right; sin = sinister, left

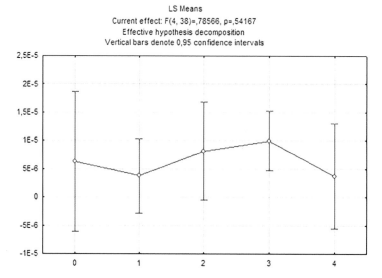

Fig. As/Ca age. Graphical representation of the As/Ca ratio in various age groups (ascaage). Age groups: 0—infants, 1—up to age 10, 2—up to age 20, 3—up to age 40, 4—up to age 60.

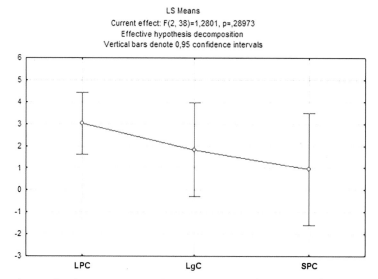

Fig. As, cult. Graphical representation of As concentrations (μg/g of bone) in the Neolithic cultures (Linear Pottery Culture—LPC; Lengyel Culture—LgC; and Stroked Pottery Culture—SPC).

BARIUM *(Ba)*

Over 90% of Ba in the body is found in bone tissue (Curzon and Cutress 1983; WHO 1990; Fischer et al. 2014). Despite this, its physiological importance with regards to bone metabolism has not been explained. Barium should be judged in relation to Ca (Fischer et al. 2014).

The average Ba concentration in bone for the Neolithic population (N = 46) was estimated to be 171.86 ± 96.15 μg/g (tab. 1).

The highest bone Ba concentrations were seen in the 20-40 year old age group, comprised of 6 LPC individuals (234.58 ± 151.06 μg/g) and 8 LgC individuals (182.48 ± 86.87 μg/g) (tab. Ba, age; fig. Bacaage).

These values are greater than the average Ba concentration in bone of the Neolithic population. The Ba bone concentration of the new-born infant (N = 1) in LgC (192 μg/g) was also greater than the average.

The highest Ba concentrations for LPC were seen in women (N = 6), and in children for LgC (N = 3). All SPC groups were below the average Ba concentration of the Neolithic population (tab. Ba, sex; fig. Bacult).

In the femurs of the Neolithic people, Ba had the highest metabolic activity in the 20–40-year old age group, reaching a significance level of p 0.753, and showed an association with calcium (Ba/Ca ratio p 0.751) (fig. Bacaage).

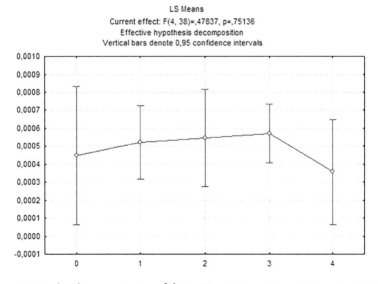

Fig. Bacaage. Graphical representation of the Ba/Ca ratio in various age groups. Age groups: 0—infants, 1—up to age 10, 2—up to age 20, 3—up to age 40, 4—up to age 60.

Tab. Ba, age. Barium concentration in bone in age groups of the Neolithic populations

	Ba									Ba/Ca		
	dx µg/g Mean	dx N	dx µg/g SD	sin µg/g Mean	sin N	sin µg/g SD	aver.µg/g Mean	N	aver.µg/g SD	Mean	N	SD
LPC	178.45	26	112.14	168.41	21	85.85	178.32	27	105.80	0.0005702	27	3.48E-04
Newborn	139.05	1	0.00	141.55	1	0.00	140.30	1	0.00	0.0004956	1	0.00E+00
1–10 years	167.29	10	81.58	196.86	7	96.45	170.26	10	84.49	0.0005391	10	2.55E-04
10–20 years	163.97	7	120.97	130.06	6	49.44	167.09	7	117.82	0.0005311	7	4.04E-04
20–40 years	239.01	6	163.83	193.34	5	120.36	234.58	6	151.06	0.0007482	6	5.09E-04
40–60 years	122.87	2	7.38	114.01	1	0.00	119.35	2	2.40	0.0003719	2	2.04E-05
Undef		0		155.97	1	0.00	155.97	1	0.00	0.0005581	1	0.00E+00
LgC	185.95	12	89.24	179.84	10	114.00	186.88	12	94.94	0.0006062	12	2.78E-04
Newborn	215.71	1	0.00	168.02	1	0.00	191.87	1	0.00	0.0006323	1	0.00E+00
1–10 years	233.29	2	99.92	290.31	2	187.16	261.80	2	143.54	0.0008463	2	3.51E-04
10–20 years		0			0			0			0	
20–40 years	184.80	8	91.78	164.34	6	92.16	182.48	8	86.87	0.0005914	8	2.56E-04
40–60 years	70.71	1	0.00	63.76	1	0.00	67.24	1	0.00	0.0002188	1	0.00E+00
Undef		0			0			0			0	
SPC	127.09	7	29.66	115.29	7	30.80	121.19	7	25.81	0.0003779	7	9.32E-05
Newborn		0			0			0			0	
1–10 years	108.93	1	0.00	104.92	1	0.00	106.93	1	0.00	0.0003420	1	0.00E+00
10–20 years	186.69	1	0.00	132.95	1	0.00	159.82	1	0.00	0.0005529	1	0.00E+00
20–40 years	109.08	3	8.85	112.02	3	39.38	110.55	3	22.74	0.0003346	3	6.62E-05
40–60 years	133.40	2	13.73	116.56	2	46.24	124.98	2	29.99	0.0003734	2	7.62E-05
Undef		0			0			0			0	

LPC—Linear Pottery Culture; LgC—Lengyel Culture; SPC—Stroked Pottery Culture; dx = dexter, right; sin = sinister, left

Tab. Ba, sex. Barium concentration in bone with regard to sex of the Neolithic populations

	Ba									Ba/Ca		
	dx µg/g Mean	dx N	dx µg/g SD	sin µg/g Mean	sin N	sin µg/g SD	aver.µg/g Mean	N	aver.µg/g SD	Mean	N	SD
LPC	178.45	26	112.14	168.41	21	85.85	178.32	27	105.80	5.70E-04	27	3.48E-04
Children	163.88	13	77.62	183.83	10	86.69	166.27	13	78.90	5.26E-04	13	2.37E-04
Females	245.21	6	157.69	199.57	5	113.83	240.28	6	144.89	7.65E-04	6	4.91E-04
Males	209.10	3	175.19	150.31	2	7.99	201.58	4	140.73	6.78E-04	4	4.84E-04
Undef	102.64	4	18.98	99.95	4	20.37	101.30	4	19.56	3.13E-04	4	5.39E-05
LgC	185.95	12	89.24	179.84	10	114.00	186.88	12	94.94	6.06E-04	12	2.78E-04
Children	227.43	3	71.38	249.54	3	150.00	238.49	3	109.23	7.75E-04	3	2.77E-04
Females	139.62	5	96.32	104.36	4	57.34	136.00	5	87.08	4.31E-04	5	2.52E-04
Males	214.15	2	4.87	235.12	1	0.00	218.54	2	11.06	7.16E-04	2	6.95E-06
Undef	211.36	2	146.65	198.62	2	144.79	204.99	2	145.72	6.81E-04	2	4.11E-04
SPC	127.09	7	29.66	115.29	7	30.80	121.19	7	25.81	3.78E-04	7	9.32E-05
Children	108.93	1	0.00	104.92	1	0.00	106.93	1	0.00	3.42E-04	1	0.00E+00
Females	111.27	2	17.56	83.56	2	0.44	97.41	2	9.00	3.00E-04	2	2.78E-05
Males	150.42	2	51.28	144.92	2	16.93	147.67	2	17.18	4.81E-04	2	1.02E-04
Undef	128.66	2	20.43	122.58	2	37.72	125.62	2	29.08	3.71E-04	2	7.93E-05

LPC — Linear Pottery Culture; LgC — Lengyel Culture; SPC — Stroked Pottery Culture; dx = dexter, right; sin = sinister, left

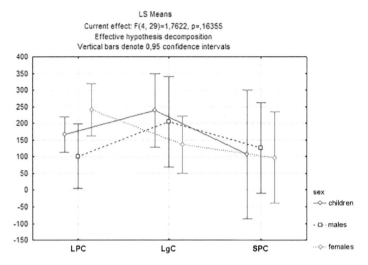

Fig. Bacult. Graphical representation Ba (μg/g of bone) in various cultures and sex groups

CHROMIUM (Cr)

Trivalent Cr is an essential trace element that has several roles in the metabolism of lipids and sugars (Martin 2000; Beattie and Avenell 1992).

Some forms of hexavalent Cr may induce oxidative stress and have a cytotoxic effect on bone cells. When water enriched with Cr salts is consumed during gestation, the developing foetuses have impaired ossification, most notably in the parietal and caudal bones. This indicates accelerated resorption and reduced bone formation (Kanojia et al. 1998).

In vitro studies have shown that Cr may induce osteolysis, increase bone resorption, and reduce new bone formation (Sansone et al. 2013).

The average Cr concentration in femoral bones of individuals (N = 46) of the Neolithic populations was 9.34 ± 5.15 μg/g (tab. 1).

The Cr concentration in the bone of children of the LPC (N = 13) and SPC (N = 1) were above the mean value of the Neolithic population. Conversely, LgC children (N = 3) had concentrations below the population average (tab. Cr, sex).

The Cr bone concentrations of those under 10 years of age were above the average of the Neolithic population, while the lowest Cr concentration in bone was found in the new-born LgC infant (tab. Cr, age).

Cr passes through the placenta and its concentration rises in the foetus during the 2nd and 7th month (Underwood 1977; Smrčka 2005).

In Neolithic populations, Cr showed the highest metabolic activity in the femurs of children under 10 years of age, which was also apparent in the ratio to calcium Cr/Ca (fig. Crcaage). The new-born LgC infant was noted to have a Cr deficiency. The main source of Cr in the Neolithic is believed to be honey.

Tab. Cr, sex. Chromium concentration in bone with regard to sex of the Neolithic populations

	Cr									Cr/Ca		
	dx μg/g Mean	dx N	dx μg/g SD	sin μg/g Mean	sin N	sin μg/g SD	aver.μg/g Mean	N	aver.μg/g SD	Mean	N	SD
LPC	9.550	26	4.602	9.003	21	4.614	9.640	27	4.432	3.08E-05	27	1.43E-05
Children	9.338	13	3.352	9.343	10	3.391	9.445	13	3.344	3.01E-05	13	1.07E-05
Females	10.434	6	6.867	10.244	5	7.164	10.323	6	6.409	3.20E-05	6	1.96E-05
Males	5.202	4	0.992	4.745	4	1.549	4.974	4	1.235	1.53E-05	4	3.32E-06
Undef	14.497	3	0.863	12.712	2	0.896	13.913	4	0.996	4.64E-05	4	4.00E-06
LgC	9.992	12	8.388	9.241	10	7.209	9.739	12	7.549	3.25E-05	12	2.55E-05
Children	7.656	3	5.527	8.049	3	5.510	7.853	3	5.482	2.71E-05	3	2.11E-05
Females	9.403	5	12.445	9.838	4	11.470	9.165	5	11.231	2.93E-05	5	3.65E-05
Males	12.795	2	4.303	8.696	2	0.915	10.746	2	2.609	3.81E-05	2	1.42E-05
Undef	12.168	2	5.619	11.524	1	0.000	13.000	2	4.442	4.31E-05	2	1.71E-05
SPC	7.916	7	2.350	7.137	7	2.522	7.526	7	2.168	2.35E-05	7	7.24E-06
Children	8.256	1	0.000	10.930	1	0.000	9.593	1	0.000	3.07E-05	1	0.00E+00
Females	7.590	2	0.766	7.338	2	0.445	7.464	2	0.605	2.30E-05	2	1.87E-06
Males	7.439	2	4.880	7.056	2	3.585	7.248	2	4.232	2.16E-05	2	1.29E-05
Undef	8.547	2	2.677	5.121	2	1.583	6.834	2	2.130	2.25E-05	2	9.05E-06

LPC — Linear Pottery Culture; LgC — Lengyel Culture; SPC — Stroked Pottery Culture; dx = dexter, right; sin = sinister, left

Tab. Cr, age. Chromium concentration in bone in age groups of the Neolithic populations

	Cr									Cr/Ca		
	dx µg/g Mean	dx N	dx µg/g SD	sin µg/g Mean	sin N	sin µg/g SD	aver.µg/g Mean	N	aver.µg/g SD	Mean	N	SD
LPC	9.550	26	4.602	9.003	21	4.614	9.640	27	4.432	0.0000308	27	1.43E-05
Newborn	6.783	1	0.000	7.697	1	0.000	7.240	1	0.000	0.0000256	1	0.00E+00
1–10 years	10.184	10	3.394	10.797	7	2.839	10.409	10	3.198	0.0000332	10	1.00E-05
10–20 years	7.942	7	4.270	5.983	6	3.253	7.511	7	4.177	0.0000237	7	1.39E-05
20–40 years	11.031	6	6.159	10.896	5	6.333	10.893	6	5.659	0.0000337	6	1.73E-05
40–60 years	8.945	2	9.107	2.054	1	0.000	8.833	2	9.267	0.0000286	2	3.10E-05
Undef		0		13.346	1	0.000	13.346	1	0.000	0.0000478	1	0.00E+00
LgC	9.992	12	8.388	9.241	10	7.209	9.739	12	7.549	0.0000325	12	2.55E-05
Newborn	2.446	1	0.000	2.156	1	0.000	2.301	1	0.000	0.0000076	1	0.00E+00
1–10 years	10.261	2	4.513	10.996	2	2.937	10.629	2	3.725	0.0000368	2	1.80E-05
10–20 years		0			0			0			0	
20–40 years	8.251	8	5.781	7.181	6	4.962	8.157	8	5.352	0.0000272	8	1.88E-05
40–60 years	30.929	1	0.000	25.184	1	0.000	28.056	1	0.000	0.0000913	1	0.00E+00
Undef		0			0			0			0	
SPC	7.916	7	2.350	7.137	7	2.522	7.526	7	2.168	0.0000235	7	7.24E-06
Newborn		0			0			0			0	
1–10 years	8.256	1	0.000	10.930	1	0.000	9.593	1	0.000	0.0000307	1	0.00E+00
10–20 years	10.440	1	0.000	6.240	1	0.000	8.340	1	0.000	0.0000289	1	0.00E+00
20–40 years	8.197	3	2.340	6.872	3	2.798	7.535	3	2.494	0.0000228	3	7.40E-06
40–60 years	6.060	2	2.929	6.087	2	2.214	6.074	2	2.572	0.0000184	2	8.39E-06
Undef		0			0			0			0	

LPC — Linear Pottery Culture; LgC — Lengyel Culture; SPC — Stroked Pottery Culture; dx = dexter, right; sin = sinister, left

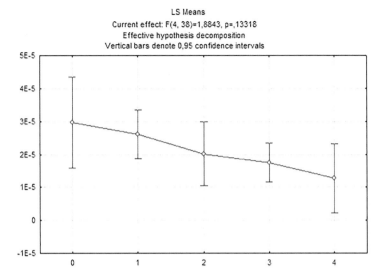

Fig. Cr/Ca age. Graphical representation of the Cr/Ca ratio in various age groups. Age groups: 0—infants, 1—up to age 10, 2—up to age 20, 3—up to age 40, 4—up to age 60.

COBALT (Co)

Co is an essential trace element, being a core component of vitamin B12. As vitamin B12 cannot be synthesised endogenously and must come directly from dietary sources, there are no dietary recommendation related directly to Co. Co is not known to have any other physiological function (Dermience et al. 2015).

The average Co concentration in the femoral bones of individuals (N = 46) of the Neolithic populations was 1.95 ± 1.32 µg/g (tab. 1).

The highest Co concentrations in bones were found in new-borns of the LPC (N = 1) (3.48 µg/g) and of the LgC (N = 1) (4.85 µg/g) (tab. Co, age).

The group of LPC children aged under 10 (N = 10) exhibited bone Co concentrations above the Neolithic population average (2.024 ± 0.944 µg/g), which persisted in individuals (0–4.7 µg/g) of the 10–20 year old age group (N = 7). In the LgC and SPC, the Co concentrations in the bones of children under the age of 10 were below the Neolithic population average (fig. Cocaage).

Between the 14 children and 14 adults, there were significant changes in Co concentrations, with a 5% significance level (tab. Co, sex; fig. Cocaage). The lowest bone Co concentrations were detected in males.

Evident from the Co concentrations in bone, it can be said that in the Neolithic, this element was important for both infants and children under 10 years of age.

Tab. Co, sex. Cobalt concentration in bone with regard to sex of the Neolithic populations

	Co									Co/Ca		
	dx µg/g Mean	dx N	dx µg/g SD	sin µg/g Mean	sin N	sin µg/g SD	aver.µg/g Mean	N	aver.µg/g SD	Mean	N	SD
LPC	2.026	26	1.516	1.801	21	1.014	2.097	27	1.521	6.77E-06	27	5.22E-06
Children	2.078	13	0.924	1.954	10	0.865	2.104	13	0.932	6.69E-06	13	3.06E-06
Females	1.706	6	1.465	1.660	5	1.088	1.629	6	1.229	5.11E-06	6	3.98E-06
Males	1.189	4	0.407	1.041	4	0.154	1.115	4	0.278	3.51E-06	4	1.18E-06
Undef	3.557	3	3.573	2.905	2	1.984	3.759	4	2.926	1.28E-05	4	1.01E-05
LgC	2.122	12	1.767	1.460	10	0.466	1.919	12	1.188	6.40E-06	12	3.98E-06
Children	3.651	3	3.079	1.986	3	0.479	2.818	3	1.776	9.44E-06	3	5.86E-06
Females	1.434	5	0.529	1.157	4	0.231	1.412	5	0.543	4.57E-06	5	1.50E-06
Males	1.273	2	0.114	1.259	2	0.244	1.266	2	0.179	4.46E-06	2	1.22E-06
Undef	2.397	2	1.803	1.498	1	0.000	2.491	2	1.670	8.34E-06	2	5.97E-06
SPC	1.468	7	0.254	1.342	7	0.160	1.405	7	0.202	4.39E-06	7	8.55E-07
Children	1.851	1	0.000	1.613	1	0.000	1.732	1	0.000	5.54E-06	1	0.00E+00
Females	1.318	2	0.065	1.268	2	0.093	1.293	2	0.014	3.98E-06	2	4.25E-08
Males	1.257	2	0.066	1.233	2	0.070	1.245	2	0.068	3.68E-06	2	1.34E-07
Undef	1.636	2	0.197	1.390	2	0.165	1.513	2	0.181	4.93E-06	2	1.06E-06

LPC—Linear Pottery Culture; LgC—Lengyel Culture; SPC—Stroked Pottery Culture; dx = dexter, right; sin = sinister, left

Tab. Co, age. Cobalt concentration in bone in age groups of the Neolithic populations

| | Co | | | | | | | | | Co/Ca | | |
	dx µg/g Mean	dx N	dx µg/g SD	sin µg/g Mean	sin N	sin µg/g SD	aver.µg/g Mean	N	aver.µg/g SD	Mean	N	SD
LPC	2.026	26	1.516	1.801	21	1.014	2.097	27	1.521	0.0000068	27	5.22E-06
Newborn	3.373	1	0.000	3.587	1	0.000	3.480	1	0.000	0.0000123	1	0.00E+00
1–10 years	2.010	10	0.935	1.746	7	0.775	2.024	10	0.944	0.0000064	10	2.88E-06
10–20 years	2.339	7	2.398	1.398	6	0.451	2.317	7	2.401	0.0000075	7	8.27E-06
20–40 years	1.702	6	1.467	1.674	5	1.077	1.632	6	1.227	0.0000051	6	3.98E-06
40–60 years	1.309	2	0.417	0.939	1	0.000	1.290	2	0.444	0.0000041	2	1.69E-06
Undef		0		4.307	1	0.000	4.307	1	0.000	0.0000154	1	0.00E+00
LgC	2.122	12	1.767	1.460	10	0.466	1.919	12	1.188	0.0000064	12	3.98E-06
Newborn	7.179	1	0.000	2.512	1	0.000	4.845	1	0.000	0.0000160	1	0.00E+00
1–10 years	1.887	2	0.548	1.723	2	0.210	1.805	2	0.379	0.0000062	2	2.20E-06
10–20 years		0			0			0			0	
20–40 years	1.633	8	0.924	1.219	6	0.246	1.648	8	0.920	0.0000055	8	3.11E-06
40–60 years	1.448	1	0.000	1.331	1	0.000	1.390	1	0.000	0.0000045	1	0.00E+00
Undef		0			0			0			0	
SPC	1.468	7	0.254	1.342	7	0.160	1.405	7	0.202	0.0000044	7	8.55E-07
Newborn		0			0			0			0	
1–10 years	1.851	1	0.000	1.613	1	0.000	1.732	1	0.000	0.0000055	1	0.00E+00
10–20 years	1.776	1	0.000	1.507	1	0.000	1.641	1	0.000	0.0000057	1	0.00E+00
20–40 years	1.326	3	0.151	1.264	3	0.075	1.295	3	0.094	0.0000039	3	3.01E-07
40–60 years	1.334	2	0.042	1.242	2	0.057	1.288	2	0.007	0.0000039	2	1.21E-07
Undef		0			0			0			0	

LPC—Linear Pottery Culture; LgC—Lengyel Culture; SPC—Stroked Pottery Culture; dx = dexter, right; sin = sinister, left

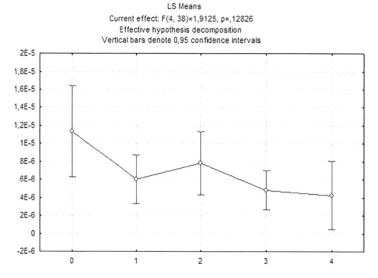

Fig. Co/Ca age. Graphical representation of the Co/Ca ratio in various age groups (Cocaage). Age groups: 0—infants, 1—up to age 10, 2—up to age 20, 3—up to age 40, 4—up to age 60.

COPPER (Cu)

The average Cu concentration in the femoral bones of individuals (N = 46) of the Neolithic populations was 6.67 ± 3.63 µg/g (tab. 1).

The concentration of Cu in bone was higher in children across all Neolithic cultures when compared with adult females and males (10% significance level).

With regard to children of the Neolithic cultures, the highest Cu levels were found in LgC children (8.90 ± 2.27 µg/g) (N = 3), and Cu was also in proportion to Ca (5% significance level; LgC > LPC > SPC; tab. Cu, sex; fig. Cucacult).

Infants from the LPC (N = 1) (9.36 µg/g) and the LgC (N = 1) (10.06 µg/g) exhibit the highest Cu concentrations in bone (tab. Cu, age; fig. Cucaage).

The lowest bone Cu concentrations in the Neolithic were observed in individuals aged about 60 years old (tab. Cu, age).

The highest metabolic activity of Cu was detected in new-borns and children under 10 years of age.

Tab. Cu, sex. Copper concentration in bone with regard to sex of the Neolithic populations

	dx μg/g Mean	dx N	dx μg/g SD	sin μg/g Mean	sin N	sin μg/g SD	aver.μg/g Mean	N	aver.μg/g SD	Mean	N	SD
	Cu									**Cu/Ca**		
LPC	7.094	26	3.936	7.162	21	4.461	7.308	27	4.068	2.33E-05	27	1.31E-05
Children	8.438	13	2.999	7.793	10	2.869	8.483	13	2.997	2.69E-05	13	9.25E-06
Females	6.633	6	6.333	7.559	5	8.222	6.843	6	6.883	2.16E-05	6	2.22E-05
Males	4.169	4	1.701	4.465	4	1.660	4.317	4	1.659	1.36E-05	4	5.96E-06
Undef	6.089	3	2.015	8.411	2	2.865	7.178	4	2.725	2.42E-05	4	1.04E-05
LgC	6.487	12	3.254	5.255	10	2.848	6.210	12	3.176	2.08E-05	12	1.13E-05
Children	9.280	3	2.486	8.509	3	2.410	8.895	3	2.268	3.02E-05	3	1.02E-05
Females	4.544	5	2.147	3.303	4	1.951	4.252	5	2.113	1.36E-05	5	6.07E-06
Males	6.045	2	0.915	4.474	2	1.258	5.260	2	1.086	1.86E-05	2	6.28E-06
Undef	7.601	2	6.297	4.864	1	0.000	8.030	2	5.691	2.69E-05	2	2.03E-05
SPC	5.283	7	2.078	4.697	7	1.689	4.990	7	1.828	1.57E-05	7	6.69E-06
Children	6.431	1	0.000	6.620	1	0.000	6.525	1	0.000	2.09E-05	1	0.00E+00
Females	4.015	2	0.596	3.714	2	0.172	3.864	2	0.212	1.19E-05	2	6.54E-07
Males	5.419	2	1.961	4.375	2	0.099	4.897	2	1.030	1.45E-05	2	3.31E-06
Undef	5.842	2	4.063	5.041	2	3.317	5.442	2	3.690	1.82E-05	2	1.37E-05

LPC — Linear Pottery Culture; LgC — Lengyel Culture; SPC — Stroked Pottery Culture; dx = dexter, right; sin = sinister, left

Tab. Cu, age. Copper concentration in bone in age groups of the Neolithic populations

	Cu									Cu/Ca		
	dx μg/g Mean	dx N	dx μg/g SD	sin μg/g Mean	sin N	sin μg/g SD	aver.μg/g Mean	N	aver. μg/g SD	Mean	N	SD
LPC	7.094	26	3.936	7.162	21	4.461	7.308	27	4.068	0.0000233	27	1.31E-05
Newborn	9.500	1	0.000	9.221	1	0.000	9.361	1	0.000	0.0000331	1	0.00E+00
1–10 years	8.674	10	3.327	8.091	7	3.253	8.816	10	3.263	0.0000278	10	9.70E-06
10–20 years	6.080	7	1.342	5.652	6	1.092	6.030	7	1.299	0.0000190	7	4.73E-06
20–40 years	6.466	6	6.464	7.493	5	8.272	6.732	6	6.966	0.0000212	6	2.25E-05
40–60 years	3.417	2	0.752	2.734	1	0.000	3.379	2	0.805	0.0000106	2	3.30E-06
Undef		0		10.436	1	0.000	10.436	1	0.000	0.0000373	1	0.00E+00
LgC	6.487	12	3.254	5.255	10	2.848	6.210	12	3.176	0.0000208	12	1.13E-05
Newborn	11.420	1	0.000	8.699	1	0.000	10.060	1	0.000	0.0000332	1	0.00E+00
1–10 years	8.209	2	2.343	8.414	2	3.400	8.312	2	2.872	0.0000288	2	1.39E-05
10–20 years		0			0			0			0	
20–40 years	5.453	8	3.210	3.850	6	1.789	5.335	8	3.203	0.0000178	8	1.10E-05
40–60 years	6.387	1	0.000	3.925	1	0.000	5.156	1	0.000	0.0000168	1	0.00E+00
Undef		0			0			0			0	
SPC	5.283	7	2.078	4.697	7	1.689	4.990	7	1.828	0.0000157	7	6.69E-06
Newborn		0			0			0			0	
1–10 years	6.431	1	0.000	6.620	1	0.000	6.525	1	0.000	0.0000209	1	0.00E+00
10–20 years	8.716	1	0.000	7.386	1	0.000	8.051	1	0.000	0.0000279	1	0.00E+00
20–40 years	4.456	3	2.059	3.658	3	0.888	4.057	3	1.428	0.0000123	3	4.23E-06
40–60 years	4.234	2	0.286	3.949	2	0.504	4.091	2	0.109	0.0000123	2	1.25E-07
Undef		0			0			0			0	

LPC – Linear Pottery Culture; LgC – Lengyel Culture; SPC – Stroked Pottery Culture; dx = dexter, right; sin = sinister, left

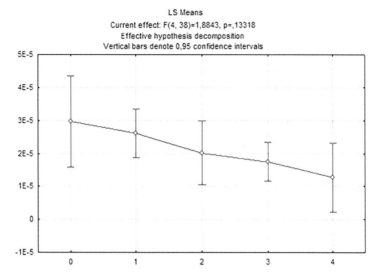

Fig. Cu/Ca age. Graphical representation of the Cu/Ca ratio in various age groups (Cucaage). Age groups: 0—infants, 1—up to age 10, 2—up to age 20, 3—up to age 40, 4—up to age 60.

CALCIUM (Ca)

The primary function of Ca in bone metabolism is the formation of hydroxy-apatite, while also having a vital role in numerous processes throughout the body. Ca deficiency leads to a reduction of the inorganic bone component and bone density; a long term deficiency may result in pathologies such as rickets, osteomalacia, and osteoporosis (Dermience et al. 2015).

The average concentration of Ca in bone of the 46 individuals of the Neolithic cultures was 313 ± 22 mg/g (tab. 1).

In the LPC, adults had higher Ca content in bones than the children and infant. The highest Ca concentrations were found in males (N = 4) (323 ± 22 mg/g). In the SPC, the highest Ca concentrations were also detected in males (N = 2) (338 ± 62 mg/g).

The lowest bone Ca concentration was seen in the LPC infant (283 mg/g). The highest Ca concentration was found in individuals, aged approx. 60 years old, of LPC (N = 2) (322 ± 24 mg/g) and SPC (N = 2) (333 ± 12 mg/g) (p 0.532) (tab. Ca, age; fig. Caage).

In the Moravian Painted Ware Culture (LgC), in all age categories, there was a stable concentration of Ca (~300 mg/g,) which was below the overall population average.

The lowest Ca concentrations were detected in LgC males (N = 2) (289 ± 39 mg/g).

Tab. Ca, sex. Calcium concentration in bone with regard to sex of the Neolithic populations

	Ca								
	dx µg/g Mean	dx N	dx µg/g SD	sin µg/g Mean	sin N	sin µg/g SD	aver.µg/g Mean	N	aver.µg/g SD
LPC	317684.3	26	22612.3	316746.2	21	22441.0	315398.2	27	20473.5
Children	316834.4	13	23745.3	311885.6	10	23819.9	314682.6	13	20122.4
Females	320041.2	6	18383.9	328672.9	5	22199.6	321709.8	6	20782.0
Males	325519.4	4	33436.8	320504.3	4	12539.4	323011.9	4	22462.4
Undef	306206.8	3	12029.6	303716.8	2	34336.3	300642.8	4	18418.9
LgC	306680.9	12	21293.5	294320.9	10	45151.7	301778.7	12	24764.2
Children	301888.2	3	29326.4	300367.8	3	38614.0	301128.0	3	32024.1
Females	308321.6	5	23610.4	297187.1	4	34006.8	305735.4	5	24495.6
Males	323592.4	2	680.0	255025.5	2	79159.9	289308.9	2	39240.0
Undef	292856.6	2	770.9	343305.9	1	0.0	305332.7	2	18414.7
SPC	321201.9	7	22340.7	324152.5	7	21691.2	322677.2	7	17418.5
Children	312219.5	1	0.0	313078.1	1	0.0	312648.8	1	0.0
Females	335813.7	2	10937.4	313765.1	2	10853.0	324789.4	2	42.2
Males	336255.4	2	10274.1	339317.8	2	22605.5	337786.6	2	6165.7
Undef	296027.7	2	23261.2	324911.8	2	37345.5	310469.8	2	30303.4

LPC—Linear Pottery Culture; LgC—Lengyel Culture; SPC—Stroked Pottery Culture; dx = dexter, right; sin = sinister, left

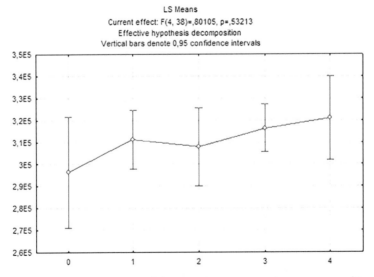

LS Means
Current effect: $F_{(4, 38)}=,80105$, p=,53213
Effective hypothesis decomposition
Vertical bars denote 0,95 confidence intervals

Fig. Ca age. Graphical representation of the Ca proportion in various age groups (Caage). Age groups: 0—infants, 1—up to age 10, 2—up to age 20, 3—up to age 40, 4—up to age 60.

Tab. Ca, age. Calcium concentration in bone in age groups of the Neolithic populations

	Ca								
	dx µg/g Mean	dx N	dx µg/g SD	sin µg/g Mean	sin N	sin µg/g SD	aver.µg/g Mean	N	aver.µg/g SD
LPC	317684.3	26	22612.3	316746.2	21	22441.0	315398.2	27	20473.5
Newborn	279583.7	1	0.0	286533.7	1	0.0	283058.7	1	0.0
1–10 years	316545.4	10	20579.7	309736.3	7	22570.2	313882.6	10	18449.8
10–20 years	319575.3	7	26913.1	324540.5	6	15594.2	319953.3	7	19193.7
20–40 years	323855.6	6	22729.1	324620.9	5	19678.8	321928.7	6	21001.3
40–60 years	317297.3	2	17992.3	347198.1	1	0.0	321591.9	2	24065.7
Undef		0		279437.4	1	0.0	279437.4	1	0.0
LgC	306680.9	12	21293.5	294320.9	10	45151.7	301778.7	12	24764.2
Newborn	316761.4	1	0.0	290105.5	1	0.0	303433.5	1	0.0
1–10 years	294451.6	2	37259.4	305498.9	2	53142.3	299975.2	2	45200.9
10–20 years		0			0			0	
20–40 years	308670.9	8	21261.9	288760.1	6	54477.6	301327.3	8	25804.1
40–60 years	305138.3	1	0.0	309544.6	1	0.0	307341.5	1	0.0
Undef		0			0			0	
SPC	321201.9	7	22340.7	324152.5	7	21691.2	322677.2	7	17418.5
Newborn		0			0			0	
1–10 years	312219.5	1	0.0	313078.1	1	0.0	312648.8	1	0.0
10–20 years	279579.6	1	0.0	298504.6	1	0.0	289042.1	1	0.0
20–40 years	333181.3	3	17931.4	326914.4	3	22825.8	330047.8	3	4592.2
40–60 years	328535.2	2	644.0	338370.8	2	23944.8	333453.0	2	12294.4
Undef		0			0			0	

LPC—Linear Pottery Culture; LgC—Lengyel Culture; SPC—Stroked Pottery Culture; dx = dexter, right; sin = sinister, left

The lower bone Ca concentrations in males, females and children of the Moravian Painted Ware Culture (LgC) (fig. Cacult) in comparison to the LPC and SPC are significant, at a 5% significance level (tab. Ca, sex).

LEAD (Pb)

Pb accumulates in bone during foetal development, and even at low levels can have a detrimental effect on bone metabolism. Pb causes growth retardation

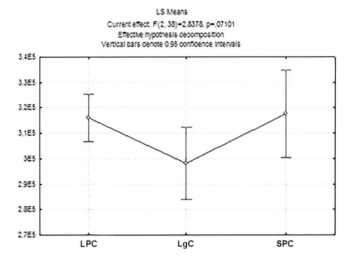

LS Means
Current effect: $F_{(2, 38)} = 2,8378$, p=,07101
Effective hypothesis decomposition
Vertical bars denote 0.95 confidence intervals

Fig. Ca, cult. Graphical representation of the changes in calcium concentration in bone in the Neolithic cultures (Linear Pottery Culture — LPC; Lengyel Culture — LgC; and Stroked Pottery Culture — SPC).

through the restriction of endochondral ossification. The reduction of bone minerals may cause osteoporosis.

Surprisingly, Pb stimulates chondrogenesis; this not beneficial however, because the cartilage persists while bone formation is reduced (Zuscik et al. 2007). In hydroxyapatite crystals, Ca is replaced by Pb (Dermience et al. 2015).

The average Pb concentration in bones of the Neolithic population (N = 46) is 0–3,6 µg/g (tab. 1).

The highest Pb concentration in bone was found in the LPC infant (6.18 µg/g). The 10 LPC children aged under 10, had significantly lower Pb concentrations (1.57 ± 1.23 µg/g), indicating a decrease in the accumulation of Pb in the cartilage after birth. The second increase in Pb concentration in femurs was seen in the 10–20 age group (fig. Pb/Ca age).

The Pb concentrations in the femoral bone of LPC children (N = 13) (1.8 ± 1.7 µg/g), in LgC children (N = 3) (0–3.5 µg/g), and the SPC child (N = 1) (1.5 µg/g) were above the Neolithic population average (1.2 µg/g) (tab. Pb, age).

The Pb concentration in the adult LPC and LgC groups was below the average for Neolithic population. There was a significant difference between children and adult, at significance level of 0.01 for Pb, and 0.01% for Pb/Ca (fig. Pb/Ca age, tab. 2).

The activity of Pb in bone metabolism was greatest in infants under 1 year of age, children under 10 years of age, and also males and females aged ~20 years old (tab. Pb, sex).

Tab. Pb, sex. Lead concentration in bone with regard to sex of the Neolithic populations

	Pb									Pb/Ca		
	dx μg/g Mean	dx N	dx μg/g SD	sin μg/g Mean	sin N	sin μg/g SD	aver.μg/g Mean	N	aver.μg/g SD	Mean	N	SD
LPC	1.4954	26	2.9518	0.9972	21	1.6151	1.5716	27	2.9213	5.20E-06	27	9.94E-06
Children	1.7618	13	1.6801	1.6653	10	1.9961	1.8064	13	1.7242	5.84E-06	13	5.97E-06
Females	0.1021	6	0.1905	0.2493	5	0.3451	0.1549	6	0.2517	4.81E-07	6	7.93E-07
Males	0.0998	4	0.1995	0.0088	4	0.0177	0.0543	4	0.1086	1.87E-07	4	3.75E-07
Undef	4.9883	3	7.9592	1.5028	2	2.0392	4.4504	4	6.6017	1.52E-05	4	2.24E-05
LgC	0.6023	12	1.3789	0.5900	10	1.0996	0.6411	12	1.2234	2.25E-06	12	4.49E-06
Children	1.5987	3	2.4985	1.2860	3	1.8270	1.4423	3	2.1615	5.29E-06	3	8.14E-06
Females	0.0004	5	0.0009	0.3967	4	0.7934	0.1589	5	0.3553	4.85E-07	5	1.08E-06
Males	0.0297	2	0.0419	0.0000	2	0.0000	0.0148	2	0.0210	5.67E-08	2	8.02E-08
Undef	1.1852	2	1.5171	0.4552	1	0.0000	1.2709	2	1.3959	4.31E-06	2	4.83E-06
SPC	1.0019	7	1.1627	0.3205	7	0.5487	0.6612	7	0.6714	2.05E-06	7	2.07E-06
Children	1.7157	1	0.0000	1.2929	1	0.0000	1.5043	1	0.0000	4.81E-06	1	0.00E+00
Females	0.0843	2	0.1192	0.0000	2	0.0000	0.0421	2	0.0596	1.30E-07	2	1.84E-07
Males	1.9048	2	1.9934	0.4618	2	0.6531	1.1833	2	0.6701	3.52E-06	2	2.05E-06
Undef	0.6598	2	0.2560	0.0135	2	0.0191	0.3367	2	0.1375	1.11E-06	2	5.52E-07

LPC—Linear Pottery Culture; LgC—Lengyel Culture; SPC—Stroked Pottery Culture; dx = dexter, right; sin = sinister, left

Tab. Pb, age. Lead concentration in bone in age groups of the Neolithic populations

	Pb									Pb/Ca		
	dx μg/g Mean	dx N	dx μg/g SD	sin μg/g Mean	sin N	sin μg/g SD	aver.μg/g Mean	N	aver.μg/g SD	Mean	N	SD
LPC	1.4954	26	2.9518	0.9972	21	1.6151	1.5716	27	2.9213	0.0000052	27	9.94E-06
Newborn	5.7493	1	0.0000	6.6145	1	0.0000	6.1819	1	0.0000	0.0000218	1	0.00E+00
1–10 years	1.5362	10	1.3097	1.2282	7	1.1617	1.5685	10	1.2323	0.0000049	10	3.91E-06
10–20 years	2.3779	7	5.2249	0.2562	6	0.3987	2.3115	7	5.2488	0.0000077	7	1.78E-05
20–40 years	0.1021	6	0.1905	0.2493	5	0.3451	0.1549	6	0.2517	0.0000005	6	7.93E-07
40–60 years	0.2551	2	0.3608	0.0000	1	0.0000	0.2551	2	0.3608	0.0000008	2	1.18E-06
Undef		0		2.9447	1	0.0000	2.9447	1	0.0000	0.0000105	1	0.00E+00
LgC	0.6023	12	1.3789	0.5900	10	1.0996	0.6411	12	1.2234	0.0000023	12	4.49E-06
Newborn	0.0000	1	0.0000	0.0000	1	0.0000	0.0000	1	0.0000	0.0000000	1	0.00E+00
1–10 years	2.3980	2	2.9413	1.9290	2	2.0482	2.1635	2	2.4948	0.0000079	2	9.51E-06
10–20 years		0			0			0			0	
20–40 years	0.3040	8	0.7906	0.3403	6	0.6372	0.4207	8	0.7923	0.0000014	8	2.69E-06
40–60 years	0.0000	1	0.0000	0.0000	1	0.0000	0.0000	1	0.0000	0.0000000	1	0.00E+00
Undef		0			0			0			0	
SPC	1.0019	7	1.1627	0.3205	7	0.5487	0.6612	7	0.6714	0.0000020	7	2.07E-06
Newborn		0			0			0			0	
1–10 years	1.7157	1	0.0000	1.2929	1	0.0000	1.5043	1	0.0000	0.0000048	1	0.00E+00
10–20 years	0.8408	1	0.0000	0.0270	1	0.0000	0.4339	1	0.0000	0.0000015	1	0.00E+00
20–40 years	1.2644	3	1.7914	0.0000	3	0.0000	0.6322	3	0.8957	0.0000019	3	2.69E-06
40–60 years	0.3319	2	0.2310	0.4618	2	0.6531	0.3969	2	0.4421	0.0000012	2	1.28E-06
Undef		0			0			0			0	

LPC—Linear Pottery Culture; LgC—Lengyel Culture; SPC—Stroked Pottery Culture; dx = dexter, right; sin = sinister, left

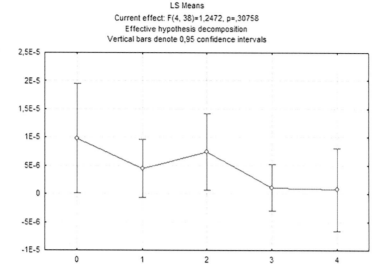

Fig. Pb/Ca age. Graphical representation of the Pb/Ca ratio in various age groups (Pbcaage). Age groups: 0—infants, 1—up to age 10, 2—up to age 20, 3—up to age 40, 4—up to age 60.

MAGNESIUM (Mg)

Mg is abundant in the human body and is essential for the function of 300 enzymes (Dermience et al. 2015). Approximately 50–60% of the 25 g present in the body is located in bone. Deficiency causes impaired bone growth, osteopenia, skeletal fragility and osteoporosis, even at low levels (Rude et al. 2009).

The average Mg concentration in the femurs of the Neolithic population (N = 46) was 1355 ± 609 µg/g (tab. 1).

The LPC (N = 27) and SPC (N = 7) populations were below the mean Mg concentration for Neolithic populations, while the LgC (N = 3) individuals were above the average level (fig. Mgcult).

Femoral Mg concentrations of LPC and SPC children were below the Neolithic population average. The concentrations seen in the three LgC children exceeds the average values (2524 ± 694 µg/g) (tab. Mg, sex). LgC newborns and children under 10 years of age had Mg concentrations above the average value.

Mg can therefore be considered metabolically active, with higher levels during growth periods, and particularly during intrauterine growth and up to the age of 10.

Tab. Mg, sex. Magnesium concentration in bone with regard to sex of the Neolithic populations.

	Mg									Mg/Ca		
	dx µg/g Mean	dx N	dx µg/g SD	sin µg/g Mean	sin N	sin µg/g SD	aver.µg/g Mean	N	aver.µg/g SD	Mean	N	SD
LPC	1263.52	26	629.24	1199.60	21	615.02	1240.81	27	594.13	3.96E-03	27	1.90E-03
Children	1268.50	13	806.18	1311.25	10	846.64	1277.42	13	780.51	4.07E-03	13	2.42E-03
Females	1205.91	6	463.66	1050.80	5	353.87	1207.08	6	479.55	3.83E-03	6	1.76E-03
Males	1497.86	4	373.25	1278.50	4	186.46	1388.18	4	262.62	4.35E-03	4	1.12E-03
Undef	1044.74	3	334.09	855.62	2	108.58	1025.03	4	266.54	3.43E-03	4	9.71E-04
LgC	1728.70	12	665.68	1777.43	10	747.86	1733.52	12	670.98	5.75E-03	12	2.11E-03
Children	2565.38	3	544.45	2482.66	3	845.84	2524.02	3	694.31	8.29E-03	3	1.42E-03
Females	1455.46	5	552.81	1427.23	4	645.00	1468.38	5	561.26	4.89E-03	5	2.14E-03
Males	1472.49	2	503.78	1480.21	2	425.38	1476.35	2	464.58	5.04E-03	2	9.22E-04
Undef	1412.96	2	34.89	1656.95	1	0.00	1467.79	2	112.43	4.80E-03	2	7.84E-05
SPC	1135.54	7	171.28	1157.60	7	215.34	1146.57	7	189.34	3.55E-03	7	5.52E-04
Children	1246.98	1	0.00	1316.56	1	0.00	1281.77	1	0.00	4.10E-03	1	0.00E+00
Females	1170.55	2	19.65	1079.62	2	12.66	1125.08	2	3.49	3.46E-03	2	1.12E-05
Males	1154.17	2	330.97	1248.41	2	421.38	1201.29	2	376.18	3.57E-03	2	1.18E-03
Undef	1026.17	2	163.14	1065.31	2	171.90	1045.74	2	167.52	3.36E-03	2	2.12E-04

LPC — Linear Pottery Culture; LgC — Lengyel Culture; SPC — Stroked Pottery Culture; dx = dexter, right; sin = sinister, left

Tab. Mg, age. Magnesium concentration in bone in age groups of the Neolithic populations.

	Mg									Mg/Ca		
	dx µg/g Mean	dx N	dx µg/g SD	sin µg/g Mean	sin N	sin µg/g SD	aver.µg/g Mean	N	aver.µg/g SD	Mean	N	SD
LPC	1263.52	26	629.24	1199.60	21	615.02	1240.81	27	594.13	0.0039648	27	1.90E-03
Newborn	789.10	1	0.00	798.60	1	0.00	793.85	1	0.00	0.0028045	1	0.00E+00
1–10 years	1402.77	10	882.45	1481.72	7	976.09	1400.49	10	859.16	0.0044721	10	2.65E-03
10–20 years	1209.19	7	466.56	1112.12	6	282.94	1179.79	7	356.38	0.0037397	7	1.32E-03
20–40 years	1239.43	6	461.01	1066.02	5	357.37	1230.18	6	476.03	0.0038955	6	1.74E-03
40–60 years	1066.98	2	34.81	1085.80	1	0.00	1065.53	2	32.76	0.0033188	2	1.46E-04
Undef		0		932.40	1	0.00	932.40	1	0.00	0.0033367	1	0.00E+00
LgC	1728.70	12	665.68	1777.43	10	747.86	1733.52	12	670.98	0.0057521	12	2.11E-03
Newborn	2480.40	1	0.00	2254.09	1	0.00	2367.24	1	0.00	0.0078015	1	0.00E+00
1–10 years	2607.88	2	762.91	2596.94	2	1162.98	2602.41	2	962.94	0.0085304	2	1.92E-03
10–20 years		0			0			0			0	
20–40 years	1549.68	8	330.17	1602.32	6	398.12	1568.57	8	335.80	0.0052432	8	1.26E-03
40–60 years	650.79	1	0.00	712.40	1	0.00	681.60	1	0.00	0.0022177	1	0.00E+00
Undef		0			0			0			0	
SPC	1135.54	7	171.28	1157.60	7	215.34	1146.57	7	189.34	0.0035540	7	5.52E-04
Newborn		0			0			0			0	
1–10 years	1246.98	1	0.00	1316.56	1	0.00	1281.77	1	0.00	0.0040997	1	0.00E+00
10–20 years	910.81	1	0.00	943.75	1	0.00	927.28	1	0.00	0.0032081	1	0.00E+00
20–40 years	1228.79	3	138.26	1273.93	3	241.00	1251.36	3	188.15	0.0037881	3	5.31E-04
40–60 years	1052.29	2	186.89	1010.56	2	85.01	1031.42	2	135.95	0.0031028	2	5.22E-04
Undef		0			0			0			0	

LPC—Linear Pottery Culture; LgC—Lengyel Culture; SPC—Stroked Pottery Culture; dx = dexter, right; sin = sinister, left

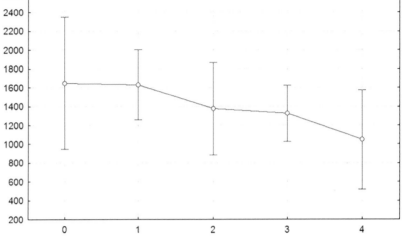

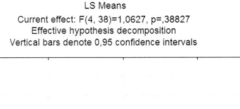

Fig. Mgage. Graphical representation of the proportion of Mg (μg/g of bone) in various age groups. Age groups: 0—infants, 1—up to age 10, 2—up to age 20, 3—up to age 40, 4—up to age 60.

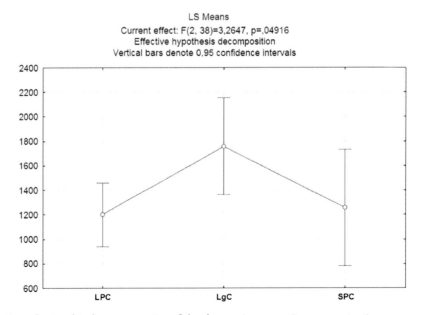

Fig. Mg, cult. Graphical representation of the changes in magnesium concentration (μg/g in bone) in the Neolithic cultures (Linear Pottery Culture—LPC; Lengyel Culture—LgC; and Stroked Pottery Culture—SPC).

NICKEL *(Ni)*

Ni is essential for the majority anaerobic micro-organisms. In rats and goats Ni reduces growth, reproductive ability and glucose in plasma. In addition, it also influences the distribution of other elements such as Ca, Fe and Zn (Nielsen 1995).

The average bone concentration of Ni of the Neolithic populations (N = 46) of Moravia is 14.8 ± 4.6 µg/g (tab. 1).

The highest concentrations were detected in the unidentified LPC (N = 4) (18 µg/g) and LgC individuals (N = 2), and in the LgC children (N = 3) (17.3 µg/g).

The Ni bone concentration of Neolithic Moravian males can be compared in the following manner: LgC > SPC > LPC.

The lowest bone concentration of Ni was found in LPC males (N = 4) (10.6 ± 0.34 µg/g). LgC males (N = 2) had a significantly higher concentration of Ni (13.4 ± 0.8 µg/g) compared to males of the LPC (N = 4)(10.5 ± 0.34 µg/g), with a 5% significance level. There was also a significance in the Ni to calcium ratio (4.70 E-05 in LgC and 3.29 E-05 in LPC) (tab. Ni, sex, tab. 2).

Infants of the LPC (N = 1) (19.9 µg/g) and LgC (N = 1)(24.1 µg/g) exhibited concentrations above the Neolithic population average, with this age group having the highest concentrations of Ni in bone (fig. Nicaage, tab. Ni, age).

The raised Ni concentrations in femoral bones of the Neolithic indicate its metabolic activity in new-born infants.

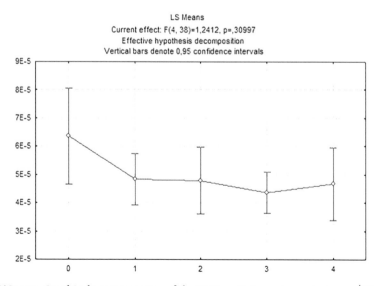

Fig. Ni/Ca age. Graphical representation of the Ni/Ca ratio in various age groups (Nicaage). Age groups: 0—infants, 1—up to age 10, 2—up to age 20, 3—up to age 40, 4—up to age 60.

Tab. Ni, sex. Nickel concentration in bone with regard to sex of the Neolithic populations

	Ni									Ni/Ca		
	dx μg/g Mean	dx N	dx μg/g SD	sin μg/g Mean	sin N	sin μg/g SD	aver.μg/g Mean	N	aver.μg/g SD	Mean	N	SD
LPC	14.196	26	4.796	13.997	21	5.064	14.567	27	5.211	4.66E-05	27	1.81E-05
Children	14.983	13	5.013	14.212	10	4.618	15.018	13	5.024	4.78E-05	13	1.61E-05
Females	14.158	6	6.008	14.150	5	4.783	13.776	6	5.300	4.29E-05	6	1.71E-05
Males	10.922	4	0.802	10.192	4	0.540	10.557	4	0.335	3.29E-05	4	3.48E-06
Undef	15.231	3	4.299	20.154	2	9.713	18.297	4	6.731	6.20E-05	4	2.64E-05
LgC	15.991	12	5.047	14.590	10	3.720	15.660	12	4.495	5.21E-05	12	1.51E-05
Children	18.444	3	7.619	16.104	3	4.266	17.274	3	5.942	5.76E-05	3	1.94E-05
Females	14.824	5	4.101	14.275	4	5.004	14.644	5	4.200	4.78E-05	5	1.28E-05
Males	13.722	2	0.587	13.083	2	1.079	13.403	2	0.833	4.70E-05	2	9.25E-06
Undef	17.499	2	7.536	14.325	1	0.000	18.038	2	6.774	5.99E-05	2	2.58E-05
SPC	14.257	7	1.387	13.764	7	0.768	14.010	7	1.046	4.37E-05	7	5.71E-06
Children	15.252	1	0.000	14.043	1	0.000	14.647	1	0.000	4.68E-05	1	0.00E+00
Females	14.297	2	0.165	13.956	2	0.386	14.127	2	0.110	4.35E-05	2	3.34E-07
Males	13.136	2	1.043	12.884	2	0.617	13.010	2	0.830	3.85E-05	2	1.75E-06
Undef	14.840	2	2.498	14.312	2	0.840	14.576	2	1.669	4.74E-05	2	1.00E-05

LPC — Linear Pottery Culture; LgC — Lengyel Culture; SPC — Stroked Pottery Culture; dx = dexter, right; sin = sinister, left

Tab. Ni, age. Nickel concentration in bone in age groups of the Neolithic populations

	Ni									Ni/Ca		
	dx μg/g Mean	dx N	dx μg/g SD	sin μg/g Mean	sin N	sin μg/g SD	aver.μg/g Mean	N	aver. μg/g SD	Mean	N	SD
LPC	14.196	26	4.796	13.997	21	5.064	14.567	27	5.211	0.0000466	27	1.81E-05
Newborn	19.742	1	0.000	20.090	1	0.000	19.916	1	0.000	0.0000704	1	0.00E+00
1–10 years	14.644	10	5.411	13.347	7	4.909	14.672	10	5.441	0.0000465	10	1.65E-05
10–20 years	13.493	7	3.632	11.993	6	2.529	13.327	7	3.706	0.0000420	7	1.31E-05
20–40 years	14.007	6	6.106	14.218	5	4.718	13.729	6	5.332	0.0000428	6	1.72E-05
40–60 years	12.217	2	1.359	10.357	1	0.000	11.992	2	1.676	0.0000376	2	8.03E-06
Undef		0		27.022	1	0.000	27.022	1	0.000	0.0000967	1	0.00E+00
LgC	15.991	12	5.047	14.590	10	3.720	15.660	12	4.495	0.0000521	12	1.51E-05
Newborn	27.233	1	0.000	21.024	1	0.000	24.128	1	0.000	0.0000795	1	0.00E+00
1–10 years	14.050	2	0.487	13.644	2	0.288	13.847	2	0.388	0.0000466	2	5.73E-06
10–20 years		0			0			0			0	
20–40 years	14.362	8	3.640	12.696	6	1.624	14.321	8	3.682	0.0000478	8	1.31E-05
40–60 years	21.660	1	0.000	21.415	1	0.000	21.537	1	0.000	0.0000701	1	0.00E+00
Undef		0			0			0			0	
SPC	14.257	7	1.387	13.764	7	0.768	14.010	7	1.046	0.0000437	7	5.71E-06
Newborn		0			0			0			0	
1–10 years	15.252	1	0.000	14.043	1	0.000	14.647	1	0.000	0.0000468	1	0.00E+00
10–20 years	16.607	1	0.000	14.906	1	0.000	15.756	1	0.000	0.0000545	1	0.00E+00
20–40 years	13.217	3	0.900	13.465	3	0.917	13.341	3	0.892	0.0000405	3	3.24E-06
40–60 years	14.144	2	0.382	13.502	2	0.257	13.823	2	0.319	0.0000415	2	2.49E-06
Undef		0			0			0			0	

LPC—Linear Pottery Culture; LgC—Lengyel Culture; SPC—Stroked Pottery Culture; dx = dexter, right; sin = sinister, left

SODIUM (Na)

Hyponatremia has proven links in the development of osteoporosis, and an increased risk of fractures. Due to this, in clinical medicine monitoring of hyponatremia is recommended, particularly in the elderly and postmenopausal women. Hyponatremia directly influences bone metabolism, it stimulates osteoclast proliferation and may mobilise Na stores in bones (Dermience et al. 2015).

The average Na concentration in the femoral bones in the 46 individuals of the Neolithic cultures was 2170 ± 656 µg/g (tab. 1).

In the Neolithic cultures, differences in bone Na concentrations were found between sexes and age groups. In the LPC children (N = 13) and its successive SPC, there was the lowest concentration of Na in bone (1782–1800 µg/g).

In contrast, the Na concentration in bone of the children (N = 3) (2502 ± 398 µg/g) of the Moravian Painted Ware Culture (LgC), was above the average level of the Neolithic population (p 0.077) (tab. Na, sex; fig. Nacult).

The Na concentrations in bone were higher in infants under 1 year of age and in the maturus age group (ages 40-60).

Based on Na analysis in femurs, it is presumed that groups with an increased risk of osteoporosis were infants, children, and 40-60-year-old age group, particularly in the Moravian Painted Ware Culture (LgC).

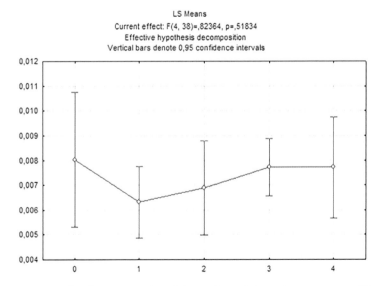

Fig. Na/Ca age. Graphical representation of the Na/Ca ratio in various age groups (Nacaage). Age groups: 0—infants, 1—up to age 10, 2—up to age 20, 3—up to age 40, 4—up to age 60.

Tab. Na, sex. Sodium concentration in bone with regard to sex of the Neolithic populations

	Na									Na/Ca		
	dx µg/g Mean	dx N	dx µg/g SD	sin µg/g Mean	sin N	sin µg/g SD	aver.µg/g Mean	N	aver.µg/g SD	Mean	N	SD
LPC	1953.15	26	470.68	1999.46	21	542.72	1963.26	27	485.13	6.25E-03	27	1.58E-03
Children	1747.66	13	411.99	1880.45	10	601.51	1782.55	13	481.11	5.73E-03	13	1.81E-03
Females	2090.34	6	211.95	1997.09	5	373.42	2061.79	6	270.51	6.41E-03	6	7.70E-04
Males	2254.22	4	788.18	2377.92	4	641.26	2316.07	4	710.97	7.13E-03	4	1.90E-03
Undef	2167.77	3	354.06	1843.45	2	282.57	2049.99	4	386.57	6.81E-03	4	1.16E-03
LgC	2625.10	12	880.25	2636.96	10	1042.50	2595.76	12	910.26	8.76E-03	12	3.55E-03
Children	2493.99	3	471.72	2510.34	3	351.23	2502.17	3	398.52	8.42E-03	3	1.86E-03
Females	3129.82	5	1161.12	3375.92	4	1278.71	3147.35	5	1178.46	1.06E-02	5	4.80E-03
Males	2008.96	2	433.61	1904.79	2	298.39	1956.88	2	366.00	6.91E-03	2	2.20E-03
Undef	2176.10	2	98.08	1525.33	1	0.00	1996.07	2	156.52	6.56E-03	2	9.09E-04
SPC	2251.26	7	600.45	2200.19	7	388.16	2225.72	7	359.34	6.89E-03	7	9.79E-04
Children	1861.65	1	0.00	1738.84	1	0.00	1800.24	1	0.00	5.76E-03	1	0.00E+00
Females	2305.22	2	232.79	2454.03	2	237.53	2379.62	2	235.16	7.33E-03	2	7.25E-04
Males	2048.85	2	266.97	2390.07	2	568.61	2219.46	2	417.79	6.58E-03	2	1.36E-03
Undef	2594.52	2	1250.03	1987.13	2	140.18	2290.82	2	554.92	7.33E-03	2	1.07E-03

LPC—Linear Pottery Culture; LgC—Lengyel Culture; SPC—Stroked Pottery Culture; dx = dexter, right; sin = sinister, left

Tab. Na, age. Sodium concentration in bone in age groups of the Neolithic populations

	Na									Na/Ca		
	dx µg/g Mean	dx N	dx µg/g SD	sin µg/g Mean	sin N	sin µg/g SD	aver. µg/g Mean	N	aver. µg/g SD	Mean	N	SD
LPC	1953.15	26	470.68	1999.46	21	542.72	1963.26	27	485.13	0.0062516	27	1.58E-03
Newborn	2064.12	1	0.00	2068.33	1	0.00	2066.23	1	0.00	0.0072996	1	0.00E+00
1–10 years	1689.72	10	444.84	1734.18	7	605.44	1692.93	10	491.01	0.0054752	10	1.92E-03
10–20 years	1896.98	7	152.88	2135.67	6	348.44	2005.97	7	217.50	0.0062842	7	7.04E-04
20–40 years	2280.57	6	591.56	2173.94	5	705.46	2230.59	6	606.87	0.0069035	6	1.65E-03
40–60 years	2429.16	2	206.86	2453.62	1	0.00	2471.85	2	146.50	0.0077250	2	1.03E-03
Undef		0		1643.65	1	0.00	1643.65	1	0.00	0.0058820	1	0.00E+00
LgC	2625.10	12	880.25	2636.96	10	1042.50	2595.76	12	910.26	0.0087622	12	3.55E-03
Newborn	2991.76	1	0.00	2753.83	1	0.00	2872.79	1	0.00	0.0094676	1	0.00E+00
1–10 years	2245.10	2	270.87	2388.60	2	397.23	2316.85	2	334.05	0.0078970	2	2.30E-03
10–20 years		0			0			0			0	
20–40 years	2700.87	8	1064.72	2685.34	6	1375.82	2634.15	8	1118.54	0.0089405	8	4.32E-03
40–60 years	2412.25	1	0.00	2726.55	1	0.00	2569.40	1	0.00	0.0083601	1	0.00E+00
Undef		0			0			0			0	
SPC	2251.26	7	600.45	2200.19	7	388.16	2225.72	7	359.34	0.0068900	7	9.79E-04
Newborn		0			0			0			0	
1–10 years	1861.65	1	0.00	1738.84	1	0.00	1800.24	1	0.00	0.0057580	1	0.00E+00
10–20 years	1710.61	1	0.00	2086.25	1	0.00	1898.43	1	0.00	0.0065680	1	0.00E+00
20–40 years	2618.88	3	745.96	2322.07	3	453.14	2470.48	3	238.06	0.0074804	3	6.37E-04
40–60 years	2164.95	2	431.16	2305.00	2	448.29	2234.97	2	439.73	0.0067314	2	1.57E-03
Undef		0			0			0			0	

LPC — Linear Pottery Culture; LgC — Lengyel Culture; SPC — Stroked Pottery Culture; dx = dexter, right; sin = sinister, left

Fig. Na/Ca, cult. Graphical representation of the changes in sodium concentration in bone in the Neolithic cultures (Linear Pottery Culture—LPC; Lengyel Culture—LgC; and Stroked Pottery Culture—SPC).

STRONTIUM (Sr)

Sr has similar chemical properties similar to that of Ca. It has a protective and curative effect on postmenopausal osteoporosis, and reduces the risk of fractures (Franěk et al. 2009).

It has not been conclusively determined whether Sr is an essential element, or if an excess of inorganic Sr salts is detrimental to bone health.

The average Sr concentration in bone of the Neolithic population (N = 46) was 301 ± 80.82 µg/g (tab. 1).

In the Neolithic cultures, the highest Sr concentrations of 421.85 ± 89.85 µg/g was found in children of the LgC, aged 1–10 (N = 3). There was a significant difference in Sr concentrations between children and adult males, at significance level of 10% (tab. Sr, sex; fig. Srage).

Bone Sr concentrations in infants and children up to 10 years of age, of both the LPC and LgC were greater than the average values for Neolithic populations. The highest Sr concentrations were found in 10-year-old children (N = 2) of the LgC (436.5 ± 121.9 µg/g).

The lowest Sr concentrations in bone were detected in males (N = 2), approx. 60 years old, of the LPC at 212.39 ± 1.2 µg/g, 2 unidentified LgC individuals (215.8 ± 19.2 µg/g), and 4 LPC males (241.9 ± 56.8 µg/g) (tab. Sr, age).

In Neolithic femoral bones, Sr was metabolically active in children of up to 10 years of age. It was also in proportion to Ca concentrations in infants of up to 1 year of age (tab. Sr, age; fig. Srcaage).

Tab. Sr, sex. Strontium concentration in bone with regard to sex of the Neolithic populations

	Sr									Sr/Ca		
	dx µg/g Mean	dx N	dx µg/g SD	sin µg/g Mean	sin N	sin µg/g SD	aver. µg/g Mean	N	aver. µg/g SD	Mean	N	SD
LPC	301.44	26	77.22	299.49	21	90.77	300.96	27	78.07	9.59E-04	27	2.56E-04
Children	320.19	13	73.55	321.81	10	81.30	319.55	13	72.12	1.01E-03	13	2.12E-04
Females	317.74	6	94.54	306.82	5	133.37	315.56	6	105.82	9.96E-04	6	3.82E-04
Males	248.29	4	49.03	235.59	4	64.68	241.94	4	56.77	7.48E-04	4	1.58E-04
Undef	258.51	3	68.09	297.40	2	5.06	277.66	4	53.28	9.30E-04	4	2.12E-04
LgC	323.26	12	106.17	314.79	10	100.43	319.32	12	104.57	1.05E-03	12	3.11E-04
Children	431.35	3	89.20	412.35	3	91.58	421.85	3	89.85	1.39E-03	3	1.59E-04
Females	311.21	5	76.68	277.43	4	40.84	310.02	5	77.62	1.02E-03	5	2.47E-04
Males	302.08	2	152.06	282.37	2	163.11	292.23	2	157.58	9.82E-04	2	4.11E-04
Undef	212.43	2	14.35	236.35	1	0.00	215.87	2	19.22	7.06E-04	2	2.04E-05
SPC	272.43	7	41.32	269.22	7	28.52	270.82	7	28.18	8.40E-04	7	8.42E-05
Children	280.90	1	0.00	271.21	1	0.00	276.05	1	0.00	8.83E-04	1	0.00E+00
Females	288.29	2	14.94	255.54	2	7.59	271.92	2	3.67	8.37E-04	2	1.14E-05
Males	288.76	2	62.94	298.46	2	31.59	293.61	2	47.27	8.71E-04	2	1.56E-04
Undef	235.99	2	47.91	252.66	2	34.50	244.33	2	6.71	7.92E-04	2	9.89E-05

LPC – Linear Pottery Culture; LgC – Lengyel Culture; SPC – Stroked Pottery Culture; dx = dexter, right; sin = sinister, left

Tab. Sr, age. Strontium concentration in bone in age groups of the Neolithic populations

	Sr									Sr/Ca		
	dx µg/g Mean	dx N	dx µg/g SD	sin µg/g Mean	sin N	sin µg/g SD	aver.µg/g Mean	N	aver.µg/g SD	Mean	N	SD
LPC	301.44	26	77.22	299.49	21	90.77	300.96	27	78.07	0.0009587	27	2.56E-04
Newborn	301.78	1	0.00	300.45	1	0.00	301.12	1	0.00	0.0010638	1	0.00E+00
1–10 years	329.66	10	75.87	337.36	7	85.08	329.29	10	73.41	0.0010458	10	2.06E-04
10–20 years	273.37	7	58.61	268.30	6	63.86	275.72	7	59.35	0.0008625	7	1.86E-04
20–40 years	311.79	6	101.18	307.04	5	133.12	312.68	6	109.39	0.0009875	6	3.93E-04
40–60 years	227.43	2	20.09	181.45	1	0.00	212.39	2	1.19	0.0006624	2	5.33E-05
Undef				300.97	1	0.00	300.97	1	0.00	0.0010771	1	0.00E+00
LgC	323.26	12	106.17	314.79	10	100.43	319.32	12	104.57	0.0010532	12	3.11E-04
Newborn	413.35	1	0.00	371.77	1	0.00	392.56	1	0.00	0.0012937	1	0.00E+00
1–10 years	440.35	2	124.21	432.64	2	119.59	436.50	2	121.90	0.0014409	2	1.89E-04
10–20 years		0			0			0			0	
20–40 years	294.42	8	90.74	280.45	6	78.56	292.17	8	91.44	0.0009648	8	2.71E-04
40–60 years	229.74	1	0.00	228.10	1	0.00	228.92	1	0.00	0.0007448	1	0.00E+00
Undef		0			0			0			0	
SPC	272.43	7	41.32	269.22	7	28.52	270.82	7	28.18	0.0008403	7	8.42E-05
Newborn		0			0			0			0	
1–10 years	280.90	1	0.00	271.21	1	0.00	276.05	1	0.00	0.0008829	1	0.00E+00
10–20 years	269.87	1	0.00	228.27	1	0.00	249.07	1	0.00	0.0008617	1	0.00E+00
20–40 years	271.04	3	65.83	286.25	3	30.99	278.65	3	44.46	0.0008439	3	1.30E-04
40–60 years	271.55	2	38.61	263.14	2	18.34	267.35	2	10.13	0.0008029	2	6.00E-05
Undef		0			0			0			0	

LPC—Linear Pottery Culture; LgC—Lengyel Culture; SPC—Stroked Pottery Culture; dx = dexter, right; sin = sinister, left

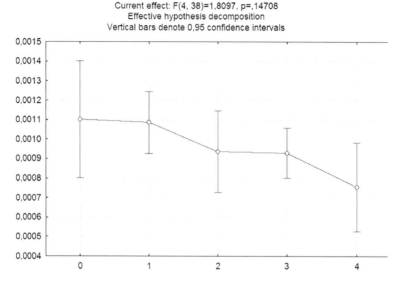

Fig. Sr/Ca age. Graphical representation of the Sr/Ca ratio in various age groups (Srcaage). Age groups: 0—infants, 1—up to age 10, 2—up to age 20, 3—up to age 40, 4—up to age 60.

ZINC (Zn)

Zn is crucial for the organism, having a role in over 200 enzymatic processes. Its effect on bone metabolism is similar to that of a growth hormone, as proven by Ovesen et al. (2001). Zn deficiency leads to growth retardation, bone anomalies, and osteopenia.

Disrupted bone development is demonstrated through abnormal development of ribs, vertebrae, agenesis of long bones, cleft palate and impaired ossification (Beattie and Avenell 1992).

The average Zn concentration in femoral bones of the Neolithic population (N = 46) was 108.01 ± 54,20 µg/g (tab. 1).

Across all LPC age groups, Zn concentrations were within the range of mean values of the population.

In the LPC and LgC, children had higher Zn concentrations in bone than adults.

The highest Zn concentration in bone was detected in the LgC infant (317.8 µg/g) (tab. Zn, age). The LgC children (N = 3) also showed high levels of Zn in the sampled femoral bone (155.7 ± 140 µg/g) (tab. Zn, sex).

Zn exhibited the highest metabolic activity in the femurs of infants under 1 year of age (fig. Zncaage) and was in proportion to Ca concentrations.

Tab. Zn, sex. Zinc concentration in bone with regard to sex of the Neolithic populations

| | Zn | | | | | | | | | Zn/Ca | | |
	dx µg/g Mean	dx N	dx µg/g SD	sin µg/g Mean	sin N	sin µg/g SD	aver. µg/g Mean	N	aver. µg/g SD	Mean	N	SD
LPC	96.60	26	44.76	104.32	21	43.88	101.25	27	46.12	3.21E-04	27	1.45E-04
Children	104.79	13	57.53	104.38	10	37.03	108.64	13	56.10	3.45E-04	13	1.74E-04
Females	91.76	6	36.14	120.48	5	74.30	103.11	6	51.52	3.23E-04	6	1.69E-04
Males	84.02	4	22.34	85.71	4	21.34	84.87	4	21.82	2.62E-04	4	6.02E-05
Undef	87.55	3	15.13	100.84	2	2.52	90.83	4	14.00	3.03E-04	4	4.78E-05
LgC	130.40	12	103.87	97.05	10	49.84	112.51	12	72.12	3.74E-04	12	2.37E-04
Children	186.29	3	185.70	125.11	3	95.13	155.70	3	140.40	5.17E-04	3	4.60E-04
Females	127.64	5	92.62	84.78	4	14.52	105.20	5	49.08	3.44E-04	5	1.58E-04
Males	92.12	2	7.75	88.09	2	14.48	90.11	2	11.11	3.17E-04	2	8.14E-05
Undef	91.74	2	2.04	79.89	1	0.00	88.42	2	2.66	2.90E-04	2	2.62E-05
SPC	125.00	7	64.43	127.69	7	71.92	126.35	7	51.42	3.98E-04	7	1.80E-04
Children	129.00	1	0.00	129.94	1	0.00	129.47	1	0.00	4.14E-04	1	0.00E+00
Females	97.41	2	15.33	97.20	2	2.79	97.31	2	9.06	3.00E-04	2	2.79E-05
Males	178.86	2	117.50	104.53	2	7.70	141.69	2	62.60	4.21E-04	2	1.93E-04
Undef	96.74	2	43.89	180.21	2	150.04	138.47	2	96.96	4.63E-04	2	3.58E-04

LPC — Linear Pottery Culture; LgC — Lengyel Culture; SPC — Stroked Pottery Culture; dx = dexter, right; sin = sinister, left

Tab. Zn, age. Zinc concentration in bone in age groups of the Neolithic populations

	Zn									Zn/Ca		
	dx µg/g Mean	dx N	dx µg/g SD	sin µg/g Mean	sin N	sin µg/g SD	aver.µg/g Mean	N	aver. µg/g SD	Mean	N	SD
LPC	96.60	26	44.76	104.32	21	43.88	101.25	27	46.12	0.0003214	27	1.45E-04
Newborn	65.26	1	0.00	133.57	1	0.00	99.41	1	0.00	0.0003512	1	0.00E+00
1–10 years	116.43	10	61.17	106.87	7	41.21	116.55	10	62.02	0.0003689	10	1.91E-04
10–20 years	80.88	7	20.44	89.12	6	18.06	83.67	7	18.19	0.0002608	7	5.01E-05
20–40 years	91.63	6	36.22	119.95	5	74.71	102.82	6	51.71	0.0003222	6	1.69E-04
40–60 years	83.04	2	13.72	75.48	1	0.00	83.58	2	12.96	0.0002621	2	5.99E-05
Undef		0		99.05	1	0.00	99.05	1	0.00	0.0003545	1	0.00E+00
LgC	130.40	12	103.87	97.05	10	49.84	112.51	12	72.12	0.0003737	12	2.37E-04
Newborn	400.71	1	0.00	234.89	1	0.00	317.80	1	0.00	0.0010474	1	0.00E+00
1–10 years	79.08	2	0.07	70.21	2	4.29	74.64	2	2.18	0.0002511	2	3.06E-05
10–20 years		0			0			0			0	
20–40 years	89.23	8	9.47	84.32	6	13.17	86.55	8	9.97	0.0002894	8	4.40E-05
40–60 years	292.09	1	0.00	89.27	1	0.00	190.68	1	0.00	0.0006204	1	0.00E+00
Undef		0			0			0			0	
SPC	125.00	7	64.43	127.69	7	71.92	126.35	7	51.42	0.0003975	7	1.80E-04
Newborn		0			0			0			0	
1–10 years	129.00	1	0.00	129.94	1	0.00	129.47	1	0.00	0.0004141	1	0.00E+00
10–20 years	127.78	1	0.00	286.30	1	0.00	207.04	1	0.00	0.0007163	1	0.00E+00
20–40 years	138.07	3	107.78	93.11	3	18.02	115.59	3	61.84	0.0003494	3	1.84E-04
40–60 years	102.01	2	8.83	99.13	2	0.07	100.57	2	4.45	0.0003021	2	2.45E-05
Undef		0			0			0			0	

LPC — Linear Pottery Culture; LgC — Lengyel Culture; SPC — Stroked Pottery Culture; dx = dexter, right; sin = sinister, left

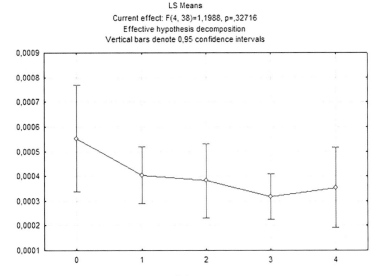

Fig. Zn/Ca age. Graphical representation of the Zn/Ca ratio in various age groups. Age groups: 0—infants, 1—up to age 10, 2—up to age 20, 3—up to age 40, 4—up to age 60.

IRON (Fe)

The average Fe concentration in femurs of the Neolithic population (N = 46) was 0–1457 µg/g.

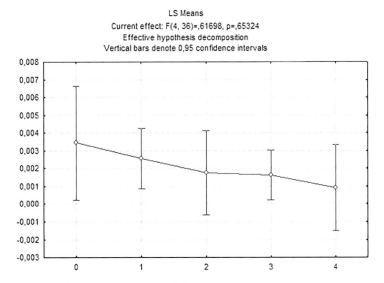

Fig. Fe/Ca age. Graphical representation of the Fe/Ca ratio in various age groups. Age groups: 0—infants, 1—up to age 10, 2—up to age 20, 3—up to age 40, 4—up to age 60.

Tab. Fe, sex. Iron concentration in bone with regard to sex of the Neolithic populations

	Fe									Fe/Ca		
	dx µg/g Mean	dx N	dx µg/g SD	sin µg/g Mean	sin N	sin µg/g SD	aver.µg/g Mean	aver. N	aver. µg/g SD	Mean	N	SD
LPC	2177.09	26	5455.05	1649.70	21	4585.95	2155.06	27	5241.04	0.0070527	27	1.72E-02
Newborn	584.37	1	0.00	899.38	1	0.00	741.88	1	0.00	0.0026209	1	0.00E+00
1–10 years	935.19	10	605.66	966.16	7	919.72	1018.01	10	672.75	0.0032118	10	2.16E-03
10–20 years	3137.72	7	6645.14	329.90	6	393.03	3001.90	7	6677.46	0.0101303	7	2.27E-02
20–40 years	4002.38	6	9214.23	4551.16	5	9440.66	3926.11	6	8915.23	0.0125722	6	2.86E-02
40–60 years	344.85	2	238.80	306.17	1	0.00	377.39	2	192.78	0.0011993	2	6.89E-04
Undef		0		1939.77	1	0.00	1939.77	1	0.00	0.0069417	1	0.00E+00
LgC	833.37	12	1208.08	343.11	10	296.88	802.57	12	1169.82	0.0027030	12	4.00E-03
Newborn	832.62	1	0.00	256.48	1	0.00	544.55	1	0.00	0.0017946	1	0.00E+00
1–10 years	1063.48	2	1121.29	647.48	2	552.57	855.48	2	836.93	0.0030972	2	3.26E-03
10–20 years		0			0			0			0	
20–40 years	847.42	8	1432.39	294.60	6	213.36	898.57	8	1405.49	0.0029799	8	4.77E-03
40–60 years	261.42	1	0.00	112.02	1	0.00	186.72	1	0.00	0.0006075	1	0.00E+00
Undef		0			0			0			0	
SPC	258.17	7	175.33	214.08	7	203.17	236.12	7	157.87	0.0007433	7	5.15E-04
Newborn		0			0			0			0	
1–10 years	457.69	1	0.00	643.54	1	0.00	550.61	1	0.00	0.0017611	1	0.00E+00
10–20 years	325.83	1	0.00	210.21	1	0.00	268.02	1	0.00	0.0009273	1	0.00E+00
20–40 years	252.59	3	229.66	150.45	3	102.83	201.52	3	83.30	0.0006103	3	2.50E-04
40–60 years	132.94	2	55.78	96.73	2	48.72	114.83	2	52.25	0.0003417	2	1.44E-04
Undef		0			0			0			0	

LPC = Linear Pottery Culture; LgC = Lengyel Culture; SPC = Stroked Pottery Culture; dx = dexter, right; sin = sinister, left

Tab. Fe, age. Iron concentration in bone in age groups of the Neolithic populations

	Fe									Fe/Ca		
	dx µg/g Mean	dx N	dx µg/g SD	sin µg/g Mean	sin N	sin µg/g SD	aver.µg/g Mean	aver. N	aver.µg/g SD	Mean	N	SD
LPC	2177.09	26	5455.05	1649.70	21	4585.95	2155.06	27	5241.04	7.05E-03	27	1.72E-02
Children	816.29	13	574.30	819.57	10	806.40	886.64	13	642.29	2.81E-03	13	2.06E-03
Females	4004.11	6	9213.37	4594.11	5	9415.75	3944.87	6	8905.75	1.26E-02	6	2.86E-02
Males	781.81	4	1176.80	345.48	4	510.25	563.65	4	843.17	1.90E-03	4	2.94E-03
Undef	6280.20	3	10222.56	1047.72	2	1261.55	5184.09	4	8632.66	1.76E-02	4	2.92E-02
LgC	833.37	12	1208.08	343.11	10	296.88	802.57	12	1169.82	2.70E-03	12	4.00E-03
Children	986.52	3	804.00	517.15	3	451.25	751.84	3	618.43	2.66E-03	3	2.42E-03
Females	473.71	5	699.56	211.05	4	204.27	492.29	5	692.59	1.53E-03	5	2.10E-03
Males	224.08	2	104.41	250.85	2	216.41	237.47	2	56.00	8.42E-04	2	3.08E-04
Undef	2112.06	2	2839.57	533.73	1	0.00	2219.45	2	2687.70	7.55E-03	2	9.26E-03
SPC	258.17	7	175.33	214.08	7	203.17	236.12	7	157.87	7.43E-04	7	5.15E-04
Children	457.69	1	0.00	643.54	1	0.00	550.61	1	0.00	1.76E-03	1	0.00E+00
Females	85.15	2	11.80	165.25	2	145.63	125.20	2	66.92	3.85E-04	2	2.06E-04
Males	170.45	2	2.73	117.93	2	18.73	144.19	2	10.73	4.27E-04	2	2.40E-05
Undef	419.13	2	131.95	144.33	2	93.17	281.73	2	19.39	9.09E-04	2	2.62E-05

LPC = Linear Pottery Culture; LgC = Lengyel Culture; SPC = Stroked Pottery Culture; dx = dexter, right; sin = sinister, left

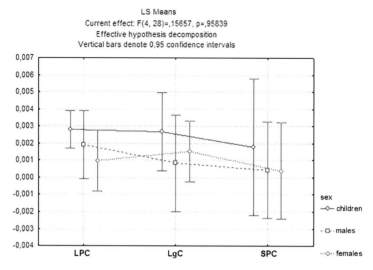

Fig. Fe/Ca, cult. Graphical representation of the changes in the Fe/Ca ratio in bone in the Neolithic cultures (Linear Pottery Culture—LPC; Lengyel Culture—LgC; and Stroked Pottery Culture—SPC) and sex groups.

The Fe bone concentrations in the children and infants of all Neolithic cultures (fig. Fecult; fig. Fecacult) were higher than in females. The Fe/Ca ratio had a significance level of 10%.

In the Neolithic, Fe was metabolically active in new-born infants and children up to 10 years of age (fig. Feage).

Note: Fe is a significant diagenetic contaminator: the woman no. 5 (aged 20-25) and the unidentified individual no. 43 (aged 18-21) had to be excluded due to their abnormally high values.

CONCLUSION

Trace element concentrations in Neolithic individuals (N = 46) from the LPC, LgC, and SPC were determined from samples taken from femoral bone. Concurrently, their ratio to Ca was also calculated.

In group 0, comprising of 2 infants under 1 year of age, the highest concentrations of the following elements were measured: Co; Cr; Cu; K; Mg; Ni; Pb; Zn.

In group 1, comprising of 13 children aged 1-10, the highest trace element concentrations in bone were detected for: Sr.

In group 2, comprising of 8 adolescents aged 10-20, the highest trace element concentrations in bone were detected for: Cd; Fe; Mg.

In group 3, comprising of 17 individuals aged 20-40, the highest trace element concentrations in bone were detected for these elements: As; Ba; V.

In group 4, comprising of 5 individuals aged 40–60, the highest trace element concentrations in bone were detected for these elements: Ca; Cr; Na.

Supposing periods featuring the highest trace element concentrations in bone are those when bone metabolism is most pronounced, then the period of priority with regard to metabolic activity is between 10 and 20 years of age. In this age range, 17 trace elements are involved, and surprisingly, rare-earth elements are also included; these were previously considered to be ballast bone.

The second most metabolically active period is the first year of life, when 10 trace elements seem to be involved in bone metabolism. In other age groups, usually the same number of trace elements are involved.

We realise that the trace element concentrations in individual bones are dependent on age and sex. The examination of metabolic activity during growth in the Neolithic Age is of crucial importance for comparison with the present times, and the burdens of a changing environment.

13. CONCLUSION: THE LIFESTYLE AND MORBIDITY OF THE LENGYEL CULTURE

VÁCLAV SMRČKA

For the purposes of the study in this book, a total of 1088 Neolithic skeletons of the Lengyel Culture (LgC) from regions in Western Hungary (Barány and Tolna counties) and the Czech Republic (Moravia region) were examined from the available aspects.

From analyses conducted by the work groups for the individual chapters, it follows that in the Lengyel Culture (LgC) focus should be given to age groups, as in these, differences in grave goods, social stratification, morbidity and dietary habits are observed. While the lifestyle of this culture was similar in the described geographic locations, differences were discovered on comparison of the age groups with the Early Neolithic cultures. For this reason, we have divided the life cycle in LgC into age groups similar to those of anthropological age classification: 1. Infants up to age 1; 2. Children under 14 years of age; 3. Juvenis up to age 20; 4. Adultus up to age 40; 5. Maturus up to age 60. The differences between the males and females of the latter two groups were also noted.

At multicultural burial sites, the LgC was compared to Early Neolithic cultures (LPC and SPC) (Price 2000; Zalai-Gaál 1982; Pavlů 2000).

In this comparison, other Central European regions were also taken into consideration (Pavlů and Zápotocká 2007; Bickle and Whittle 2013; Verhagen et al. 2021).

For the description of lifestyle in each group, the results of carbon and nitrogen isotope analyses were utilised, along with diet reconstruction, trace element content in bone health assessment, the archaeological description of the environment, and the morbidity for the corresponding ages.

Morbidity, the palaeopathological profile of LgC, was determined through the macroscopic description of diseases in bones, and considers the examined regions, in addition to previous analyses (Regöly-Mérei 1960; Regöly-Mérei 1962; Ubelaker 2006; Zoffmann and Hajdu 2013). In special instances histological findings and X-rays were incorporated.

13.1 THE LIFE CYCLE IN THE LENGYEL CULTURE AGE GROUPS

13.1.1 INFANTS

The infants group comprised of individuals under 1 year of age. Prenatally, infants are nourished through placental blood.

Infants of the LgC from Moravia (N = 3) had higher Co, Cu, Mg, Ni, Sr and Zn concentrations in their bones. These, as well as other elements (Pb), are important for normal bone growth and for the transformation of cartilage to bone.

Lengyel women, given their smaller stature, would experiences difficulties delivering a child with a larger head due to be a narrow pelvis; such instances would lead to death in childbirth or soon after delivery.

Köhler (chapter 3) documented two such cases in graves 474 and 4414 from the Alsónyék collection.

A special case was identified in the unborn foetus in grave no. 10 in Villánykővesd (chapters 6, 7) ($\delta^{15}N$ 10.75 ± 0.03; $\delta^{13}C$ –20.07 ± 0.06).

The foetus suffered from a liver disease as proven by trace element analysis (chapter 6), and macroscopic identification of pelvic and endocranial periostitis (chapter 3).

Its mother, aged 36–40, also in grave no. 10 ($\delta^{15}N$ 11.10; $\delta^{13}C$ –20.49) was not local. Her $\delta^{15}N$ values point to sources of animal protein from fish.

In the compact parts of the foetus's femurs, the Cd concentration was high due to the displacement of Zn and Mn from the disease-affected liver (Noel et al. 2004).

An osteological examination of the foetus identified intracranial and pelvic periostitis. From trace element concentrations, it can be claimed that the unborn foetus suffered from a liver disease.

13.1.2 CHILDREN

This group encompasses individuals up to 14 years of age.

At four years of age, a child would be weaned, which can be observed in C and N isotope changes.

In Zengővárkony, 6 individuals (1 male, 3 females and 2 children) were available for sampling, which represent approximately 10% of the analysed skeletons (6/59).

The younger of these children from grave no. 340 ($\delta^{15}N$ 14.27 ± 0.02; $\delta^{13}C$ –18.94 ± 0.03) was between 1 and 5 years of age. Its variation in the graph in comparison to the other individuals may have been caused by it being breastfed.

Another child, Infans aged 4–5 (from grave no. 331) ($\delta^{15}N$ 9.27; $\delta^{13}C$ –19.75) exhibited different values and it is apparent that it was no longer being breast-fed. From the stated stable C, and N isotope data, it can be assumed that in the Lengyel Culture weaning occurred around age 4.

In Villánykővesd, 9 individuals (3 males, 2 females and 4 children) were available for sampling, representing approximately 39% of the analysed skeletons (9/23).

The youngest child aged 1–1.5, from grave no. 19 ($\delta^{15}N$ 12.98 ± 0.04; $\delta^{13}C$ –18.97 ± 0.01) holds an eccentric position in the graph. It is presumed that the child was being breast-fed.

Another child, aged 8.5, from grave no. 15 ($\delta^{15}N$ 9.11 ± 0.01; $\delta^{13}C$ –20.56 ± 0.01) exhibits completely different values of $\delta^{15}N$ and $\delta^{13}C$. This "children's diet" and similar stable C, N isotope values were also observed in the child from grave 12 ($\delta^{15}N$ 9.64 ± 0.00; $\delta^{13}C$ –20.26 ± 0.01), aged 12–13. This type of diet was likely common between being weaned at age 4 up to the age of 12–13.

The diet could have changed after initiation rites, which were performed on teeth as explained in chapter 3. Similar $\delta^{15}N$ and $\delta^{13}C$ values to both the individuals of the Infans group were detected in the female from grave 21, aged 53–62 ($\delta^{15}N$ 9.54; $\delta^{13}C$ –20.65).

Based on micro abrasion of teeth, it can be claimed that the diet of children of the LgC in Moravia was different from that of adults and had a high vegetal content (Jarošová et al. 2008 and chapter 8).

Children were involved in work. They would help women with sewing, as archaeologically documented by the finding of needles in child graves in Zengővárkony (Čermáková 2007; chapter 3). They aided in hide processing along with elderly women, archaeologically documented by the finding of scrapers in graves (Čermáková 2007 and chapter 3), and biologically through excessive tooth wear in a 4–5-year-old child (grave no. 331, Zengővárkony).

At ages 12–13, initiation rituals likely took place, as seen by the artificial incisions in teeth (16 types of incisions, see classification 3.6). Subsequently, the diet changed to one of adolescents

Analysis of stable strontium *isotopes* in the Hungarian Lengyel settlements showed that migrant women who arrived at the settlements also brought children with them (1/6 in Zengővárkony aged 4–5; 2/5 in Villánykövésd aged 1–1.5 and 12–13).

13.1.3 JUVENIS

Individuals up to age 20.

On comparison of dental pathology in juvenile individuals aged 15 to 20, no dental caries were found either in LgC or SPC (I-CE as well as F-CE = 0) (Jarošová et al. 2008 and chapter 8). This may have been the result of ground soluble silicate minerals present in flour (conveyed in person by Jambor

2019). These would aid the formation of crystals in dental enamel along with a yet undocumented element.

The diet of this age group exhibited the greatest differences in composition between LgC and LPC Neolithic cultures as determined by stable C, N isotope analysis. The diet of the Juvenis group differed from the diet of infants and children (chapters 5, 6, 10, 12).

13.1.4 ADULTUS

Individuals up to 40 years of age.

In this group, individuals aged between 20-30 years old exhibited a higher prevalence of sarcomas due to an increased sensitivity to carcinogens (Strouhal and Němečková 2008). In the Lengyel Culture, a multiple myeloma was documented in Mauer, Vienna (Strouhal and Němečková 2008).

13.1.5 MATURUS

Individuals up to 60 years of age.

In this group, hide processing was the predominant occupation of elderly women as archaeologically documented by scrapers (Čermáková 2007) and biologically by excessive tooth wear (Smrčka et al. 2018).

13.1.6 MALES

Men were tasked with hunting, but bows would only be used sporadically; the men did not have enlarged bone rims on second phalanges which are typical for hunting with bows. Harpoons and nets would be used for fishing, which is evidenced biologically through tooth deformation, by rims on proximal phalanges (chapter 9), and findings of grave goods (Čermáková 2007).

With regard to the analysis of stable strontium isotopes in Hungarian settlements, men were the most mobile constituent group in the population. Their increased mobility could explain the prevalence of female over male skeletons in the settlements in Hungary and in Moravia.

Of the 6 migrants (3 males, 2 females, 1 child) in Zengővárkony, a male, aged 48-58, from grave 5 suffered from spondylosis in the whole spine with 3-5 mm osteophytes. The second male, aged 40-80, from grave 99, had large rims on the proximal phalanges of his hands which indicates excessive strain on interosseous muscles of the fingers, probably from making fishing nets. The third male, aged 38-48, from grave no. 325, suffered from spina ventosa tuberculosis of the calcaneus and spina bifida in the sacral region.

Of the five migrants (2 males, 1 female, 2 children) in Villánykővesd, the first, in grave 22 was aged 36-43, and the second, in grave 24, aged 41-43, developed hydrocephalus in adulthood, which would have manifested as a syndrome of cognitive impairment, incontinence and gait disturbances.

The greatest work strain on men was seen in the large settlements; these strains mostly affected joints of their extremities and manifested as severe arthrotic changes.

The average height of males of the LgC in Moravia (N4) was 159.8 cm (chapter 8), in Hungarian Zengővárkony the average height of 14 males was measured at 164 cm (Zoffmann 1969-70) and in the LgC in Poland (N = 24) it was 161.4 cm (SD = 3.98) (Garłowska 2001).

13.1.7 FEMALES

It is apparent, that an occupation in which women were involved was weaving. This can be seen from the enlarged rims on the proximal phalanges of the fingers (Smrčka et al. 2018). However, weaving was to a lesser extent than in the preceding, Early Neolithic LPC and SPC cultures. Parts of clothing which would previously have been woven were being replaced by leather. Some individuals would carry out specialised tasks; there is biological (tooth wear) and archaeological (scrapers in graves) evidence (chapter 3.1.2, Čermáková 2007) that older women would process hides. These women would be assisted by children.

Women adorned themselves with copper ornaments, earrings and copper bead necklaces.

LgC females in Moravia (N8) averaged 152.7 cm (chapter 8). In Zengő-várkony, Hungary, the height of 16 females averaged at 151 cm (Zoffmann 1969-70), however shorter statures as low as 145 cm were not uncommon. In Poland, the average height of LgC females (N = 22) was found to be 152.3 cm (SD = 3.58) (Garłowska 2001).

13.2 DIFFERENCES OF THE LgC LIFESTYLE FROM THE EARLY NEOLITHIC LPC AND SPC CULTURES

13.2.1 METAL

The Lengyel Culture differed from the preceding LPC and SPC cultures with the introduction of metal, copper. Copper's primary use was in the manufacturing of jewellery for women

In several instances (graves no. 87, 88a, and 88b), copper corrosion was found on the mastoids of skulls. In Zengővárkony, in grave no. 88, copper corrosion was detected on the first three neck vertebrae, likely from a copper bead necklace. Copper beads were also archaeologically confirmed in

10 graves in Zengővárkony (25%) by Čermáková (2007). She stated, that if the deceased had several items of jewellery, then one of them was always comprised of beads, and that copper ornaments were associated with richly furnished female burials.

13.2.2 AGGRESSION IN THE LENGYEL CULTURE

The initial 400 years of development of the Lengyel Culture were not affected by any critical influences as Barna (2015) recorded from the internal development of the Sormás-Török-földek site.

Gradually, fear of being attacked developed among the settlement populations. In the counties of Barány and Tolna, Bartók and Gáti (2014) documented the existence of defence structures related to rondels, which therefore means rondels can no longer be considered to be solely places of religious rites.

Aggression can manifest in various forms. Men were attacked, such as the 36–42-year-old man from grave no. 314 in Zengővárkony (Smrčka et al. 2018); he had lived with a penetrating wound in the left parietal region for a few months after the initial trauma. Acts of aggression were not limited to those against men; a woman from Alsónyék, with a depression of the left parietal bone described by Köhler (chapter 3) managed to defend herself at the cost of a fracture of her left forearm.

Similarly, in LgC in Moravia, injured women were found: in Střelice, a woman aged 50–90 (in grave H1/12) with a perimortem stellate fracture with a central circular fragment 30 mm in diameter on the border between her right parietal and frontal bones was described (fig. 9, chapter 9), and also in Předmostí-Dluhonice (126/1/2006), a woman aged 20–40 (Schenk et al. 2007). Evidence of violence was also documented in LgC in Poland by Garłowska (2001), where 11.5% of adult individuals, predominantly men, were affected.

These resulted from aggressive clashes between settlements. The common denominator between them being similar wounds inflicted with a Lengyel shoe-last axe (Smrčka et al. 2018). On impact, it would create an oval opening approximately 30 mm in diameter.

Makkay (2000) originally termed execution in the Lengyel Culture mass grave at the Esztergályhorváti site as "The Early War."

In September 1994, archaeologist Judith P. Barna of the Balaton Museum in Keszthely, discovered a late Neolithic mass grave in Esztergályhorváti during a rescue excavation. The site lay in the Kis-Balaton region south of the Zala river valley. In a pit, 1.8 × 2.3 m, there were 38 males of all age categories over 16 (Makkay 2000). Ceramic fragments pointed to an early stage of the Lengyel Culture, with radiocarbon data from seven individuals dated the grave at 4940–4720 B.C. (95.4% probability) (Barna 2015).

An execution at the Esztergályhorváti site was clearly identified by Zoff-mann (2007) in individual no. 3:

It is a 50-60-year-old man, who suffered a large, 20 × 7 mm, penetrating wound in the left parietal bone. The edges are sharp, with fragments displaced intracranially. Further injuries were present: one measuring 9 × 5 mm on the left side of the skull, and another on the left side of the occipital squama in the sagittal direction (20 × 8 mm). It splits the upper and lower arch into 14 mm and 16 mm pieces respectively. All the injuries have sharp edges without any signs of healing, and it is clear that such blows must have caused damage to the brain.

Zsuzsanna K. Zoffmann (2007, 56) concluded that all the individuals in the grave were men. "Over the pit a ritual fire was lit. The fatal injuries were inflicted with a weapon ± 30 mm wide. The men were killed as execution of an enemy."

This description of the injuries says everything. The male had two wounds from hand to hand combat, but the injury in the occipital region indicates an execution.

Aggressive behaviour in the LgC can be traced to the origins and is further evidenced during its westward expansion at comparable sites such as Frieb-ritz (Austria), Bajč-Ragona and Ružindol-Borová (Slovakia). Unfortunately, in Džbánice in Moravia, the skeletal materials have not been recovered.

Friebritz 1, Austria, is a small burial site of 10 crouched skeletons were uncovered. Signs of aggression were identified (Neugebauer-Maresch 2005, 225) in a couple (male, aged 20–30; female, aged 18–25) buried in an unusual manner. The findings show that both were killed by arrows. The man, who lay at the bottom of the grave suffered a serious jaw injury while still alive. His hands seem to have been bound. Both individuals appear to bear signs of cannibalism. According to Vencl (1999, 64), this burial gives evidence of a massacre, likely an attack on a village while men were gone. This Friebritz burial appears to strongly resemble the one near Lake Balaton.

Victims of an unusual massacre were found at the Ružindol-Borová site near Trnava, Slovakia, which dates to the early Lengyel period. It contained the remains of 18 individuals, among which were infants, children, men, and women, all buried in a circular pit 60 m in diameter. It suggests an unfinished rondel which could have contained 60–70 people. The injuries found on the remains provide evidence of a brutal murderous attack. There are unhealed injuries on the bones and bite marks from animals, which clearly indicate acts of aggression (Němejcová-Pavúková 1995, 214, 215; 1997, 95–99; Jakab 1997, 193–218; Makkay 2000, 43; Neubauer, and Trnka 2005, 223).

Another find similar to the aforementioned instances was discovered in Slovakia at the Bajč-Ragona site, dated to the Ludanice group, which is considered to be the last developmental phase of the Lengyel Culture. In a 2.7 m deep pit outside the settlement, six skeletons were found (Točík 1991, 301–317). The grave goods and signs on the skeletons correspond with the previously described sites.

Evidence of executions, even in the Early Neolithic populations, is not uncommon in the German LPC (5600–4900 B.C.).

Signs of aggression were described in Talheim (Price et al. 2006), Herxheim (Spatz 1998; Zeeb-Lanz 2009), Wiederstedt (Meyer et al. 2015) and in Schletz-Asparn, Austria (Windl 2001).

In a mass grave in Halberstadt, Mayer et al. (2018) found multiple wounds, mostly inflicted on the dorsal aspect of the skull (12.92%). These affected the posterior portion of the parietal bone and the superior part of the occipital region and signify an execution.

13.2.3 DIET, MOBILITY AND BONE HEALTH IN LgC

The reason for changes in food strategies of the Moravian Neolithic must be tied with climatic fluctuation. In the period of expansion of the Lengyel Culture in Moravia, there was a slight decrease in temperatures and rainfall compared to the preceding Neolithic stages of LPC and SPC. This led to lower yields of cereal crops, while forested areas expanded (Ložek 1980, Pavúk 1991). This fact was reflected in the rise of hunting (Ambros 1986) in Hungary noted by Bököny (1974).

DIET OF THE LENGYEL CULTURE COMPARED WITH THAT OF THE EARLY NEOLITHIC

The changes in Upper Neolithic food strategy in both Hungary and Moravia is an example of the populations' adaptation to the natural environment. While in the older LPC culture the vegetal component prevailed (meat constituted only about 25%), in LgC about 50% of the consumed diet consisted of meat as is evident from the microabrasion of tooth enamel. Further differences were found on comparing tooth microabrasion in adults and children. It appears that children had a different diet compared to the adult members of the LgC population, with them consuming a greater proportion of vegetal foods (Jarošová et al. 2008c, 113). These results correspond to the osteological analyses of animals; at LgC sites there are a greater proportion of young cattle, sheep and goats, as well as a comparative increase in the proportion of pig bones. These animals would have been bred solely for meat (Jarošová et al. 2008c, 119; Dreslerová 2006; Bököny 1974). Therefore, a change in food strategy in favour of increased meat consumption, from both domestic and wild animal sources, from 5% of the Lower Neolithic to 50–60% of LgC (Pavúk

1991; Bököny 1974) was seen. These changes, traceable through tooth micro-abrasion and archeozoological finds, were also evidenced in the stable nitrogen and carbon isotopes, and in the trace element contents of bone samples. The LPC diet was based on the wheat type C3 photosynthetic cycle (Tauber 1981), which was typical of LPC. In the Hungarian and Moravian LgC, the diet was also based on the C3 cycle, but included the addition of a diet based on the millet type C4 photosynthetic cycle, as in the instance of the male from grave 24 in Villánykővesd. He had been ill, and millet could have been used therapeutically. In LgC stable isotopes indicate an increase in the animal component of the diet across the population.

In LgC, significant differences of 10% appear in the diets of children and women; on comparison between the age groups, the difference between infants and juvenis in the $\delta^{15}N$ animal component of the diet is at a 1% significance level. The differences between infants and children, and between infants and adults are at a 10% significance level.

The change in dietary strategies were also confirmed by multielement analyses of trace elements. Trace elements affect the development of crystals responsible for the physical qualities of dental enamel (Ghadimi 2013). In the Hungarian burial sites of the Lengyel Culture, high concentrations of elements that reduce caries risk (Sr, Al, Fe) were found, as were low concentrations of trace elements that promote caries and periodontal disease (Cu, Mn, Cd). These results show why there was a low caries incidence in LgC.

Trace elements have proven to be of great importance in the formation of dental enamel in the Neolithic, not only in early childhood but also during Juvenis age. Throughout the Neolithic, in all observed cultures (LPC, LgC and SPC), dental caries are absent in the Juvenis age group (chapter 8).

At the Hungarian site of Zengővárkony, a place where copper and obsidian were manufactured and distributed (Dombay 1960), trace elements antimony (Sb), cadmium (Cd) and vanadium (V) were found in bones. Antimony is the first element released during copper extraction. The aforementioned elements proved the contamination of individuals, and the subsequent accumulation of these trace elements in bones during copper processing.

In the Moravian Neolithic sites, where a comparison of bone health between Neolithic cultures (LPC, LgC and SPC) using trace elements was conducted, a lower concentration of calcium was found in males of the Lengyel Culture. In this culture, males consumed milk to a lesser extent than the remaining population (chapters 5 and 10). Another possible explanation for the lower bone calcium concentration could have been a higher consumption of meat by LgC men, causing at increased magnesium (Mg) concentration in bone deposits and a subsequent displacement of calcium.

In Neolithic Moravia, certain correlated trace element groups were prominent within the various age groups of the population. In infants, there were the following elements: Co, Cu, Mg, Ni, Pb, Sr, Zn. In children aged 1–14: Sr. In the Juvenis group, aged 14–20, the following trace elements were active in bones: Mg, Cu. In adults aged 20–40 there were As, Ba and V; and in the Maturus group, aged 40–60, Ca and Na were active in femoral bones.

The mobility of the Lengyel population was investigated using stable strontium isotopes. In the Lengyel Culture sites in Hungary, mobility varied between the settlements. In the Belvárdgyula settlement no migration was discovered, meaning the population was local, while in Zengővárkony and Villánykővesd migration exceeded 50% (chapter 5).

Borič and Price (2013) unequivocally proved that in earliest phases of the Neolithic in southern Europe, perhaps paradoxically, farming communities were significantly more mobile than local foraging populations.

There is a greater variance of strontium ratios at this time among females in comparison with males, suggesting that woman came to these sites from Neolithic communities as part of ongoing social exchange. There was spread of Neolithic communities through south-eastern Europe, from the south and south-east, to the north and northwest. In some LgC settlements, the migration was 55–60%, while in others the mobility was not evident.

In Zengővárkony, 6 out of 11 individuals who were analysed for strontium isotopes (6/11) were determined to have been nonlocal. It can therefore be supposed that mobility at this site was 55%.

In Vilánykövesd, 5 out of 8 individuals who were analysed for stable strontium isotopes (5/8) was determined to have been nonlocal, and it can therefore be supposed that mobility at this site was 62.5%.

On analysis of randomly selected individuals, it was discovered that the population at the Belárdgyula site was likely local.

Overall, the wave of LgC migration was heading northwesterly at a similiar rate as the LPC at the onset of the Neolithic. The comparison of the mobility of Neolithic cultures in Moravia shows that the mobility of LgC in Moravia is similar to that of LPC (40%), although the migration pressure was reduced by approximately 10% compared to Hungary. The mobility of SPC, the successor of LPC in Moravia, is lower than in both cultures. This finding would agree with the view of archaeologists that it was passively pushed by the LgC to areas of present-day Bohemia and northern Moravia (Pavlů and Zápotocká 2007). The pattern of LgC migration is evidenced not only by the results of Sr isotopes, but also by congenital malformations of the skull (see chapter 3).

In conclusion, it can be speculated that the Lengyel Culture adapted well to the changing climate. It enhanced its food sources through hunting. However, its expansion westward carried with it signs of aggression, in both interpersonal and interpopulation conflicts.

In the Upper Neolithic, the formed Lengyel Culture expanded westwards to regions inhabited by peoples with stroked pottery. Along the Danube, it reached Austria (Lenneis et al. 1995), and further north on crossing the Morava river it occupied the whole of Moravia (Podborský et al. 1993) stopping at the foothills of the Bohemian-Moravian Highlands (Českomoravská vysočina). The people with stroked pottery withdrew from southern Moravia to the north reaching Lesser Poland. Yet, it is beyond doubt that part of the population merged with the newcomers and gradually assimilated themselves (Pavlů and Zápotocká 2007, 105).

13.2.4 OCCUPATIONS IN LgC

The division of labour was specified according to gender and age, as it has already been mentioned with the age groups, but also according to site.

The daily occupation at the settlement was surely related to the providing of food sources and the preparation of food. From the viewpoint of biological evidence, these tasks can be associated with the osteophytes and Schmorl's nodes in the lumbar spines of women, likely a result of daily hard work on the quern-stone.

The lumbar spines and joints were also affected in males, and to a greater extent than seen in women. Some had rims on the phalanges of their fingers. From a detailed examination of the rims on proximal phalanges, in relation with grave goods, it is be possible to single out "specialist." Rims were formed by short interosseous muscles upon excessive workload (in the flexional position of the metacarpophalangeal joints), such as in making fishing nets, or in weaving in the case of women.

Even though a higher proportion of hunting is attributed to LgC, no "specialist" hunters could be identified.

Excessive activity of the superficial flexor lead to the formation of rims on intermediate phalanges, particularly if the fingers formed a hook at the interphalangeal joints and were in partial extension of the metacarpophalangeal joints. It is possible that other forms of hunting which did not involve a bow were employed in LgC.

Some women in LgC would weave and sew clothes and hides; they had rims on their proximal phalanges. Other women, usually the elderly, would process the hides. Children would assist in these tasks.

Biological evidence for children's help has been scarce, nevertheless, archaeological evidence prevails (Čermáková 2007; and chapter 3).

TEXTILE WEAVING

In the Neolithic LPC site of Vedrovice, Moravia, the presence of bone rims on the proximal phalanges of hands was identified in 80% of the female population (Dočkalová 2008). This indicates strain on interosseous muscles of the hand during textile weaving or the making of fishing nets. In the Lengyel Culture, these rims were not expressed to such an extent (chapters 3, 9).

HIDE-WORKING

The decrease in textile production was probably substituted with hide-working. This process, in which children, old females, and eventually elder males were involved, was proven both archaeologically in a gender study and biologically by augmented tooth wear inconsistent with the individuals' ages (chapter 3). The increased usage of hides as a material could have partially replaced parts of certain garments. Hide processing may have also involved "specialists."

In Zengővárkony, it was proven that Jaromír Chochol was correct when he wrote in 1964:

> We may mention one detailed issue, the clarification of which is important for our Neolithic and Eneolithic periods.
>
> In some instances, the upper front teeth from skulls of this time showed extreme abrasions; incisors, cuspids and, to a lesser extent, premolars, were abraded in a single line and plane up to the gingival line. Tooth wear in the lower jaw remains within the normal limits and is therefore comparably less. Either this is a manifestation of an extraordinarily intense chewing function limited to the upper jaw, or perhaps some developmental inferiority with minute resilience to abrasion of the affected teeth. The former should make us consider what mechanism could have led to such extensive and localised tooth wear.
>
> Drawing parallels from Eskimos of recent times, similar abrasions of the upper front teeth have been noted to occur during their process of primitive hide-working; the processed area of the hide rests on lower front teeth while it is intensely honed and softened by rubbing against the upper front teeth. This effect on teeth documented in Eskimos has a striking similarity to our finds. (Chochol 1964)

The greatest workload on women was likely in the Neolithic chert mines, as per information from Mauer and the Krumlov Forest. It is possible that labour in some mines was involuntary, as can be inferred from the burials in Mauer and the Krumlov Forest (Oliva 2007).

WORK IN NEOLITHIC MINES

The extent of the work load in mines is evidenced by an adult female, buried in grave no. 1, embedded in a Neolithic chert mine (Mauer, Vienna 23). She had a right humeral fracture, which healed by formation of a callus, and deformation of the distal end of the right radius, which had also been previously fractured. It is possible the unfavourable conditions and presence of carcinogens (e.g. radon) in the mines had an impact on the woman's health and were responsible for her developing a plasmacytoma, multiple myeloma, which proved fatal.

In LgC, notable repercussions of manual labour were found on the skeletons of two women buried in a mining pit in the Krumlov Forest. These women ranked among the shortest in the Neolithic period in Moravia and their skeletons showed osteophytes, Schmorl's nodes, porotic hyperostosis, Harris lines, and evidence of pronounce muscle strength on bone insertion points, demonstrating the effects of long-term physical exertion and periods of distress. One factor that cannot be excluded is their involvement in chert mining in the Krumlov Forest (Tvrdý 2010). These stresses on the spine from flexion and lateral rotation result from lifting of heavy weights and can be expected in pre-historic hunters, farmers, as well as stone cutters.

DIFFERENCES IN OCCUPATIONS BETWEEN SITES

It seems that the division into distinct specialisations was not limited to differentiation within the LgC society, but also at individual sites. This fact is inferred from trace element and stable isotope analyses. In Zengővárkony, the concentration of antimony in femoral bones was higher than those of Villánykővesd. Antimony is released during copper processing. This corresponds with Dombay's hypothesis (1960) that it was a distribution and processing centre of copper and obsidian.

On the other hand, the Villánykővesd and Belvárdgyula sites specialised in agriculture and animal breeding. This is also shown by the trace element analyses. The population of Belvárdgyula was local.

13.2.5 ARTIFICIAL DEFORMATION OF TEETH

In the Hungarian LgC burial sites of Villánykővesd, Zengővárkony and Belvárdgyula artificial deformations of teeth were discovered in males, females, and also children. We presume that these artificial dental incisions were performed at initiation rituals during childhood, around 12–13 years of age (chapter 3).

These artificial incisions necessitated a skilled specialist due to the fine nature of the cuts. It is likely they were created using an obsidian blade approximately 500 times sharper than a modern surgeon's scalpel (*American Medical Association News* 1984; Disa et al. 1993).

13.3 PATHOLOGICAL PROFILE OF THE LENGYEL CULTURE IN VARIOUS REGIONS

13.3.1 CONGENITAL DEFECTS

At the Hungarian burial sites in the Barány and Tolna counties: Zengővárkony (Zoffmann 1969-70), Villánykővesd (Zoffmann 1968), and Mórágy (Zoffmann 2004), congenital defects affecting the cranial sutures of the skull were identified: *scaphocephaly*, *plagiocephaly* and *hydrocephalus*. Cranial suture defects (craniosynostoses) occur in 1/2500 births.

The most prevalent aetiology of craniosynostoses within LgC would be genetic, with less common causes including vitamin D deficiency and multiple birth pregnancies (Lewis 2018; Kiliç Safak et al. 2020).

The shape of the skull depends on which sutures closes prematurely. Early closure of the sagittal suture (57% of cases) results in frontal and occipital expansion. The skull becomes long and narrow (*scaphocephaly*). Premature unilateral closure of the coronal sutures results in an asymmetric flattening of skull (*plagiocephaly*) (Sadler 2015, 148).

One of the important discoveries of molecular biology was the role of fibroblast growth factor (FGF) and its receptors (FGFRs). Mutations of these receptors (FGFR1 & FGFR2) often consist of the substitution of a single amino-acid and are associated with specific types of craniosynostoses. A mutation of the TWIST gene, which encodes a transcription factor regulating proliferation, leads to a premature termination of the sutura coronalis and the subsequent craniosynostosis, plagiocephaly (Sadler 2011, 149).

The high incidence of congenital skull defects accompanied the Lengyel population on its migration west to present-day Poland.

However, in Poland different congenital skull defects occurred; congenital *meningocele* and *torticollis* which were discovered by Garłowska (2001). She studied the northern branch of the Lengyel Culture in Poland at the Osłonky site in Kujawy. Through an analysis of 92 individuals, she created a pathological profile of the population between 4300 and 4000 B.C. Congenital defects also occurred in the spine: *sacralisation, spina bifida occulta, spondylolysis.* These affected the Lengyel population to a lesser extent than defects of the skull.

In the Barány county, Hungary, rare defects such as the *congenital amputation at the wrist* in a man, aged 30-59, in grave no. 345 in Zengővárkony was documented (Smrčka et al. 2018).

In Moravia, Czech Republic, from the comparison of LgC with early Neolithic cultures (Chapter 9), it follows that the early Neolithic LPC spine was more susceptible to congenital fusion of the frontal aspects of cervical vertebrae, seen in the case of a male, aged 65–90 from Brno, Starý Lískovec (K806/obj. 7727/2008). This fusion was categorised as *Klippel-Feil syndrome* with prevalence of 16%. Aside from the congenital cervical spine deformities in LPC, a case of *spina bifida* was observed in a young female, aged 15–17 from Mašovice (grave no. 1/613/2003). Spina bifida had a prevalence of 20% (chapter 9).

13.3.2 DEGENERATIVE JOINT DISEASES

Degenerative joint diseases are most frequently observed in paleopathology (Steinbock 1976; Ortner and Putschar 1981; Rogers and Waldron 1987; Roberts and Manchester 1995). They are conditional on genetic predisposition and strong mechanical stress, along with microtraumas, sex, age and climate.

In the Lengyel Culture, men were more susceptible to arthrotic, degenerative changes in the spine (*osteophytosis; Schmorl's nodes*) and limb joints when compared with women. In the Hungarian Alsónyék-Bátaszék site, Köhler (chapter 3) *osteoarthrotic changes* were found in 43% of males and 33% of females. Similar results were observed in the LgC of the Kujawy region, Poland, several centuries later (4300–4000 B.C.) with 40% of males and 30% females affected (Garłowska 2001).

Roberts and Manchester (1995) recognised primary osteoarthritic changes associated with increasing age (p. 101) and secondary changes in previously affected joints. At the same time, they point out the relationship between occupation and arthritis (p. 110–113).

From this viewpoint, there is an apparent difference in the incidence of spinal osteophytes in the lumbar region and Schmorl's nodes in the thoracic region within the LgC compared to early Neolithic cultures.

Köhler (chapter 3) described *lumbar osteophytosis* in Alsónyék-Bátaszék, Hungary, in 37.79% (75/199) of males and 33% (84/252) of women. In LgC of the Kujawy region in Poland, osteophytosis was found in 27.7% (8/30) of males and 25.9% (7/27) of females (Garłowska 2001).

In both cases, vertebral osteophytosis was greater in males, indicating a greater workload on the lumbar spine.

In Moravia, Czech Republic, the comparison of LgC with early Neolithic cultures showed the greatest incidence of osteophytes in the lumbar region, and therefore also the greatest workload, in LPC females (25%).

This labour model of the early Neolithic with greater workload burden on women, likely from agriculture, was only preserved in the smaller LgC sites, such as Villánykővesd.

In the large settlements we find arthritic changes, even in their most severe forms. Men were predominately affected, such as the case of severe *coxarthrosis* in a Maturus age group male from Alsónyék-Bátaszék, grave no. 808 (Köhler, chapter 3), and another male, aged 30–50 from grave no. 355 in Zengővárkony (chapter 3) with *gonarthrosis*, and *rhizartrosis* of the small joints of the hand which merged into ankyloses of interphalangeal muscles (PIP joints). Repeated work strain caused nodules on flexor tendons. These blocked the movement of flexor tendons (trigger-finger) and in combination with rhizarthrosis led to PIP joint ankylosis (Smrčka and Dylevský 1998, 134–140) as documented in Alsónyék-Bátaszék in grave no. 5115 by Köhler (chapter 3).

13.3.3 TRAUMA

Injuries of women in mines stand out among traumas identified in the Lengyel Culture. An adult female, grave no. 1 (inv. no. 22239) in Mauer, Vienna (District XXIII) was buried in a chert quarry; she had a fractured right humerus which had healed by callus formation and a previous fracture of the right radius (*Colles' fracture*). She died later from myeloma. She was buried with grave goods (Strouhal and Němečková 2008).

Another possible work-related injury may be the poorly healed *ulnar neck fracture* (fig. 11a, b; chapter 9) of a female, aged 35–40 found in a chert mine in Krumlov Forest (grave 2a/2002) (chapter 9). The fracture had not been immobilized, fragments were not reduced, and a false joint had formed (Oliva 2007).

Yet how different the discovery in Krumlov Forest was from the burial in Mauer! A female skeleton was buried 6 metres deep in a firmly crouched position with a dislocated arm, and at the depth of 7 metres, there lay another female skeleton in an outstretched position with her arms folded behind her head.

This female had an infant skeleton on her chest and stomach. According to the archaeologist (Oliva 2007), these were ritually sacrificed individuals, despite the absences of traces of violence on their bones. These graves are the deepest to have been discovered from Central-European prehistory and lacked the usual grave goods. A small collection of dog bones was discovered above the head of the deeper of the two skeletons, however these bones did not make up a complete skeleton. Some pieces of the skeleton may have remained in the unexcavated part of the backfill. Radiometric dating of the upper skeleton GrA-22839: 5380 ± 50BP confirmed the Late Lengyel origin of the human remains. This described situation of sacrificed individuals was the first of its kind in Central European prehistoric mines. Up until this discovery, LgC remains have only been found as individual bones or regular burials with grave goods.

A special group of traumas comprised of cranial wall with *impression fractures* and penetrating injuries.

Traumas on the skulls of the women from Střelice and Předmostí-Dluhonice correspond to strikes from the side with a blunt instrument, probably a shoe-adze or a stone. These subsequently resulted in the star-shaped fracture seen in Střelice (fig. 9; chapter 9) and the break lines at the sides of the impact area, as in Předmostí-Dluhonice (fig. 10; chapter 9).

In Polish LgC, traumatic changes were documented in 11.5% of adult individuals, particularly in males (Garłowska 2001).

In Hungarian LgC, *penetrating skull injuries* were identified, as in the case of the male, aged 36–42 in Zengővárkony (grave 314) (Smrčka et al. 2018) whose injury had started the regeneration process.

These traumatic injuries inflicted by a Lengyel shoe-last axe shed light on social relationships and provide evidence of interpersonal and interpopulation aggression.

In Alsónyék-Bátaszék, Hungary, Köhler (chapter 3) described an oval shaped depression, 22 × 16 mm, on the left parietal bone of a female of mature age (grave no. 4132). The left radius and ulna of the female were also fractured. It cannot be ruled out that these two injuries arose from the same incident and are evidence of defensive wounds she received when she raised her arm to defend herself from attack.

In long bones, both fractures of particular bones and *multiple injuries* were documented.

From the Lengyel (LgC) period in Moravia, Czech Republic, multiple injuries were found on the skeleton of a young man in Mašovice-Pšeničné (fig. 8; chapter 9). They are suggestive of the stoning a lying person to death or the burying of him with rocks within the six weeks of his death, when bones can still be broken in this specific way.

13.3.4 NONSPECIFIC INFLAMMATIONS

Periostitis is an inflammatory process on the periosteal bone surface that manifests as pitting, longitudinal striation, and an eventual plaque-like film on new bone formation on the surface of the compact bone (Roberts 2012, 172).

In LgC, periostitis was predominately found in tibias, endocranially, on pelvic bones and ribs. Several periostitides affecting multiple bones were also identified.

The greatest incidence of *periostitis* was seen in *tibias*. Due to stagnation of blood in the lower extremities, bacteria could accumulate in the lower leg region (Steinbock 1976).

In Zengővárkony, Hungary, periostitides had a prevalence of 2.7% (1/37) on the right side and 5.3% (2/38) on the left.

Endocranial periostitides provide information about the state of the inflammatory condition of membranes covering the brain and the spinal cord (Roberts 2012, 178). These periostitides could have been caused by a bacterial or viral infection which most frequently occured in the winter and spring (Patterson 1993).

In LgC of Villánykővesd, Hungary, the prevalence of endocranial periostitis was 28% (2/7).

There were two instances of periostitis in children:

The first was an unborn child in grave 10 (fig. 6b; chapter 3). Besides striated endocranial new bone formation, the foetus also had periostitis in the pelvis. The foetus suffered from liver disease (see chapter 6).

The second case was in a child, aged 1–1.5, from grave 19 (fig. 6a; chapter 3). The new bone formation is rippled, which corresponds to the bacterial character of a granuloma on the meningeal coverings of the brain. It is presumed that it was a case of brucella meningitis.

In a Slavic female with endocranial periostitis, parvovirus was discovered (Mühlemann et al. 2018a). It may however have been an instance of hepatitis B considering the affection of liver (Mühlemann et al. 2018b), or another viral infection.

In grave 98–292–1529 in Belvárdgyula, alongside a woman, aged 40–60, a long goat/sheep bone with striated new bone formation was found (fig. 4a; chapter 3). In the lumbar spine region of the woman, a periosteal reaction in the superior frontal part of two lumbar vertebrae indicate symptoms of brucellosis (fig. 4b; chapter 3). In the region of anulus fibrosus, fixation was present (Capasso 1999). Large osteophytes result from tendon osseous metaplasia. Periostitis found in the goat bone also corroborate the signs of brucellosis in the woman's spine. This woman also suffered from cribra orbitalia in the left orbit.

In another grave in Belvárdgyula (no. 98–243–1231), a male aged 20–40 with osteoporosis with "fish vertebra" was described. Traits of osteolytic lesions (fig. 5a; chapter 3) of the impression of the anulus fibrosus in a layer of compact bone in the superior frontal aspect of lumbar vertebrae were also present. In the chipped-off part on the right, new formation under the uncovered segment of the plate is apparent.

Many individuals in Belvárdgyula likely suffered from *brucellosis*, as visible in the *rib periostitis* (fig. 7a) of a female, aged 40–60, from grave no. 98–83–408, who had multiple periostitis. In this instance, it also occurred in the pelvic region (fig. 7b).

Signs of brucella periostitis can also be observed in the ribs of a male, aged 20–40, from grave no. 98–379–2387, where there are small elongated neoformations and impressions of the pleura (fig. 9). In this male, anaemia manifesting as type 2 cribra orbitalia was also identified.

In grave no. 98–73, an unidentified, likely male, individual with right cribra orbitalia, periostitis in proximal phalanges was seen (fig. 8b).

In a male, aged 30–37, from Villánykővesd (grave no. 23), a vertebral lesion was found; tuberculosis or brucellosis cannot be excluded. Adler (2000) wrote that in instances of brucellosis, the occurrence of osteoporosis is lower, which would correspond with this case.

It can be concluded that the LgC population suffered from periostitis of the skeleton, with at least 5 cases associated with brucellosis in Belvárdgyula (where periostitis in a goat was identified in grave no. 292) and a further 3 cases in Villánykővesd.

13.3.5 SPECIFIC INFLAMMATIONS

In terms of specific inflammations, tuberculosis is highly significant for the Neolithic and for LgC.

With increasing population density in the large settlements, *various forms of tuberculosis* are observed in the Lengyel Culture: the typical Pott's disease of the spine was documented at Alsónyék-Bátaszék (Köhler et al. 2014), and tuberculosis of the small bones of the foot in Zengővárkony (Smrčka et al. 2018). The latter we believe was facilitated by the accumulation of people and animals in larger settlements. Only 5% of tuberculosis manifested as the osseous type. These typical forms were not verified through DNA analysis. The verification of the tubercular forms of periostitis in the ribs is advisable and will be conducted in the near future.

Tuberculosis in the male, aged 30–35 from grave no. 4027 in Alsónyék (Köhler, chapter 3) is one of the oldest paleopathologically documented instances of spinal tuberculosis (gibbus) in Hungary and Central Europe. In the Tisza Culture of the Late Neolithic, tuberculosis was found in Hódmezővásárhely-Gorzsa (4970–4594 B.C.) (Masson et al. 2015a), and in Vésztö-Mágor through DNA analysis of tooth pulp (Pósa et al. 2012).

In terms of differential diagnostics, it is difficult to distinguish tubercular lesions from brucella lesions (Adler 2000, 154–155).

13.3.6 ANAEMIA

Environmental factors affect the physiological balance of both the individual and the whole population. When the environment deteriorates, the physiological balance is affected and leads to cascade of changes. The consequences of these changes—stress markers—can be observed in both dental enamel (*hypoplasia*) and in bone (*Harris lines, cribra orbitalia*).

Cribra orbitalia, also known as *usura orbitae* (Möller-Christensen 1961) and *hyperostosis spongiosa orbitae* (Hengen 1971), refers to a process of bone destruction and formation in the anterior portion of the orbit roof. This causes the bone structure to become porous, almost spongy in appearance. It was described by Welcker (1888) and classified by Hengen (1971). The most commonly recognised types are porotic, cribrotic and trabecular.

These changes are frequently encountered in children and are well documented in prehistoric as well as historical populations (Ubelaker et al. 2006). In LgC in Alsónyék (Köhler, chapter 3), the prevalence of cribra orbitalia in children was 47.83% (24/46) in left orbit and 58% (21/36) in right orbit.

In the Polish LgC (Garłowska 2001), the prevalence in the 0–15 age group was 77.8% (7/9) and among juveniles (ages 15–20) it was 66.7% (6/9).

These results clearly demonstrate a higher frequency of cribra orbitalia, signifying greater dietary and immunological stresses on the LgC children in Poland.

A high prevalence of orbital cribra was detected in adult individuals from the Western European LPC populations by Ash et al. (2016) and was explained by a low intake of animal protein in their diet.

Much like the diet of adults in LPC, the diet of children up to the age of 15 had a proportionally higher vegetal component. The high prevalence in LgC children in Poland could therefore also be associated with a lower intake of animal protein.

The relationship of cribra orbitalia to dietary trends and natural conditions in the East and West could also be demonstrated by comparing LgC males and females.

In LgC females from Alsónyék (Köhler, chapter 3) the prevalence of cribra orbitalia in left orbit was 15.78% (24/152) and 15.88% (20/126) in right orbit. In LgC females in Poland, the prevalence was 15.8% (3/19). It is clear that the prevalence of cribra orbitalia in both regions was similar, just like dietary and nutritional stress.

In LgC males from Alsónyék (Köhler, chapter 3) the prevalence in left orbit was 12.23% (17/138) and 11.76% (12/102) in right orbit, while in LgC males in Poland, the prevalence was 23.1% (8/26). Thus, males in the north-west LgC regions suffered from greater dietary and immunological stresses than those in the east (Garłowska 2001).

It is therefore apparent that even within the Lengyel population there were differences in the prevalence of cribra orbitalia; the difference in stress factors arising from natural condition in the east and west forced the population to adapt to them.

13.3.7 BENIGN TUMOURS

Among the benign tumours occurring in the LgC were osteomas (N = 3): in flat cranial bones in Villánykővesd (grave no. 24, male aged 41–45) and Alsónyék (grave no. 614, female, Maturus) (Köhler, chapter 3), and in a humerus (grave no. 6244). Osteomas only occurred in their solitary form, with no cases of multiple osteomatosis documented, as would be seen in Gardner's syndrome.

In the female, aged 62–75 in grave no, 341, Zengővárkony, widened and deepened impressions of vessels with depression too large for Pacchionian arachnoid granulation were found. Regöly-Merei (1960, 1962) described these changes as a tumour (Zoffmann 1969–70). This find in grave no. 341 was compared to a mediaeval trepanation with a diagnosed calvarial meningioma from Sedlčany (Smrčka et al. 2003), and it was concluded that this was also an instance of advanced *meningioma* (Smrčka et al. 2018; Campillo 1977, 143–163).

13.3.8 MALIGNANT TUMOURS

The occurrence of malignant tumours in the Neolithic is undoubtedly related to the presence or rise in risk factors from the outer environment (Strouhal and Němečková 2008, 165; Finch 2018).

Thus far, the only malignant tumour in the Lengyel Culture was diagnosed by Eugen Strouhal (Strouhal and Jungwirth 1970; Strouhal and Kritscher 1990; Strouhal 1991) in an adult female buried in grave no. 1 (deposited with inv. no. 22239) in Vienna-Mauer (Vienna XXIII District) dating to beginning of the 4th millennium B.C. She was found among six graves embedded in Neolithic chert mines (2 males, 3 females, 2 children), excavated by J. Bayer between 1924 and 1930 (Ruttkay 1970). It was a primary bone tumour of haematopoietic origin, either myeloma multiplex or plasmacytoma (formerly referred to as Kahler's disease). It is caused by mutated plasma cells spreading haematogenously to various locations on the axial skeleton. Tumour cells secrete lymphoma kinase, which stimulates osteoclastic activity in trabecular bone, leading to the formation of osteolytic lesions. During an X-ray examination, the image of the skull revealed clusters of small holes resembling Swiss cheese. A similar perforated character was observed in the cervical vertebrae, rib, scapula, pelvic bone fragments and to a lesser extent in clavicular bones (Strouhal and Němečková 2008, 95–100).

13.3.9 SPREADING OF ZOONOSES AND THE BEGINNINGS OF THE DECLINE OF THE NEOLITHIC LIFESTYLE

The Lengyel herd comprised of cattle, sheep, goats and pigs. Neolithic farmers could have contracted some infections, such as tuberculosis from cows' milk, or brucellosis from goats' milk.

INTRODUCTION OF MILK INTO THE DIET

In the Neolithic, milk was an important innovation, while at the same time being a key factor in the transmission of zoonoses to the human population. Archaeological research has shown that dairy farming originated around 8000 B.C. in the Middle East. However, direct evidence of the preserved organic remains of milk on ceramics from Anatolia only dates to the 7th millennia B.C. (Evershed et al. 2008).

MYCOBACTERIUM TUBERCULOSIS

Of the infections specific for the Neolithic and LgC, tuberculosis was of crucial significance. While its original ties to the human population date to distant time in mankind's history, it was not until the Neolithic that the circumstances were optimal for the disease to thrive. A growing population, settled lifestyle, and the domestication of cattle were all driving factors in spreading the disease (Donoghue 2009).

For instance, in the Tripillia Culture, animals were kept on the ground floor of the house while people inhabited the floor above them (Videnko 2003). This close contact between people and animals led to easy transmission of zoonoses.

Palaeopathological finds of tuberculosis from Neolithic era in the Near East, Jordan (El-Najjar et al. 1997; Ortner 1979) and Israel (Hershkovitz et al. 2008; Zias 1998) demonstrate that tuberculosis was present in the Levant when these populations were transitioning to agriculture (Lazaridis et al. 2016). At the same time, tuberculosis would follow the individual strands of spreading agriculture—to Africa, documented by a find from Predynastic Egypt (Strouhal 1987), to Asia with a find in Iraq (Ortner 1999) and to Europe, seen in several finds: Neolithic Germany (Morse 1967; Manchester 1991), France (Dastugue and de Lumley 1976), Neolithic Poland (Gladykowska-Rzeczycka 1999), Sweden (Nuorala et al. 2004) and Denmark (Bennike 1999).

Biomolecular identification will provide clarification on the relationship between the spreading of tuberculosis, and the movement of animals and people in the Neolithic associated with the introduction of dairying (Müller et al. 2014).

BRUCELLA MELITENSIS

The accumulation of people and animals together in large Neolithic settlements led to the spreading of other infections, such as brucellosis. Goat populations were a suitable brucella reservoirs (Fournié et al. 2017).

Goat breeding spread in the middle of the 7th millennium B.C. (Merrett 2004). In most Neolithic sites of this time, male goats were being slaughtered. This changing paradigm to a focus on meat production augmented the transmission of brucellosis. Brucellosis is transmitted from female goats through their vaginal secretions. As the carriers of the disease, they are responsible for the spread of the pathogen throughout their fertile life. It is possible that the butchering of male goats started due to the fact that brucellosis infections manifests predominantly in males. In the larger settlements, the mixing of herds led to the spread of brucellosis. The pathogens in a herd could die out in smaller settlements more easily than larger ones (Fournié et al. 2017).

From the viewpoint of differential diagnostics, it is difficult to make a distinction between tubercular and brucellar lesions (Adler 2000). It has to be considered that sooner or later an increasing number of brucellosis cases will be diagnosed within the Lengyel Culture. In the macroscopically described occurrences of brucellosis from the Hungarian sites of Belvárdgyula (N = 5) and Villánykövesd (N = 3), and in particular those with periostitis, verification through DNA analyses and genomic methods would be appropriate.

YERSINIA PESTIS

A plague pandemic may have played its part in the Neolithic decline (Kristiansen 2014). Genomic analysis led to the discovery of the oldest occurrence of plague in a human population in Sweden, in the Neolithic TRB—Funnel Beaker Culture, 4900 B.C. The plague pandemic most likely originated in large settlements and spread along trade routes. It is a possible cause of the fall of the mega settlements of the Trypillia Culture (4800–3000 B.C.) in today's Moldavia, Romania and Ukraine (Rascovan et al. 2019).

It can be concluded, that in the large settlements of the Lengyel Culture, key factors linked to Neolithic decline started to appear, within which zoonoses could have played a part. This role is confirmed by the spread of tuberculosis and the suspected transmission of brucellosis. The spread of plague in the Lengyel Culture has not yet been proven, but it cannot be excluded considering the pandemics in Northern Europe and Asia, as well as the probable outbreaks in the nearby Tripyllia Culture (Rascovan et al. 2019).

APPENDIX: METHODOLOGY

PROCESSING OF THE SPECIMENS FOR MULTIELEMENTARY ANALYSIS

Fragments of bones were cleansed of the rest of soil, washed with deionized water and leached with formic acid to remove diagenetically influenced fractions. After thorough washing with deionized water and subsequent drying, the bone specimens were ground in an agate mortar to the size of analytic fineness. Concurrently with the bone material, specimens of soils were taken at the site. The soils were sieved through a sieve with 2-mm spaces and dried to the constant weight in the laboratory.

CHEMICAL ANALYSIS
MARTIN MIHALJEVIČ

The dose of 0.2 g bone specimen was put in a 50 ml calibrated flask with 5 ml of concentrated HNO_3 and dissolved by gentle heating on a hotplate at ca 80 °C. After cooling, the flasks were topped up with deionized water. With each series of 10 specimens, a blind test was prepared. Common mineralization of soil was performed as follows: The dose of 0.2 g soil in a platinum dish was annealed in a furnace (Linn, FRG) up to the temperature of 450 °C. After cooling, the specimen was poured over with 10 ml of concentrated HF and 0.5 ml of concentrated $HClO_4$ and digested in a fume. Subsequently, the rest was dissolved in water in a dish and placed in a 100 ml calibrated flask with 2 ml HNO_3 added. For preparation of the solutions, Merck brand acids and deionized water from a MilliQPlus appliance (Millipore, USA) were used.

The contents of Ca, Mg, K, Fe and Na in mineralized specimens were established through flame atomic absorption spectrometry (Spectra AA 200 HT, Varian Australia) under the conditions recommended by the manufacturer.

The contents of V, Cr, Co, Ni, As, Y, Cd, Ba, Pb, U, La, Ce, Pr, Nd, Sm, Eu, Gd, Tb, Dy, Ho, Er, Tm, Yb and Lu in mineralized specimens were established through mass spectrometry with induction-bound plasma (PQ 3, VG Elemental, Great Britain) under the following conditions: output ICP 1350 W, measurement mode "peak jump," measurement time 3 × 50 s, parameter of ion optics optimized with [115]In, gas flows 13.5 l/min cooling, 0.7 l/min additional, 0, 65 l/min nebulizer, internal standards In, Re, Sc.

For calibration of the measurements, Astasol brand solutions (Analytika, Czech Republic) were used.

The method had been tested on certified reference bone material NIST SRM 1486.

STATISTICAL ANALYSIS
MARTIN HILL

Respecting the skewed distribution and non-constant variance in most dependent variables, these were transformed by power transformations to attain data symmetry and homoscedasticity prior further processing (see Meloun et al. 2000). The homogeneity and distribution of the transformed data and residuals was checked by residual analysis as described elsewhere (Meloun et al. 2004, Meloun et al. 2002). The ANOVA model was used for evaluation of the relationships between concentration of elements, location (Villánykövesd vs. Zengővárkony), and matrix (bone vs. enamel). The model consisted of Subject factor explaining inter-individual variability, between-subject factor Location, within-subject factor Matrix, and Location × Matrix interaction. F represents the Fisher's statistic and p designates statistical significance for the factors and interaction. Statistical software Statgraphics Centurion, version 18 from Statgraphic Technologies, Inc. (The Plains, Virginia, USA) was used for the statistical analysis.

BIBLIOGRAPHY

Acsádi, G., and J. Nemeskéri. 1970. *History of Human Life Span and Mortality*. Budapest: Akadémia Kiadó.

Adler, C. P. 2000. *Bone Diseases*. Berlin: Springer Verlag.

Alfrey, A. C., G. H. Le Gendre, and W. D. Kaehry. 1976. "The Dialysis Encephalopathy Syndrome." *New England Journal of Medicine* 294:184–88.

Allentoft, M. E., M. Sikora, K.-G. Sjögren, et al. 2015. "Population Genomics of Bronze Age Eurasia." *Nature* 522:167–72.

Ambros, C. 1986. "Tierknochenfunde aus Siedlungen der Lengyel-Kultur in der Slowakei." In *Internationales Symposium über die Lengyel-Kultur in der Slowakei, Nové Vozokany 5.-9. November 1984*, edited by V. Némejcová-Pavúková, 11–18. Nitra: AÚ SAV.

American Medical Association News 1984, November 2:21.

Ames, K. M. 2010. "On the Evolution of the Human Capacity for Inequality and/or Egalitarianism." In *Pathways to the Power: New Perspectives on the Emergence of Social Inequality*, edited by T. D. Price and G. M. Feinman, 15–44. New York: Springer.

Andel, T. H. van, and C. N. Runnels. 1995. "The Earliest Farmers in Europe." *Antiquity* 69:481–500.

Angel, J. L. 1966. "Porotic Hyperostosis, Anemias, Malarias, and Marshes in the Prehistoric Eastern Mediterranean." *Science* 153:760–63.

Ash, A., M. Francken, I. Pap, Z. Tvrdý, J. Wahl, and R. Pinhasi. 2016. "Regional Differences in Health, Diet and Weaning Patterns amongst the First Neolithic Farmers of Central Europe." *Scientific Reports* 6:29458.

Bálek, M., and V. Podborský. 2001. "Začátky letecké archeologie na jižní Moravě." In *50 let archeologických výzkumů Masarykovy univerzity na Znojemsku*, edited by V. Podborský, 69–94. Brno: Masarykova univerzita.

Bancroft, J. D., and M. Gamble. 2002. *Theory and Practice of Histological Techniques*. Edinburgh: Churchill Livingstone.

Bándi, G., É. Petres, and B. Maráz. 1979. "Baranya megye története az őskorban." In *Baranya megye története az őskortól a honfoglalásig*, edited by G. Bándi, 7–220. Pécs: Baranya Megyei Levéltár.

Bánffy, E., and G. Goldmann. 2003. "Újkőkori világ." In *Magyar régészet az ezredfordulón*, edited by Z. Visy, 112–117. Budapest: Teleki László Alapítvány.

Bánffy, E., A. Osztás, K. Oross, et al. 2016. "The Alsónyék Story: Towards the History of a Persistent Place." *Bericht der Römisch-Germanischen Kommission* 94:283–318.

Barker, G. 2009. *The Agricultural Revolutinon in Prehistory. Why did Foragers Become Farmers?* Oxford: Oxford University Press.

Barna, J. 2011. "A lengyeli kultúra kialakulása a Dny-Dunántúlon." Ph.D. diss. ELTE, Hungary.

Barna, J. 2015. "Socio-historical Background of Cultural Changes in South-Western-Hungary as Reflected by Archaeological Data during Post-LBK Times." *Anthropologie* 53:399–412.

Barnes, E. 1994. *Developmental Defects of the Axial Skeleton in Paleopathology*. Niwot: University Press of Colorado.

Barnes, E. 2012. *Atlas of Developmental Field Anomalies of the Human Skeleton: A Paleopathology Perspective*. Hoboken, NJ: John Wiley.

Barron, M. L., M. S. Rybchyn, S. Ramesh, et al. 2017. "Clinical, Cellular, Microscopic and Ultrastructural Studies of a Case of Fibrogenesis Imperfecta Ossium." *Bone Research* 5:16057–78.

Bárta, J. 1983. "Pohrebisko a praveké sídlisko v jaskyni Dúpna diera pri Slatinke nad Bebravou." *Študijné zvesti AÚ SAV* 20:15–37.

Bartík, J. 2015. "Sídelní a socioekonomické aspekty lengyelské kultury v prostoru nejzápadnější Moravy." Ph.D. diss. Brno.

Bartík, J., and R. Bíško. 2013. "Fenomén výšinného osídlení na přelomu neolitu a eneolitu v prostoru nejzápadnější Moravy." In *Otázky neolitu a eneolitu našich krajín*, edited by I. Cheben and M. Soják. Nitra: AÚ SAV.

Bartucz, L. 1966. *A praehistorikus trepanáció és orvostörténeti vonatkozású sírleletek.* Budapest: Országos Orvostörténeti Könyvtár.

Bayliss, A., N. Beavan, D. Hamilton, et al. 2016. "Peopling the Past: Creating a Site Biography in the Hungarian Neolithic." *Bericht der Römisch-Germanischen Kommission* 94:3–91.

Beattie, J. H., and A. Avenell. 1992. "Trace Element Nutrition and Bone Mtabolism." *Nutrition Research Reviews* 5:167–88.

Becker, U. 2002. *Slovník symbolů.* Prague: Portál.

Belcredi, L., M. Čižmář, P. Košturík, M. Oliva, and M. Salaš. 1989. *Archeologické lokality a nálezy okresu Brno-venkov.* Tišnov: Okresní muzeum Brno-venkov.

Bender, G. 1999. *Gerincbetegségekről. Differenciáldiagnosztikai problémák a mozgásszervi betegségekben.* Budapest: Golden Book Kiadó.

Bennike, P. 1999. "Facts or Myths? A Re-evaluation of Cases of Diagnosed Tuberculosis in Denmark." In *Tuberculosis, Past and Present*, edited by G. Pálfi et al., 511–18. Budapest: Golden Book; Szeged: Tuberculosis Foundation.

Bentley, R. A., P. Bickle, L. Fibiger, et al. 2012. "Community Differentiation and Kinship among Europe's First Farmers." *Proceedings of the National Academy of Sciences U.S.A.* 109:9326–30.

Bentley, R. A., and C. Knipper 2005. "Geographical Patterns in Biologically Available Strontium, Carbon and Oxygen Isotope Signatures in Prehistoric SW Germany." *Archaeometry* 47: 629–44.

Bentley, R. A., T. D. Price, J. Lüning, D. Gronenborn, J. Wahl, and P. D. Fullagar. 2002. "Prehistoric Migration in Europe: Strontium Isotope Analysis of Early Neolithic Skeletons." *Current Anthropology* 43:799–804.

Beranová, M. 2015. *Jídlo a pití v pravěku a středověku.* Prague: Academia.

Berg, F. 1956. "Ein neolithisches Schädelnest aus Poigen." *Archaeologia Austriaca* 19-20:70–76.

Bernert, Z. 2005. "Paleoantropológiai programcsomag." *Folia Anthropologica* 3:71–74.

Bertók G., and C. Gáti. 2011. "Neue angaben zur Spätneolitschen siedlungstruktur in Südosttransdanubien." *Acta Archeologica Scientiarum Hungaricae* 62:1–28.

Bertók, G., and C. Gáti. 2014. *Old Times—New Methods.* Budapest: Archaeolingua.

Bertók, G., C. Gáti, and R. Lóki. 2008. "Elözetes jelentés a Belvárdgyula határában (Baranya megye) talált késö neolitikus település és körárok." *Ősrégészeti levelek* 10:5–16.

Bickle, P., R. A. Bentley, and M. Dočkalová. 2014. "Early Neolithic Lifeways in Moravia and Western Slovakia: Comparing Archaeological, Osteological and Isotopic Data from Cemetery and Settlement Burials of the Linearbandkeramik (LBK)." *Anthropologie* 52:35–72.

Bickle, P., and A. Whittle. 2013. *The First Farmers of Central Europe: Diversity in LBK Lifeways.* Oxford: Oxbow Books; Oakville, CT: David Brown.

Bíró, T. K. 2003a. "A termelő gazdálkodás kezdetei Magyarországon." In *Magyar régészet az ezredfordulón*, edited by Z. Visy, 99. Budapest: Teleki László Alapítvány.

Bíró, T. K. 2003b. "A késő neolitikum a Dunántúlon." In *Magyar régészet az ezredfordulón*, edited by Z. Visy, 102-103. Budapest: Teleki László Alapítvány.

Bocherens, H. 1992. "Biogéochimie isotopique (^{13}C, ^{15}N, ^{18}O) et paléontologie des vertébrés: applications à l'étude des réseaux trophiques révolus et des paléoenvironnements." Ph.D. diss. Université Paris VI.

Bocquet-Appel, J.-P., and D. Bar-Yosef, eds. 2008. *The Neolithic Demographic Transition and Its Consequences.* Dordrecht: Springer.

Bökönyi, S. 1974. *History of Domestic Mammals in Central and Eastern Europe.* Budapest: Akadémiai Kiadó.

Boldsen, J. L., G. R. Milner, L. W. Konigsberg, and J. W. Wood. 2002. "Transition Analysis: A New Method for Estimating Age from Skeletons." In *Paleodemography. Age Distribution from Skel-*

etal Samples, edited by R. D. Hoppa and J. W. Vaupel, 73–106. Cambridge: Cambridge University Press.

Bollongino, R., O. Nehlich, M. P. Richards, et al. 2013. "2000 Years of Parallel Societes in Stone Age Central Europe." *Science* 342:479–81.

Borić, D., and T. D. Price. 2013. "Strontium Isotopes Document Greater Human Mobility at the Start of the Balkan Neolithic." *Proceedings of the National Academy of Sciences U.S.A.* 110: 3298–303.

Bouzek, J. 1979. *Objevy ve středomoří.* Prague: Odeon.

Bouzek, J. 1996. "Sibily." *Religio* 4:121–26.

Bouzek, J., and Z. Kratochvíl. 1994. *Od mýtu k logu.* Prague: Hermann & synové.

Broadbent, B. H. Sr., B. H. Broadbent Jr, and W. H. Golden. 1975. *Bolton Standards of Dentofacial Developmental Growth.* St. Louis: Mosby.

Brothwell, D. R. 1963. *Digging up Bones: The Excavation, Treatment and Study of Human Skeletal Remains.* London: British Museum.

Brothwell, D. R. 1972. *Digging Up Bones: The Excavation, Treatment and Study of Human Skeletal Remains.* 2nd ed. London: British Museum.

Brun, L. R., A. M. Galich, E. Vega, et al. 2014. "Strontium Renalate Effect on Bone Mineral Density is Modified by Previous Biphosphonate Treatment." *Springer Plus* 3:676–83.

Brůžek, J. 2002. "A Method for Visual Determination of Sex, Using the Human Hip Bone." *American Journal of Physical Anthropology* 117:157–68.

Buchvaldek, M., L. Košnar, and A. Lippert. 2007. *Archaeological Atlas of Prehistoric Europe.* Vol. 1. Prague: Karolinum.

Buckberry, J. 2015. "The (Mis)use of Adult Age Estimates in Osteology." *Annals of Human Biology* 42:323–31.

Buttler, W., and W. Habarey. 1936. *Die bandkeramische Ansiedlung bei Köln-Lindentahl.* Berlin: De Gruyter.

Camfield, P. R., C. S. Camfield, and M. M. Cohen Jr. 2000. "Neurologic Aspects of Craniosynostosis." In *Craniosynostosis. Diagnosis, Evaluation and Management*, edited by M. Cohen and R. Mac Lean, 177–94. 2nd ed. Oxford: Oxford University Press.

Campillo, D. 1977. *Paleopatologia del Craneo en Cataluña, Valencia y Baleares.* Barcelona: Editoria Montblanc-Martin.

Capasso, L. 1999. "Brucellosis at Herculaneum (79AD)." *International Journal of Osteoarchaeology* 9:277–88.

Capasso, L., K. A. R. Kennedy, and C. Wilczak. 1998. *Atlas of Occupational Markers on Human Remains.* Teramo, IT: Edigrafital.

Čerevková, A. 2015. "Sídliště kultury s lineární keramikou v Žádovicích (okr. Hodonín)." MA thesis. Brno.

Čermáková, E. 2002. "Problémy dětství v neolitu střední Evropy." *Pravěk. Nová řada* 12:7–45.

Čermáková, E. 2007. "Postavení ženy, muže a dítěte ve společnosti tvůrců lengyelské kultury." In *Studium sociálních a duchovních struktur pravěku*, edited by E. Kazdová, and V. Podborský, 207–255. Brno: FF MU.

Čermáková, Eva. 2008. "Symbolika neolitických ženských pásů." *Acta archaeologica Opaviensia* 3:25–31.

Černá, L., and L. Sedláčková. 2017. "Brno (k. ú. Štýřice, okr. Brno-město)." *Přehled výzkumů* 58:150–53.

Červinka, I. L. 1902. *Vlastivěda moravská.* Vol. 1, *Země a lid.* Part 2, *Morava za pravěku.* Brno: Musejní spolek.

Childe, V. G. 1925. *The Dawn of European Civilization.* London: K. Paul, Trench, Trubner; New York: A. A. Knopf.

Childe, V. G. 1936. *Man Makes Himself.* London: Watts.

Chochol, J. 1964. "Význam stomatologického výzkumu pro úkoly historické antropologie." In *Některé stomatologické problémy*, edited by J. Chochol et al., 11–16. Praha: Univerzita Karlova.

Čihák, R. 1987. *Anatomie.* Prague: Grada.

Čižmář, Z. ed. 2008. *Život a smrt v mladší době kamenné*. Brno: Ústav archeologické památkové péče.

Čižmář, Z., and M. Dočkalová. 2004. "Pohřeb tři jedinců v objektu kultury s lineární keramikou z Hlubokych Mašůvek, okr. Znojmo." In *Otázky neolitu a eneolitu našich zemí 2003*, edited by M. Lutovský, 354-64. Prague: ÚAPP SČ.

Čižmář, Z., and Z. Hájek. 2008. "Znojmo-Novosady (ul. Jarošova)." In *Život a smrt v mladší době kamenné*, edited by Z. Čižmář, 12-23. Brno: Ústav archeologické památkové péče.

Čižmář, Z., P. Kalábková, E. Kazdová, and J. Kovárník. 2008. "Lid s moravskou malovanou keramikou lengyelské kultury." In *Život a smrt v mladší době kamenné*, edited by Z. Čižmář, 76-101. Brno: Ústav archeologické památkové péče.

Čižmář, Z., J. Pavúk, P. Procházková, and M. Šmíd. 2004. "K problému definování finálního stadia lengyelské kultury." In *Zwischen Karpaten und Ägäis. Neolithikum und ältere Bronzezeit. Gedenkschrift für Viera Němejcová-Pavúková*, edited by B. Hansel and E. Studeníková, 207-32. Rahden, Westfalen: Verlag Maria Leidorf.

Čižmářová, J., V. Ondruš, M. Salaš, and J. Tejral. 1996. *Pravěk Moravy*. Brno: Moravské zemské muzeum.

Cohen, M. N. 2009. "Introduction: Rethinking the Origins of Agriculture." *Current Anthropology* 50:591-95.

Cohen, M. N., and G. J. Armelagos. 1984. "Paleopathology at the Origins of Agriculture: Editor's Summation." In *Paleopathology at the Origins of Agriculture*, edited by M. N. Cohen and G. J. Armelagos, 585-601. Orlando: Academic Press.

Cohen, M. M., and R. Mac Lean, eds. 2000. *Craniosynostosis. Diagnosis, Evaluation and Management*. 2nd ed. Oxford: Oxford University Press.

Crubézy, E. 1996. "Surgery at the Origins of Agriculture: The Case of Central Europe." *Anthropologie* 34:329-32.

Curzon, M. E., and D. C. Crocker. 1978. "Relationship of Trace Elements in Human Tooth Enamel to Dental Caries." *Archives of Oral Biology* 23:647-53.

Curzon, M. E. J., and T. W. Cutress. 1983. *Trace Elements and Dental Disease*. Littleton, MA: John Wright/PDG.

Czech Geological Survey. 2018. "Geovědní Mapy 1 : 50 000." Prague: Czech Geological Survey. https://mapy.geology.cz/geocr50/.

Dastugue, J., and M. A. de Lumley. 1976. "Les maladies des hommes préhistoriques." In *La Prehistorie Francaise. Vol. 2, Les Civilisations Néolithiques et Prehistoriques de la France*, edited by J. Guilaine, 153-64. Paris: CNRS.

Demján, P. 2015. "Evidence of Social Structure of a Neolithic Community in Svodín, Southwest of Slovakia." *Anthropologie* 53:363-73.

DeNiro, M. J., and S. Epstein. 1978. "Influence of Diet on the Distribution of Carbon Isotopes in Animals." *Geochimica et Cosmochimica Acta* 42:495-506.

DeNiro, M. J., and S. Epstein. 1981. "Influence of Diet on the Distribution of Nitrogen Isotopes in Animals." *Geochimica et Cosmochimica Acta* 45:341-51.

DePaolo, D. J., and B. L. Ingram. 1985. "High-Resolution Stratigraphy with Strontium Isotopes." *Science* 227:938-41.

Dermience, M., G. Lognay, F. Mathieu, and P. Goyens. 2015. "Effects of Thirty Elements on Bone Metabolism." *Journal of Trace Elements in Medicine and Biology* 32:86-106.

Dimitrijević, S. 1968. *Sopotsko-Lenđelska kultura*. Zagreb: Filozofski fakultet Sveučilišta, Archeološki institut.

Disa, J. J., J. Vosoughi, and N. H. Goldberg. 1993. "A Comparison of Obsidian and Surgical Steel Scalpel Wound Healing in Rats." *Plastic and Reconstructive Surgery* 92:884-87.

Dočkalová, M. 2006. "Two Skeleton Graves from Neolithic Settlements in Moravia (Czech Republic)." *Anthropologie* 44:127-37.

Dočkalová, M. 2008. "Anthropology of the Neolithic population from Vedrovice (Czech Republic)." *Anthropologie* 46:239-315.

Dočkalová, M., and Z. Čižmář. 2007. "Neolithic Children Burial at Moravian Settlements in the Czech Republic." *Anthropologie* 45:31-59.

Dočkalová, M., and Z. Čižmář. 2008a. "Neolithic Settlement Burials of Adult and Juvenile Individuals in Moravia, Czech Republic." *Anthropologie* 46:37-76.

Dočkalová, M., and Z. Čižmář. 2008b. "Antropologie a pohřbívání v moravském neolitu." In *Život a smrt v mladší době kamenné*, edited by Z. Čižmář, 236-47. Brno: Ústav archeologické památkové péče.

Doležel, J. 1985. "Pravěké a raně středověké osídlení Tišnovska—předběžné výsledky povrchových průzkumů v letech 1979-1983 (okr. Blansko, Brno-venkov)." *Přehled výzkumů 1983*, 85-89. Brno: Archeologický ústav ČSAV.

Dombay, J. 1939. *A zengővárkonyi őskori telep és temető.* Budapest: Magyar Tőrténeti Múzeum.

Dombay, J. 1939-40. "A baranyavármegyei múzeum őskori agyagszobrai." In *Pécs sz. kir. város Majorossy Imre Múzeumának Értesítője*, 6-10. Pécs: Pécs sz. kir. város Majorossy Imre Múzeumának.

Dombay, J. 1958. "Kőrézkori és kora-vaskori település nyomai a pécsváradi Aranyhegyen." In *A Janus Pannonius Múzeum Évkönyve 1958*, 53-102. Pécs: A Janus Pannonius Múzeum.

Dombay, J. 1959. "Próbaásatás a Villánykővesdi kőrézkori telepen." In *A Janus Pannonius Múzeum Évkönyve 1959*, 53-73. Pécs: A Janus Pannonius Múzeum.

Dombay, J. 1960a. *Die Siedlung und das Gräberfeld in Zengővárkony. Beiträge zur Kultur des Aeneolithikums in Ungarn.* Bonn: Rudolf Habelt Verlag.

Dombay, J. 1960b. "Pécsvárad-Aranyhegy." *Archaeológiai Értesítő* 87:229.

Donoghue, H. D. 2009. "Human Tuberculosis—an Ancient Disease, as Elucidated by Ancient Microbial Biomolecules." *PLOS Pathogens* 11:1156-62.

Dreslerová, G. 2006. "Vyhodnocení zvířecích kostí z neolitického sídliště Těšetice-Kyjovice okr. Znojmo, Česká republika." *Archeologické rozhledy* 58:3-32.

Drozdová, E. 2004. *Základy osteometrie.* Brno: Nadace Universitas Masarykiana.

Duerr, H. P. 1997. *Sedna, aneb láska k životu.* Brno: Horus.

Dufek, J., D. Malyková, M. Popelka, and A. Přichystal. 2016. "Stopy dálkových kontaktů na neolitickém sídlišti v Kolíně-Šťáralce." *Archeologie ve středních Čechách* 20:935-57.

Dunbar, R. 2010. *How Many Friends Does One Person Need? Dunbar's Number and Other Evolutionary Quirks.* Cambridge, MA: Harvard University Press.

Dungl, P. 2005. *Ortopedie.* Prague: Grada.

Duruibe, J., M. Ogwuegbu, and J. Egwurugwu. 2007. "Heavy Metal Pollution and Human Biotoxic Effects." *International Journal of Physical Sciences* 2:112-18.

Dutour, O. 1986. "Enthesopathies (Lesions of Muscular Insertions) as Indicators of the Activities of Neolithic Saharan Populations." *American Journal of Physical Anthropology* 71:221-24.

Eliade, M. 2004. *Pojednání o dějinách náboženství.* Prague: Argo.

El-Najjar, M., A. Al-Shiyab, and I. Al-Sarie. 1997. "Cases of Tuberculosis at 'Ain Ghazal, Jordan." *Paléorient* 22:123-128.

El-Najjar, M. Y., M. V. DeSanti, and L. Ozebek. 1978. "Prevalence and Possible Etiology of Dental Enamel Hypoplasia." *American Journal of Physical Anthropology* 48:185-92.

Eriksen, E. F., D. W. Axelrod, and F. Melsen. 1994. *Bone Histomorphometry.* New York: Raven Press.

Éry, K., A. Kralovánszky, and J. Nemeskéri. 1963. "Történeti népességek rekonstrukciójának reprezentációja (A Representative Reconstruction of Historic Population)." *Anthropologiai Közlemények* 7:41-90.

Eshed, V., A. Gopher, E. Galih, and I. Hershkovitz. 2004. "Musculoskeletal Stress Markers in Natufian Hunter-Gatherers and Neolithic Farmers in the Levant: The Upper Limb." *American Journal of Physical Anthropology* 123:303-15.

Eshed, V., A. Gopher, R. Pinhasi, and I. Hershkovitz. 2010. "Paleopathology and the Origin of Agriculture in the Levant." *American Journal of Physical Anthropology* 143:121-33.

Evershed, R. P., S. Payne, A. G. Sherratt, et al. 2008. "Earliest Date for Milk Use in the Near East and Southern Europe Linked to Cattle Herding." *Nature* 455:528-31.

Falys, C. G., and M. E. Lewis. 2010. "Proposing a Way Forward: A Review of Standardisation in the Use of Age Categories and Aging Techniques in Osteological Analysis (2004-2009)." *International Journal of Osteoarchaeology* 21:704-16.

Feinman, G. M. 2016. "Variation and Change in Archaic States. Ritual as a Mechanism of Sociopolitical Integration." In *Ritual and Archaic States*, edited by J. M. A. Murphy, 1-22. Gainesville: University Press of Florida.

Ferembach, D., I. Schwidetzky, and M. Stloukal. 1979. "Empfehlungen für die Alters- und Geschlechtsdiagnose am Skelett." *Homo* 30:1-32.

Fernández-Domínguez, E., and L. Reynolds. 2017. "The Mesolithic-Neolithic Transition in Europe: A Perspective from Ancient Human DNS." In *Times of Neolithic Transition along the Western Mediterranean*, edited by O. García-Puchol and D. C. Salazar-García, 311-38. New York: Springer.

Finch, C. E. 2018. *The Role of Global Air Pollution in Aging and Disease*. London: Academic Press.

Finlay, N. 2000. "Outside of Life: Traditions of Infant Burial in Ireland from Cillín to Cist." *World Archaeology* 31:407-22.

Fischer, A., P. Malara, and D. Wiechula. 2014. "The Study of Barium Concetration in Deciduous Teeth, Impacted Teeth, and Facial Bones of Polish Residents." *Biological Trace Elements Research* 161:32-37.

Fogel, M. L., N. Tuross, and D. W. 1989. "Nitrogen Isotope Tracers of Human Lactation in Modern and Archaeological Populations." In *Annual Report of the Director of the Geophysical Laboratory, Carnegie Institution of Washington 1988-1989*, 111-17. Washington, DC: Geophysical Laboratory.

Fojtová, M., M. Dočkalová, and I. Jarošová. 2008. "Antropologický rozbor koster ze sídlištních pohřbů moravského neolitu." *Ve službách archeologie* 1:213-21.

Fournié, G., D. U. Pfeiffer, and R. Bendrey. 2017. "Early Animal Farming and Zoonotic Disease Dynamics: Modelling Brucellosis Transmission in Neolithic Goat Populations." *Royal Society open Science* 4:1600943.

Franěk, T., R. Průša, J. Kukačka, and R. Kisel. 2009. "Stroncium v laboratorní medicíně." *Klinická biochemie a metabolismus* 17:239-44.

Frayer, D. W. 2004. "Dental Remains from Krškany and Vedrovice." *Anthropologie* 42:71-103.

Frazer, J. G. 1994. *Zlatá ratolest*. Prague: Mladá fronta.

Fuller, B. T., J. L. Fuller, D. A. Harris, and R. E. Hedges. 2006. "Detection of Breastfeeding and Weaning in Modern Human Infants with Carbon and Nitrogen Stable Isotope Ratios." *American Journal of Physical Anthropology* 129:279-93.

Furholt, M. 2021. "Mobility and Social Change: Understanding the European Neolithic Period after the Archaeogenetic Revolution." *Journal of Archaeological Research*, https://doi.org /10.1007/s10814-020-09153-x.

Gábor, O. 2008. "Kr. e. 5. századi oinochoé korsók Szajkról." *Janus Pannonius Múzeum Évkönyve* 50-52:66-82.

Gábor, O. 2009. "Oinochoe Jugs from thet 5th Century B.C. found in Szajk." In *Ex officina... Studia in honorem Dénes Gábler*, 145-60. Győr: Mursella Régészeti Egyesület.

Gábor, O., T. K. Bíró, and J. Kraft. 2000. "A mecseki bányászat története a honfoglalás koráig." *Pécsi Szemle* 4:4-15.

Gallina, Z., P. Hornok, T. Paluch, and K. Somogyi. 2010. "Előzetes jelentés az M6 AP TO 10/B és 11. számú lelőhelyrészen végzett feltárásról. Alsónyék-Bátaszék (Tolna megye) 2006-2009." *Wosinsky Mór Múzeum Évkönyve* 32:7-100.

Garłowska, E. 2001. "Disease in the Neolithic Population of the Lengyel Culture (4300-4000 B.C.) from the Kujawy Region in North-Central Poland." *Zeitschrift für Morphologie und Anthropologie* 83:43-57.

Garwin, H. M., N. V. Passalacqua, N. M. Uhl, D. R. Gipson, R. S. Overburry, and L. L. Cabo. 2012. "Developments in Forensic Anthropology: Age-at-Death Estimation." In *A Companion to Forensic Anthropology*, edited by D. C. Dirkmaat, 202-23. Wiley Online Library.

Gáti, C., and G. Bertók. 2015-16. "The Grave of the "Lady of Borjád"—A Late Neolithic Woman of High Status from Baranya County (Hungary)." *Communicationes Archaeologicae Hungariae*: 45-70.

Geisler, M., and J. Kohoutek. 1997. "Havřice (okr. Uherské Hradiště)." In *Přehled výzkumů 1993-1994*, 117-18. Brno. Archeologický ústav ČSAV.

Geisler, M., and J. Kovárník. 1983. "Pravěké sídliště u Dobšic (okr. Znojmo)." In *Přehled výzkumů 1981*, 74–76. Brno. Archeologický ústav ČSAV.

Geislerová, K., I. Rakovský, and R. Tichý. 1989. "Zu einigen Aspekten des Mährischen Neolithikums." In *Bylany: International Seminar Liblice 6–10 April 1987. Collected Papers*, editedy by J. Rulf, 299–303. Prague: Archeological Institute of the Czechoslovak Academy of Sciences.

Gerling, C. 2014. "A Multi-Isotopic Approach to the Reconstruction of Prehistoric Mobility and Economic Patterns in the West Eurasian Steppes 3500 to 300 B.C." *eTopoi. Journal for Ancient Studies* 3:1–21.

Ghadimi, E., H. Eimar, B. Marelli, S. N. Nazhat, M. Asgharian, H. Vali, and F. Tamimi. 2013. "Trace Elements Can Influence the Physial Properties of Tooth Enamel." *Springer Plus* 2:499.

Giblin, J. I., K. J. Knudson, Z. Bereczki, G. Pálfi, and I. Pap. 2013. "Strontium Isotope Analysis and Human Mobility during the Neolithic and Copper Age: A Case Study from the Great Hungarian Plain." *Journal of Archaeological Science* 40:227–39.

Gilbert, B. M., and T. W. McKern. 1973. "A Method for Aging the Female Os Pubis." *American Journal of Physical Anthropology* 38:31–38.

Gimbutas, M. 1989. *The Language of the Goddess*. San Francisco: Harper and Row.

Gladykowska-Rzeczycka, J. J. 1998. "Periostitis: Cause, Form and Frequency in Paleopathology." *Mankind Quarterly* 38:217–36.

Gladykowska-Rzeczycka, J. J. 1999. "Tuberculosis in the Past and Present in Poland." In *Tuberculosis, Past and Present*, edited by G. Pálfi et al., 561–73. Budapest: Golden Book; Szeged: Tuberculosis Foundation.

Gladykowska-Rzeczycka, J. J., and T. A. Mazurek. 2009. "Rare Case of Forearm Hypoplasia from 18th-Century Gdansk, Poland." *International Journal of Osteoarchaeology* 19:726–34.

Goodman, A. H. 1993. "On the Interpretation of Health from Skeletal Remains." *Current Anthropology* 34:281–88.

Gray, H. 1977. *Anatomy Descriptive and Surgical*. New York: Bounty Books.

Green, M. J. 1998. *Keltské mýty*. Prague: NLN.

Greenfield, H. J. 2010. "The Secondary Products Revolution: The Past, the Present and the Future." *World Archaeology* 42:29–54.

Grupe, G., T. D. Price, P. Schröter, F. Söllner, C. M. Johnson, B. L. Beard. 1997. "Mobility of Bell Baker People Revealed by Sr Isotope Ratios of Tooth and Bone: A Study of Southern Bavarian Skeletal Remains." *Applied Geochemistry* 12:517–25.

Hackett, C. J. 1981. "Microscopical Focal Destruction (Tunnels) in Exhumed Human Bones." *Medicine, Science and the Law* 21:243–64.

Hájek, Z. 2014. "Hluboké Mašůvky, Znojmo-Novosady—významná sídliště kultury s moravskou malovanou keramikou na Moravě." Ph.D. diss. Brno.

Hájek, Z., and A. Humpolová. 2010. "Žárový hrob kultury s moravskou malovanou keramikou z Vedrovic, v poloze "Za Dvorem"." *Acta Musei Moraviae—Scientiae Sociales* 95:63–90.

Hájek, Z., A. Humpolová, and A. Čerevková. 2016. "Osídlení kultury s moravskou malovanou keramikou v Nové Vsi u Oslavan (okres Brno-venkov)." *Studia Archaeologica Brunensia* 21 (2): 5–34.

Hansen, J. P. H. 1984. "The Eskimo of Greenland, A. D. 1460." Paper presented at the American Asssociation of Physical Anthropologists, Philadelphia.

Hayden, B. 2014. *The Power of Feasts from Prehistory to the Present*. Cambridge: Cambridge University Press.

Heath, J. M. 2017. *Warfare in Neolithic Europe: An Archaeological and Anthropological Analysis*. Bransley, UK: Pen and Sword; Philadelphia: Casemate Publishers.

Hedges, R. et al. 2013. "The Supra-Regional Approach." In *The First Farmers of Central Europe: Diversity in LBK Lifeways*, ed. by P. Bickle and A. Whittle, 343–84. Oxford: Oxbow Books.

Helmi, C., and S. Pruzansky. 1980. "Craniofacial and Extracranial Malformations in the Klippel-Feil Syndrome." *Cleft Palate Journal* 17:65–88.

Hengen, O. P. 1971. "Cribra Orbitalia. Pathogenesis and Probable Aetiology." *Homo* 22 (2): 57–76.

Hershkovitz, I., H. D. Donoghue, and D. E. Minnikin. 2008. "Detection and Molecular Characterization of 9000-Year-Old *Mycobacterium tuberculosis* from a Neolithic Settlemnt in the Eastern Mediterranean." *PLOS One* 3 (10): e3426.

Hillson, S. 1977. *Dental Anthropology*. Cambridge: Cambridge University Press.

Hlas, J. 2012a. "Holasovice (okr. Opava)." *Přehled výzkumů* 53:129.

Hlas, J. 2012b. "Opava (k. ú. Kylešovice, okr. Opava)." *Přehled výzkumů* 53:136.

Hlubek, L. 2011. "Opava (k. ú. Kylešovice, okr. Opava)." *Přehled výzkumů* 52:170–71.

Hodder, I. 1990. *The Domestication of Europe: Structure and Contingency in Neolithic Societies*. Cambridge, MA: Basil Blackwell.

Hodges, D. C., and R. G. Wilkinson. 1990. "Effect of Tooth Size on the Ageing and Chronological Distribution of Enamel Hypoplastic Defects." *American Journal of Human Biology* 2:553–60.

Hoogewerff, J. A., C. Reimann, H. Ueckermann, et al. 2019. "Bioavailable ^{87}Sr/^{86}Sr in European Solis. A Baseline for Provenancing Studies." *Science of the Total Environment* 672:1033–44.

Hoppa, R. D., and J. W. Vaupel, eds. 2002. *Paleodemography. Age Distribution from Skeletal Samples*. Cambridge: Cambridge University Press.

Hoppe, V., and D. Polívka. 1968. *Tuberkulóza pohybového ústrojí*. Prague: Státní zdravotnické nakladatelství.

Horňanský, J., and J. Skutil. 1950. "Hromadný hrob kultury s keramikou malovanou ve Džbánicích u Moravského Krumlova." *Obzor praehistorický* 14:333–36.

Hu, Y. C. 2012. "Arsenic Trioxide Affects Bone Remodelling by Effects on Osteoblast Differentiation and Function." *Bone* 50:1406–15.

Huang, M. H. S., J. S. Gruss, S. K. Clarren, et al. 1996. "The Differential Diagnosis of Posterior Plagiocephaly: True Lambdoid Synostosis Versus Positional Molding." *Plastic and Reconstructive Surgery* 98:765–774.

Humpolová, A. 1992. "Žárové pohřby v kultuře s moravskou malovanou keramikou." *Pravěk Nová řada* 2:61–75.

Ingvarsson-Sundström, A. 2003. *Children Lost and Found: A Bioarchaeological Study of Middle Helladic Children in Asine with Comparison to Lerna*. Uppsala: ECSI.

Işcan, M. Y., S. Loth, and R. Wright. 1984. "Age Estimation from the Rib by Phase Analysis: White Males." *Journal of Forensic Sciences* 29:1094–104.

Işcan, M. Y., S. Loth, and R. Wright. 1985. "Age Estimation from the Rib by Phase Analysis: White Females." *Journal of Forensic Sciences* 30:853–63.

Jakab, J. 1997. "Analyse der menslichen Skelettreste aus der Kreisgrabenlage in Ružindol-Borová." In *Kreisgrabenanlage der Lengyel-kultur in Ružindol-Borová*, edited by V. Němejcová-Pavúková, 193–218. Bratislava: Facultas Philosophica Universitatis Comenianae Bratislavensis.

Janák, V. 1984. "Záchranný výzkum ve Velkých Hošticích (okr. Opava)." *Přehled výzkumů 1982*, 87–88. Brno. Archeologický ústav ČSAV.

Janák, V. 1985. "Třetí etapa záchranného výzkumu ve Velkých Hošticích (okr. Opava)." In *Přehled výzkumů 1983*, 109–10. Brno. Archeologický ústav ČSAV.

Janák, V. 1987. "Pokračování záchranného výzkumu ve Velkých Hošticích (okr. Opava)." *Přehled výzkumů 1984*, 22–23. Brno. Archeologický ústav ČSAV.

Janák, V. 1989. "Morava na rozhraní starého a středního eneolitu." Ph.D. diss. Opava.

Janák, V. 1990. "Východoevropské elementy v lengyelské antropomorfní plastice na Moravě a ve Slezsku." In *Pravěké a slovanské osídlení Moravy: Sborník J. Poulíkovi k 80. narozeninám*, editedy by M. Čižmář, V. Nekuda, and J. Unger, 26–37. Brno: Muzejní a vlastivědná společnost and Archeologický ústav ČSAV.

Janák, V. 1991. "Severovýchodní vlivy v Horním Slezsku v časném a starém eneolitu." *Časopis Slezského zemského muzea B* 40:97–109.

Janák, V. 1996. "Kdy "Pravěk Slezska"? (Ad marginem "Pravěkých dějin Moravy")." *Časopis Slezského muzea B* 43:193–210.

Janák, V. 1998. "Předběžné poznámky k neolitu a eneolitu Českého Slezska." In *Otázky neolitu a eneolitu našich krajín*, edited by I. Kuzma, 95–106. Nitra: Archeologický ústav SAV.

Janák, V. 2001. "Hroby hornoslezské lengyelské skupiny z Velkých Hoštic a komplex skupin se smíšenou keramickou náplní (Příspěvek k poznání postlineárního osídlení severní části střední Evropy)." *Pravěk—Supplementum* 8:325-51.

Janák, V. 2004. "Ke kontinuitě neolitického obyvatelstva na březích řeky Opavy." In *Otázky neolitu a eneolitu našich zemí*, edited by V. Janák and S. Stuchlík, 73-86. Opava: Ústav historie a muzeologie FPF Slezské univerzity v Opavě.

Jarošová, I., and M. Dočkalová. 2008a. "Dental Remains from the Neolithic Settlements in Moravia, Czech Republic." *Anthropologie* 46:77-101.

Jarošová, I., M. Dočkalová, and M. Fojtová. 2008b. "Vybrané dentální charakteristiky neolitického obyvatelstva ze sídlišť na Moravě—předběžná zpráva." *Ve službách archeologie* 1:222-41.

Jarošová, I., M. Dočkalová, M. Fojtová, G. Dreslerová, Z. Čižmář, and M. Hajnalová. 2008c. "Rekonstrukce stravy neolitického obyvatelstva z moravských sídlišť podle mikroabrazí zubů." In *Otázky neolitu a eneolitu našich krajín 2007*, edited by I. Cheben and I. Kuzma, 111-25. Nitra: Archeologický ústav SAV.

Jellinghaus, K., C. Hachmann, K. Höland, M. Bohnert, and U. Wittwer-Backhofen. 2018. "Collagen Degradation as a Possibility to Determine the Post-mortem Interval (PMI) of Animal Bones: A Validation Study Reffering to an Original Study of Boasks et al. (2014)." *International Journal of Legal Medicine* 132:753-63.

Jisl, L. 1968. "Slezsko a Ostravsko v pravěku a rané době dějinné." In *Ostravsko do roku 1848*, edited by A. Grobelný, 10-29. Ostrava: Profil.

Józsa, L. 2006. *Paleopathologia. Elődeink betegségei*. Budapest. Semmelweis Kiadó.

Juchelka, J. 2009. "Opava (k. ú. Kateřinky, Malé Hoštice, okr. Opava)." *Přehled výzkumů* 50:254.

Kala, M. 2005. *Hydrocefalus*. Prague: Galén.

Kalábková, P. 2008. "Lengyelské osídlení střední Moravy (příspěvek k vypovídacím možnostem dosavadních pramenů)." In *Moravskoslezská škola doktorských studií*, edited by Z. Měřínský and J. Klápště, 28-35. Brno: Masarykova univerzita.

Kalábková, P. 2009. "Lengyelské osídlení střední Moravy." Ph.D. diss. Brno.

Kalicz, N. 1985. *Kőkori falu Aszódon*. Petőfi Múzeum: Aszód.

Kalicz, N. 1998. *Figürliche Kunst und bemalte Keramik aus dem Neolithikum Westungarns*. Budapest: Archaeolingua.

Kalicz, N., and J. Makkay. 1972. "A neolitikus Sopot-Bicske kultúra." *Archaeologiai Értesítő* 99:3-14.

Kampa, M., and E. Castanas. 2008. "Human Health Effects of Air Pollution." *Environmental Pollution* 151:362-67.

Kanojia, R. K., M. Junaid, and R. C. Murthy. 1998. "Embryo and Fetotoxicity of Hexavalent Chromium. A Long-Term Study." *Toxicology Letters* 95:165-72.

Kazdová, E. 1994a. "Osídlení Brněnska ve středním a mladším neolitu. Kultury s vypíchanou a moravskou malovanou keramikou." *Pravěk. Nová řada* 2:43-57.

Kazdová, E. 1994b. "Sídliště s vypíchanou a moravskou malovanou keramikou v Kuřimi, okr. Brno-venkov." *Pravěk. Nová řada* 2:23-59.

Kazdová, E. 1998. "Vztahy mezi lidem s vypíchanou a moravskou malovanou keramikou." *Sborník prací filozofické fakulty brněnské univerzity M* 1:79-88.

Kazdová, E. 1999. "K úmrtí docenta PhDr. Pavla Koštuříka, CSc." *Sborník prací filozofické fakulty brněnské univerzity M* 4:9-11.

Kazdová, E. 2001a. "Importy lengyelské keramiky v prostředí kultury s vypíchanou keramikou." *Sborník prací filozofické fakulty brněnské univerzity M* 6:39-50.

Kazdová, E. 2001b. "New Observations on Problems in the Relationship between the Stroked Pottery and Lengyel Cultures." In *Zwischen Karpaten und Ägäis: Neolithikum und ältere Bronzezeit*, edited by B. Hänsel and E. Studeníková, 233-38. Rahden, Westfalen: Verlag Maria Leidorf.

Kazdová, E. 2001c. "Osídlení střední Moravy v postlineárním neolitu." *Pravěk Nová řada—Supplementum* 8:78-96.

Kazdová, E. 2002. "Antropomorfní nádoba z lengyelské kultury z Těšetic-Kyjovic, JZ Morava." In *Otázky neolitu a eneolitu našich krajín 2001*, edited by I. Cheben and I. Kuzma, 129-36. Nitra: Archeologický ústav SAV.

Kazdová, E. 2004. "Osídlení lidem s keramikou vypíchanou na Znojemsku." In *K poctě Vladimíru Podborskému. Přátelé a žáci k sedmdesátým narozeninám*, edited by E. Kazdová, Z. Měřínský, and K. Šabatová, 55-70. Brno: Masarykova univerzita.

Kazdová, E., and Z. Čižmář. 2004. "Ojedinělý import vypíchané keramiky v objektu starší fáze kultury s moravskou malovanou keramikou v Mašovicích na Znojemsku." In *Otázky neolitu a eneolitu našich zemí*, edited by V. Janák, and S. Stuchlík, 21-32. Opava: Ústav historie a muzeologie FPF Slezské univerzity v Opavě.

Kazdová, E., and V. Podborský, eds. 2007. *Studium sociálních a duchovních struktur pravěku*. Brno: Ústav archeologie a muzeologie FF MU.

Kazdová, E., and A. Přichystal. 1994. "Nová lokalita s moravskou malovanou keramikou v Brně-Kníničkách." *Pravěk. Nová řada* 4:59-64.

Kelman, B. J., and B. K. Walter. 1977. "Passage of Cadmium across the Perfused Guinea Pig Placenta." *Proceedings of the Soceity for Experimental Biology and Medicine* 156:68-71.

Kennedy, K. A. R., J. Plummer, and J. Chiment. 1986. "Identification of the Eminent Dead: Penpi a Scribe of Ancient Egypt." In *Forensic Osteology: The Recovery and Analysis of Unknow Skeletal Remains*, edited by K. Reichs, 290-307. Springfield, IL: Charles C Thomas.

Kiliç Safak, N., R. G. Taskin, and A. H. Yücel. 2020. "Morphologic and Morphometric Evaluation of the Wormian Bones." *International Journal of Morphology* 38:69-73.

Kippler, M., Y. Wagatsuma, A. Rahman, B. Nermell, L. A. Persson, R. Raqib, and M. Vahter. 2012. "Environmental Exposure to Arsenic and Cadmium during Pregnancy and Fetal Size: A Longitudinal Study in Rural Bangladesh." *Reproductive Toxicology* 34:504-11.

Klepáček, I., and Mazánek, J. 2001. *Klinická anatomie ve stomatologii*. Grada: Prague.

Köhler, K. 2012. "A késő neolitikus lengyeli kultúra népességének biológiai rekonstrukciója." Ph.D. diss. Eötvös Loránd University, Budapest.

Köhler, K., B. Mende, and A. Pósa. 2013. "The Emergence of Tuberculosis in Late Neolithic Transdanubia." *Hungarian Archaeology*. Online, Summer.

Köhler, K., G. Pálfi, E. Molnár, et al. 2014. "A Late Neolithic Case of Pott's Disease from Hungary." *International Journal of Osteoarchaeology* 24:697-703.

Komoróczy, B., S. Klanicová, S. Sázelová, and M. Vlach. 2010. "Pasohlávky (k. ú. Mušov, okr. Břeclav)." *Přehled výzkumů* 51:321-23.

Končelová, M., and P. Květina. 2015. "Neolithic Longhouse Seen as a Witness of Cultural Change in the Post-LBK." *Anthropologie* 53:431-46.

Kontopoulos, I., P. Nystrom, and L. White. 2016. "Experimental Taphonomy: Post Mortem Microstructural Modifications in *Sus scrofa domesticus* Bone." *Forensic Science International* 266:320-28.

Kósa, F., and G. Fazekas. 1978. *Forensic Fetal Osteology*. Budapest: Akademiai Kiadó.

Košturík, P. 1972. "Hrob kultury s moravskou malovanou keramikou v opevněné části neolitického sídliště v Těšeticích-Kyjovicích." *Sborník prací filozofické fakulty brněnské univerzity E* 17:55-59.

Košturík, P. 1973. *Die Lengyel Kultur in Mähren. Die jüngere mährische bemalte Keramik*. Prague: Academia.

Košturík, P. 1974. "Archeologický výzkum kultury s moravskou malovanou keramikou u Jaroměřic nad Rokytnou, okr. Třebíč." In *Přehled výzkumů 1973*, 18-20. Brno: Archeologický ústav ČSAV.

Košturík, P. 1975/76. "Stav výzkumu kultury s moravskou malovanou keramikou na Hradisku u Kramolína." *Sborník prací filozofické fakulty brněnské univerzity E* 20-21:101-13.

Košturík, P. 1977/78. "Neolitické sídliště v poloze "Kopaniny" u Nové Vsi, okr. Brno-venkov." *Sborník prací filozofické fakulty brněnské univerzity E* 22-23:77-91.

Košturík, P. 1980a. "Hrob kultury s moravskou malovanou keramikou z neolitického sídliště u Jaroměřic nad Rokytnou." *Sborník prací filozofické fakulty brněnské univerzity E* 2:65-73.

Košturík, P. 1980b. "Systematický archeologický výzkum neolitického sídliště v trati "Sutny" u Těšetic-Kyjovic v roce 1977 (okr. Znojmo)." In *Přehled výzkumů 1977*, 24. Brno: Archeologický ústav ČSAV.

Koštuřík, P. 1981. "Hradisko u Kramolína na konci neolitu a počátkem eneolitu." In *Současné úkoly československé archeologie. Valtice 17. 10.—20. 10. 1978*, 64-73. Prague: Archeologický ústav ČSAV.

Koštuřík, P. 1983a. "Poznámky k II. stupni kultury s moravskou malovanou keramikou na jihozápadní Moravě." *Sborník prací filozofické fakulty brněnské univerzity E* 28:127-160.

Koštuřík, P. 1983b. "Terénní výzkum v Sutnách u Těšetic-Kyjovic v roce 1981 (okr. Znojmo)." *Přehled výzkumů 1981*, 17-19. Brno: Archeologický ústav ČSAV.

Koštuřík, P. 1994. "Sto let od narození Viléma Grosse." *Pravěk. Nová řada* 4:391-92.

Koštuřík, P. et al. 1986. *Pravěk Třebíčska*. Brno: Muzejní a vlastivědná společnost; Třebíč: Západomoravské muzeum.

Koštuřík, P., and M. Dočkalová. 1992. "Hrob H 14 kultury s moravskou malovanou keramikou v Těšeticích-Kyjovicích, okr. Znojmo." *Sborník prací filozofické fakulty brněnské univerzity E* 37:25-42.

Kovárník, J. 1985. "Dosavadní výsledky leteckého archeologického průzkumu na jižní Moravě." In *Přehled výzkumů 1983*, 102-105. Brno: Archeologický ústav ČSAV.

Kovárník, J. 1995. "Dějiny archeologických výzkumů na jihozápadní Moravě." In *Sborník příspěvků proslovených na I. Obnoveném sjezdu Moravskoslezského archeologického klubu v Moravských Budějovicích 16.-17. srpna 1995*, edited by V. Podborský, 23-30. Brno: Masarykova univerzita.

Kovárník, J. 1996. "Přínos letecké archeologie k poznání pravěku a rané doby dějinné na Moravě (1983-1995)." *Archeologické rozhledy* 68:177-93, 273-74.

Kovárník, J. 1998. "Pravěké kruhové příkopy na Moravě. Letecká prospekce, geofyzikální měření, archeologický výzkum a interpretace." In *Ve službách archeologie. Sborník k 60. narozeninám RNDr. Vladimíra Haška, DrSc.*, edited by P. Kouřil, R. Nekuda, and J. Unger, 143-61. Brno: Archeologický ústav ČSAV.

Kovárník, J. 1999. "Běhařovice, okr. Znojmo." In V. Podborský et al., *Pravěká sociokultovní architektura na Moravě*, 25-40. Brno: Masarykova univerzita.

Kovárník, J. 2001a. "Dějiny archeologického bádání na Znojemsku." In *50 let archeologických výzkumů Masarykovy univerzity na Znojemsku*, edited by V. Podborský, 95-125. Brno: Masarykova univerzita.

Kovárník, J. 2001b. "Nové objevy pravěkých příkopů na Moravě." In *50 let archeologických výzkumů Masarykovy univerzity na Znojemsku*, edited by V. Podborský, 139-55. Brno: Masarykova univerzita.

Kovárník, J. 2004. "Nově zjištěná pravěká příkopová ohrazení na Moravě. Rondely, rondeloidy a jiné příkopy—stručné shrnutí problematiky." In *Ve službách archeologie*. Vol. 5, *Sborník k sedmdesátinám RNDr. Emanuela Opravila, CSc.*, edited by V. Hašek, R. Nekuda, and M. Ruttkay, 11-38. Brno: Muzejní a vlastivědná společnost.

Kovárník, J. 2008. "K dějinám výzkumu neolitu (a zvláště moravské malované keramiky)." In *Život a smrt v mladší době kamenné*, edited by Z. Čižmář, 4-11. Brno: Ústav archeologické památkové péče.

Král, J. 1956. "Hrob s moravskou malovanou keramikou v Brně-Králově poli." *Archeologické rozhledy* 8:9-13.

Kramberger, B. 2014. "Evaluation of Dimitrievič's Definition of the Sopot Culture in the Light of Radiocarbon Dates." *Opuscula Archaeologica* 37-38:359-70.

Kristiansen, K. 2014. "The Decline of the Neolithic and the Rise of Bronze Age Society." In *The Oxford Handbook of Neolithic Europe*, edited by C. Fowler, J. Harding, and D. Hofmann, 1-19. Oxford: Oxford University Press.

Kristiansen, K., M. E. Allentoft, K. M. Frei, et al. 2017. "Re-theorising Mobility and the Formation of Culture and Language among the Corded Ware Culture in Europe." *Antiquity* 91:334-347.

Kuča, M. 2008. "Exploitation of Raw Materials Suitable for Chipped Stone Industry Manufacture in the Moravian Painted Ware Culture in the Brno Region." *Přehled výzkumů* 49:93-107.

Kuča, M. 2009. "Neolitické osídlení jižní části Boskovické brázdy. Současný stav poznání podle průzkumů v letech 1999-2006." *Sborník prací filozofické fakulty brněnské univerzity M* 12-13: 23-48.

Kuča, M., and J. Bartík. 2013. "Příspěvek k problematice křemičitých hmot a jejich využívání v neolitu na jižní a jihozápadní Moravě." *Přehled výzkumů* 54:41–50.

Kuča, M., E. Kazdová, Š. Hladilová, M. Fišáková Nývltová, and L. Prokeš. 2010. *Těšetice-Kyjovice 7. Osídlení kultury s moravskou malovanou keramikou v prostoru mezi příkopem a vnější palisádou rondelu*. Brno: Masarykova univerzita.

Kuča, M., Kazdová, E., and A. Přichystal. 2003. "Sídliště kultury s moravskou malovanou keramikou staršího stupně v Brně-Žebětíně. Poznámky k fázi Ib kultury s MMK v brněnské kotlině." *Pravěk. Nová řada* 13:37–89.

Kuča, M., J. J. Kovář, M. Fišáková Nývltová, P. Škrdla, L. Prokeš, M. Vaškových, and Z. Schenk 2012. "Chronologie neolitu na Moravě." *Přehled výzkumů* 53:51–64.

Květina, P. 2004. "Mocní muži a sociální identita jednotlivců—prostorová analýza pohřebiště LnK ve Vedrovicích." *Archeologické rozhledy* 56:383–92.

Květina, P. 2015. *Minulost, kterou nikdo nezapsal*. Prague: Pavel Mervart.

Lai, P. and N. C. Lowell. 1992. "Skeletal Markers of Occupational Stress in the Fur Trade: A Case Study from a Hudson's Bay Company Fur Trade Post." *International of Osteoarchaeology* 2:221–34.

Langr, J., and J. Hlas. 2013. "Opava (k. ú. Kylešovice, okr. Opava)." *Přehled výzkumů* 54:150–51.

Langsjoen, O. 1998. "Diseases of the Dentition." In *The Cambridge Encyclopedia of Human Paleopathology*, edited by A. C. Aufderheide and C. Rodríguez-Martín, 393–412. Cambridge: Cambridge University Press.

Larsen, C. S. 1985. "Dental Modification and Tool-Use in the Western Great Basin." *American Journal of Physical Anthropology* 67:489–502.

Larsen, C. S. 1995. "Changes in Human Populations with Agriculture." *Annual Review of Anthropology* 24:185–213.

Lazaridis, J., D. Nadel, G. Rollefson, et al. 2016. "Genomic Insight into the Origin of Farming in the Ancient Near East." *Nature* 536:419–24.

Lee-Thorp, J. A. 2008. "On Isotopes and Old Bones." *Archaeometry* 50:925–50.

Lenneis, E., C. Neugebauer-Maresch, and E. Ruttkay. 1995. *Jungsteinzeit im Osten Österreichs*. St. Pöllten: Niederösterreichisches Pressehaus.

Lewis, M. 2018. *Paleopathology of Children. Identification of Pathological Conditions in the Human Skeletal Remains of Non-adults*. London: Academic Press.

Lichardus, J., and J. Vladár. 2003. "Gliederung der Lengyel-Kultur in der Slowakei. Ein Rückblick nach vierzig Jahren." *Slovenská archeológia* 51:195–216.

Lillie, M. 2008. "Vedrovice: Demography and Paleopathology in an Early Farming Population." *Anthropologie* 46:135–52.

Link, T. 2014. "Welche Krise? Das Ende der Linienbandkeramik aus östlicher Perspektive." In *No future? Brüche und Endekultureller Erscheinungen. Fallbeispiele aus dem 6.-2. Jahrtausend v. Chr.*, edited by T. Link and D. Schimmelpfennig, 95–111. Kerpen-Loogh: Welt und Erde Verlag.

Link, T. 2015. "New Ideas in Old Villages. Interpreting the Genesis of the Stroked Pottery Culture." *Anthropologie* 53:351–62.

Lipson, M., A. Szécsényj-Nagy, S. Mallick, et al. 2017. "Parallel Paleogenomic Transects Reveal Complex Genetic History of Early European Farmers." *Nature* 551:368–72.

Longin, R. 1971. "New Method of Collagen Extraction for Radiocarbon Dating." *Nature* 230:241–42.

Lovejoy, C. O. 1985. "Dental Wear in the Libben Population: Its Pattern and Role in the Determination of Adult Skeletal Age at Death." *American Journal of Physical Anthropology* 68:47–56.

Ložek, V. 1980. "Holocén." *Sloveská archeológia* 28:107–18.

Lukacs, J. R. 1992. "Dental Paleopathology and Agricultural Intensification in South Asia: New Evidence from Bronze Age Harappa." *American Journal of Physical Anthropology* 87:133–150.

Lüning, J. 1979. "Über der Stand der neolitischen Stilfrage in Südwestdeutschland." *Jahrbuch des römisch-germanischen Zentralmuseums* 26:75–113.

Lüning, J. 1988. "Frühe Bauern im 6. und 5. Jahrtausend v Chr." *Jahrbuch des römisch-germanischen Zentralmuseums* 35:27–93.

Mabilleau, G., R. Filmon, P. K. Petrov, M. F. Baslé, A. Sabokbar, and D. Choppard. 2010. "Cobalt, Chromium and Nickel Affect Hydroxiapatite Crystal Growth in vitro." *Acta Biomaterialia* 6:1555–60.

Macintosh, A. A., R. Pinhasi, and J. T. Stock. 2016. "Early Life Conditions and Physiological Stress following the Transition to Farming in Central/Southeast Europe: Skeletal Growth Impairment and 6000 Years of Gradual Recovery." *PLOS ONE* 11 (2): e0148468.

Maienthal, E. J., and J. K. Taylor. 1968. "Polarographic Methods in Determination of Trace Inorganics in Water." In *Trace Inorganics in Water*, edited by R. A. Baker, 172–82. Washington, DC: American Chemical Society.

Makkay, J. 2000. *An Early War. The Late Neolithic Mass Grave from Esztergályhorváti*. Budapest: J. Makkay.

Makkay, J. 2001. *Die Grabenanlagen im indogermanischen Raum*. Budapest: J. Makkay.

Malík, P. 2013. "Velké Hoštice (okr. Opava)." *Přehled výzkumů* 54:162.

Malluche, H. H., and M. C. Faugere. 1986. *Atlas of Mineralized Bone Histology*. New York: Karger.

Malville, N. J. 1997. "Enamel Hypoplasia in Ancestral Puebloan Populations from Southwestern Colorado I: Permanent Dentition." *American Journal of Physical Anthropology* 102:351–67.

Manchester, K. 1991. "Tuberculosis and Leprosy: Evidence for Interaction of Disease." In *Human Paleopathology. Current Syntheses and Future Options*, edited by D. J. Ortner, and A. C. Aufderheide, 23–35. Washington, DC: Smithsonian Institution Press.

Marie, P. J. 2006. "Strontium Ranelate: A Physiological Approach for Optimizing Bone Formation and Resorption." *Bone* 38:10–14.

Martin, A. 2000. *Apports Nutritionneles Conseillés Pour La Population Francaise*. 3rd ed. Paris: Tec & Doc Editions.

Masson, M., Z. Bereczky, E. Molnár, et al. 2015a. "7000 Year-Old Tuberculosis Cases from Hungary—Osteological and Biomolecular Evidence." *Tuberculosis* 95:S13–S17.

Masson, M., Z. Bereczky, E. Monár, et al. 2015b. "Osteological and Biomolecular Evidence of a 7000-Year Old Case of Hypertrophic Pulmonary Osteopathy Secondary to Tuberculosis from Neolithic Hungary." *PLOS ONE* 8 (10): e78252.

Mateiciucová, I. 2001. "Surovina kamenné štípané industrie v moravském neolitu." In *50 let archeologických výzkumů MU na Znojemsku*, edited by V. Podborský, 213–24. Brno: Masarykova univerzita.

Mateiciucová, I., and G. Trnka. 2004. "Die Silexartefakte aus der Siedlung mit Kreisgrabenanlage von Kamegg, Niederösterreich." In *K poctě Vladimíru Podborskému*, edited by E. Kazdová, K. Šabatová, and Z. Měřínský, 89–99. Brno: FF MU.

Matoušek, V., and M. Dufková. 1998. *Jeskyně a lidé*. Prague: NLN.

Mausch, A., and K.-H. Ziessow. 1985. "Reconstructing Linear Culture Houses. Theoretical and Practical Contributions." *Helinium* 25:58–93.

Mavropoulos, E., A. M. Rossi, A. M. Costa, C. A. Perez, J. C. Moreira, and M. Salcanha. 2002. "Studies on the Mechanism of Lead Immobilization by Hydroxyapatite." *Environmental Science and Technology* 36:1625–29.

McKern, T. W., and T. D. Stewart. 1957. *Skeletal Age Changes in Young American Males: Analysed from the Standpoint of Age Identification*. Natick (MA): Quartermaster Research & Development Center, US Army.

Meiklejohn, C., C. Schentag, A. Venema, and P. Key. 1984. "Socioeconomic Change and Patterns of Pathology and Variation in the Mesolithic and Neolithic of Western Europe: Some Sugestion." In *Paleopathology at the Origins of Agriculture*, edited by M. N. Cohen and G. J. Armelagos, 75–100. Orlando: Academic Press.

Meindl, R. S., and C. O. Lovejoy. 1985. "Ectocranial Suture Closure: A Revised Method for the Determination of Skeletal Age at Death Based on the Lateral-Anterior Sutures." *American Journal of Physical Anthropology* 68:57–66.

Meindl, R. S., C. O. Lovejoy, R. P. Mensforth, and R. A. Walker. 1985. "A Revised Method of Age Determination Using the Os Pubis, with a Review and Tests of Accuracy of Other Current Methods of Pubic Symphyseal Aging." *American Journal of Physical Anthropology* 68:29–45.

Meloun, M., J. Militký, M. Hill, and R. G. Brereton. 2002. "Crucial Problems in Regression Modelling and Their Solutions." *Analyst* 127:433–50.

Meloun, M., J. Militký, M. Hill, and R. G. Brereton. 2004. "New Methodology of Influential Point Detection in Regression Model Building for the Prediction of Metabolic Clearance Rate of Glucose." *Clinical Chemistry and Laboratory Medicine* 42:311–22.

Meloun, M., J. Militký, J. Vrbíková, S. Stanická, and J. Škrha. 2000. "Transformation in the PC-Aided Biochemical Data Analysis." *Clinical Chemistry and Laboratory Medicine* 38:553–59.

Merrett, D. C. 2004. "Bioarchaeology in Early Neolithic Iran: Assessment of Health Status and Subsistence Strategy." Ph.D. diss. Department of Anthropology, University of Manitoba, Winnipeg.

Meyer, C., C. Knipper, N. Nicklish, et al. 2015. "The Massacre Mass Grave of Schöneck-Kilianstädten Reveals New Insights into Collective Violence in Early Neolithic Central Europe." *Proceedings of the National Academy of Sciences U.S.A.* 112:11217–22.

Meyer, C., C. Lohr, D. Gronenborn, and K. W. Alt. 2018. "Early Neolithic Executions Indicated by Clustered Cranial Trauma in the Mass Grave of Halberstadt." *Nature Communications* 9:2472.

Miles, A. E. W. 1963. "The Dentition in the Assessment of Individual Age in Skeletal Material." *Human Biology* 5:191–209.

Miller, N. F., R. N. Spengler, and M. Frachetti. 2016. "Millet Cultivation across Eurasia: Origins, Spread, and the Influence of Seasonal Climate." *Holocene* 26:1566–75.

Mills, B. J. 1994. "Gender and the Reorganization of Historic Zuni Craft Production: Implications for Prehistoric Interpretation." Paper presented at the Fourth Biennial Southwest Symposium 7–8 January 1994. Tempe.

Milner, G. R., and J. L. Boldsen. 2012. "Transition Analysis: A Validation Study With Known-Age Modern American Skeletons." *American Journal of Physical Anthropology* 148:98–110.

Möller-Christensen, V., and A. T. Sandison. 1963. "Usura Orbitae (Cribra Orbitalia) in the Collection of Crania in the Anatomy Department of the Universitzy of Glasgow." *Pathologia et Microbiologia* 26:175–83.

Morse, D. 1967. "Tuberculosis." In *Diseases in Antiquity: A Survey of the Diseases, Injuries and Surgery of Early Populations*, edited by D. R. Brothwell and A. T. Sandison, 249–71. Springfield, IL: Charles C Thomas.

Motuzaite-Matuzeviciute, G., R. Staff, H. Hunt, X. Liu, and M. Jones. 2013. "The Early Chronology of Broomcorn Millet (Panicum miliaceum) in Europe." *Antiquity* 87:1073–85.

Mühlemann, B., T. C. Jones, P. de Barros Damgaard, et al. 2018b. "Ancient Hepatitis B Viruses from the Bronze Age to the Medieval Period." *Nature* 557:418–23.

Mühlemann, B., A. Margaryan, P. de Barros Damgaard, et al. 2018a. "Ancient Human Parvovirus B19 in Eurasia Reveals Its Long-Term Association with Humans." *Proceedings of the National Academy of Sciences U.S.A.* 115:7557–62.

Müller, R. C. Roberts, and T. Brown. 2014. "Biomolecular Identification of Ancient *Mycobacterium tuberculosis* Complex DNA in Human Remains from Britain and Continental Europe." *American Journal of Physical Anthropology* 153:178–89.

Mulliken, J. B., D. L. Vander Woude, M. Hansen, R. A. LaBrie, and R. M. Scott. 1999. "Analysis of Posterior Plagiocephaly: Deformational vs Synostotic." *Plastic and Reconstructive Surgery* 103:371–80.

Nansen, F. 1891. *Eskimoliv*. Kristiana: H. Aschenhoug. English translation *Eskimo Life* (1893).

Nejedlá, A. 2012. "Terénní prospekce lokalit s moravskou malovanou keramikou na Znojemsku." In *Otázky neolitu a eneolitu 2011. Sborník referátů z 30. pracovního setkání badatelů pro výzkum neolitu a eneolitu Čech, Moravy a Slovenska, Mikulov 19.–22. 9. 2011*, edited by J. Peška and F. Trampota, 107–116. Mikulov: Regionální muzeum v Mikulově; Olomouc: Archeologické centrum Olomouc.

Němec, I., V. Smrčka, M. Mihaljevič, J. Mazánek, and J. Pokorný. 2018. "Effect of Inferior Alveolar Nerve Transection on the Inorganic Component of Bone of Rat Mandible." *Folia Biologica* 64:84–96.

Němejcová-Pavúková, V. 1981. "Výsledky archeologického výskumu ve Svodíně." In *AVANS 1980*, 186-90. Nitra: Archeologický ústav SAV.

Němejcová-Pavúková, V. 1986. "Vorbericht über die Ergebnisse der systematischen Grabung in Svodín in den Jahren 1971-1983." *Slovenská archeológia* 34:133-76.

Němejcová-Pavúková, V. 1997. *Kreisgrabenanlage der Lengyel-kultur in Ružindol-Borová*. Bratislava: Facultas Philosophica Universitatis Comenianae Bratislavensis.

Nemeskéri, J., L. Harsányi, and G. Acsádi. 1960. "Methoden zur Diagnose des Lebensalters von Skelettfunden." *Anthropologischer Anzeiger* 24:70-95.

Neubauer, W., and. G. Trnka. 2005. "Totenbrauchtum." In *Zeitreise Heldenberg Geheimnisvolle Kreisgräben*, edited by F. Daim and W. Neubauer, 223-24. Horn: Verlag Berger.

Neubauer, Z. 2002. *Golem a další příběhy o kabale, symbolech a podivuhodných setkáních*. Prague: Malvern.

Neubauer, Z., and J. Hlaváček. 2002. *Slabikář hermetické symboliky & čítanka tarotu*. Prague: Malvern.

Neugebauer, C., and J. W. Neugebauer. 1977. "Befestigungsanlagen der Lengyel-Kultur am Schanzboden zu Falkenstein in Niederösterreich." *Fundberichte aus Österreich* 15:123-31.

Neugebauer-Maresch, C. 1983-1984. "Chronologie der Befestigungs- und Kutt- anlagen des Mittelneolithikums in NÖ anhand der Grabungen von Falkenstein-"Schanzboden" und Friebritz." *Mitteilungen der Anthropologischen Gesellschaft in Wien* 33-34:189-207.

Neugebauer-Maresch, C. 2005. "Tod im Kreisgraben." In *Zeitreise Heldenberg Geheimnisvolle Kreisgräben*, edited by F. Daim and W. Neubauer, 225-27. Horn: Verlag Berger.

Nielsen, F. H. 1995. "Individual Functional Roles of Metal Iones in vivo: Beneficial Metal Ions Nickel. In *Handbook of Metal Ligand Interaction in Biological Fluids Bioinorganic Medicine*, edited G. Berthon, 1:257-60. New York: Marcel Dekker.

Noddack, I. 1936. "Über die Allgegenwart der chemischen Elemente." *Angewandte Chemie* 49:835-41.

Noël, L., T. Cuérin, and M. Kolf-Clauw. 2004. "SuB.C.hronic Dietary Exposure of Rats to Cadmium Alters the Metabolism of Metals Essential to Bone Health." *Food and Chemical Toxicology* 42:1203-10.

Novotný, V. 1986. "Sex Determination of the Pelvis Bone: A Systems Approach." *Anthropologie* 24:197-206.

Nuorala, E., A. Götherström, T. Ahlström, H. D. Donaghue, M. Spigelman, and K. Lidén. 2004. "MTB complex DNA in a Scandinavian Neolithic Passage Grave." In *Molecular Palaeopathology. Ancient DNA Analyses of the Bacterial Diseases Tuberculosis and Leprosy*. Stockholm: Archaeological Research Laboratory.

Oliva, M. 2004. "Flint Mining, Rondels, Hillforts... Symbolic Works or too much Free Time?" *Archeologické rozhledy* 56:499-531.

Oliva, M. 2007. "Practical, Social, and Ritual Dimensions of the Prehistoric Landscape of Krumlovský Les." In *Studium der sozialen und geistlichen Strukturen der Urzeit*, edited by E. Kazdová and V. Podborský, 117-35. Brno: Ústav archeologie a muzeologie Filozofické fakulty Masarykovy univerzity.

Ondráček, J., and V. Podborský. 1954. "Výzkum na Cezavách u Blučiny v r. 1953." *Archeologické rozhledy* 6:630-33.

Ondreicka, P., J. Kortus, and E. Ginter. 1971. "Aluminium, Its Absorption, Distribution, and Effects on Phosphorus Metabolism." In *Intestinal Absorption of Metal Ions, Trace Elements and Radionuclides*, edited by S. C. Skoryna and D. Waldon-Edwards, 293-305. Oxford: Pergamon Press.

Ondroušková, S. 2011. "Pravěk Moravského krasu (neolit—doba stěhování národů)." M. A. thesis. Masaryk University, Brno.

Orschiedt, J., and M. N. Haidle. 2006. "The LBK Enclosure at Herxheim: Theatre of War or Ritual Centre? References from Osteoarchaeological Investigations." *Journal of Conflict Archaeology* 2:153-67.

Ortner, D. J. 1979. "Disease and Mortality in the Early Bronze Bab edh-Dhra, Jordan." *American Journal of Physical Anthropology* 51:589-97.

Ortner, D. J. 1999. "Paleopathology: Implications for History and Evolution of Tuberculosis." In *Tuberculosis. Past and Present*, edited by G. Palfi et al., 253-61. Budapest: Golden Book and Tuberculosis Foundation.

Ortner, D. J. 2003. *Identication of Pathological Conditions in Human Skeletal Remains*. Academic Press: Amsterdam.

Ortner, D. J. 2011. "What Skeletons Tell Us. The Story of Human Paleopathology." *Virchows Archiv* 459:247-254.

Ortner, D. J., and W. G. Putschar. 1981. *Identification of Pathological Conditions in Human Skeletal Remains*. Washington, DC: Smithsonian Institution Press.

Ortner, D. J., and W. G. Putschar. 1985. *Identification of Pathological Conditions in Human Skeletal Remains*. Reprint. Washington, DC: Smithsonian Institution Press.

Osztás, A., E. Bánffy, I. Zalai-Gaál, and K. Oross. 2016a. "Alsónyék-Bátaszék: Introduction to a Major Neolithic Settlement Complex in South-East Transdanubia, Hungary." *Bericht Der Römisch-Germanischen Kommission* 94:7-22.

Osztás, A., I. Zalai-Gaál, E. Bánffy, et al. 2016b. "Coalescent Community at Alsónyék: The Timings and Duration of Lengyel Burials and Settlement." *Bericht Der Römisch-Germanischen Kommission* 94:179-282.

Ovesen, J., B. Møller-Madsen, J. S. Thomsen, G. Danscher, and L. Mosekilde. 2001. "The Positive Effects of Zinc on Skeletal Strength in Growing Rats." *Bone* 29:565-570.

Palátová, H. 1999. "Bibliografie prací docenta PhDr. Pavla Košturíka, CSc." *Sborník prací filozofické fakulty brněnské univerzity M* 4:13-20.

Palliardi, J. 1888. "Předhistorické památky města Znojma." *Časopis Vlasteneckého musejního spolku v Olomouci* 5:53-58, 115-121, 150-157.

Palliardi, J. 1894. "Předhistorická sídla na Znojemsku." *Časopis Vlasteneckého musejního spolku v Olomouci* 11:91-95, tab. I (Neolithická osada u Velkých Mašovic); 128-138, tab. II-IV (Neolithická osada na Novosadech ve Znojmě).

Palliardi, J. 1897. "Die neolithischen Ansiedelungen mit bemalter Keramik in Mähren und in Niederösterreich." *Mitteilungen d. Praehistorischen Commission d. Kaiserlichen Akademie d. Wissenschaften in Wien* 1:237-264.

Palliardi, J. 1911. "Sídliště z mladší doby kamenné u Boskovštýna." *Pravěk* 7:40-48, 125-140.

Parker-Pearson, M. 2003. *The Archaeology of the Death and Burial*. Stroud, UK: Sutton.

Patterson, K. D. 1993. "Meningitis." In *The Cambridge World History of Human Disease*, edited by K. Kiple, 875-880. Cambridge. Cambridge University Press.

Pavelčík, J. 1974. "K problematice neolitu a eneolitu Českého Slezska." In *Archeologický sborník*, 22-42. Ostrava: Ostravské muzeum.

Pavelčík, J. 1994. "Osady na Kostelním Kopcu w Opavě-Jaktaři i ich miejsce w badaniach nad problematyką neolitu i eneolitu Górnego Śląska." *Przegląd Archeologiczny* 42:5-34.

Pavlů, I. 1997. *Pottery Origins: Initial Forms, Cultural Behavior and Decorative Styles*. Prague: Karolinum.

Pavlů, I. 2000. *Life on a Neolithic Site Bylany: Situational Analysis of Artefacts*. Prague: Institute of Archaeology.

Pavlů, I., and M. Zápotocká. 2007. *Archeologie pravěkých Čech. Neolit*. Prague: Archeologický ústav.

Pavúk, J. 1981. *Umenie a život doby kamennej*. Bratislava: Tatran.

Pavúk, J. 1991. "Lengyel-culture fortified settlements in Slovakia." *Antiquity* 65:348-357.

Pavúk, J. 1994. *Štúrovo. Ein Siedlungsplatz der Kultur mit Linearkeramik und der Želiezovce-Gruppe*. Nitra: Archeologický ústav SAV.

Pavúk, J. 2004. "Kommentar zu einem Rückblick nach vierzig Jahren auf die Gliederung der Lengyel-Kultur." *Slovenská archeológia* 52:139-160.

Pavúk, J., and J. Bátora. 1995. *Siedlung und Gräber der Ludanice-Gruppe in Jelšovce*. Nitra: Archaeologisches Institut der Slowakischen Akademie der Wissenschaften.

Perizonius, W. R. K., and T. J. Pot. 1981. "Diachronic Dental Research on Human Skeletal Remains Excavated in the Netherlands I." *Berichten van de Rijksdienst voor het Oudheidkundig Bodemaderzoek* 31:369-413.

Podborský, V. 1969. "Neolitické a halštatské sídliště u Těšetic-Kyjovic na Moravě." *Památky archeologické* 60:572-592.

Podborský, V. 1970. "Současný stav výzkumu kultury s moravskou malovanou keramikou." *Slovenská archeológia* 18:235-310.

Podborský, V. 1981. "Objekt s Vypíchanou Keramikou v Těšeticích III., Okr. Znojmo a Postavení Vypíchané Keramiky ve Starolengyelském Horizontu Středodunajského Neolitu." *Sborník Prací Filozofické Fakulty Brněnské Univerzity. E, Řada Archeologicko-Klasická* 26:9-28.

Podborský, V. 1984a. "Domy lidu s moravskou malovanou keramikou." *Sborník prací filozofické fakulty brněnské univerzity E* 29:27-66.

Podborský, V. 1984b. "Zpráva o počáteční fázi některých experimentů na neolitické lokalitě v Těšeticích-Kyjovicích." *Sborník prací filozofické fakulty brněnské univerzity E* 29:225-226.

Podborský, V. 1985. *Těšetice-Kyjovice 2. Figurální plastika lidu s moravskou malovanou keramikou.* Brno: Univerzita J. E. Purkyně.

Podborský, V. 1988. *Těšetice-Kyjovice 4. Rondel osady lidu s moravskou malovanou keramikou.* Brno: Univerzita J. E. Purkyně.

Podborský, V. 1995. "Vzpomínka na Jaroslava Palliardiho (20. 2. 1861-12. 3. 1922). In *Sborník příspěvků proslovených na I. Obnoveném sjezdu Moravskoslezského archeologického klubu v Moravských Budějovicích 16.-17. srpna 1995*, edited by V. Podborský, 23-30. Brno: Masarykova univerzita.

Podborský, V. 2001. "Modely funkční interpretace pravěkých rondelů." In *50 let archeologických výzkumů Masarykovy univerzity na Znojemsku*, edited by V. Podborský, 209-212. Brno: Masarykova univerzita.

Podborský, V. 2005. *František Vildomec 1878-1975, Vědomil Vildomec 1921-1998.* Brno: Ústav archeologické památkové péče—Ústav archeologie a muzeologie FF MU.

Podborský, V., ed. 1993. *Pravěké dějiny Moravy.* Brno: Muzejní a vlastivědná společnost.

Podborský, V. 2006. *Náboženství pravěkých Evropanů.* Brno: Masarykova univerzita.

Podborský, V. et al. 1999. *Pravěká sociokultovní architektura na Moravě.* Brno: Masarykova univerzita.

Podborský, V. et al. 2002. *Dvě pohřebiště s lineární keramikou ve Vedrovicích na Moravě.* Brno: Masarykova univerzita.

Podborský, V., E. Kazdová, P. Koštuřík, and Z. Weber. 1977. *Numerický kód moravské malované keramiky.* Brno: Univerzita J. E. Purkyně.

Podborský, V., E. Kazdová, J. Kovárník, et al. 2005. *Pravěk mikroregionu potoka Těšetičky/Únanovky. K problematice pravěkých sociálních struktur.* Brno: Masarykova univerzita.

Podborský, V., and J. Kovárník. 2012. *Jaroslav Palliardi 20. 2. 1861-12. 3. 1922.* Brno: Masarykova univerzita.

Podborský, V., and V. Vildomec. 1972. *Pravěk Znojemska.* Brno: Muzejní spolek.

Pósa, A., F. Maixner, A. R. Zink, et al. 2012. "Ancient Human Tooth Samples Used for TB Paleomicrobial Research." *Acta Biologica Szegediensis* 56:125-131.

Pósa, A., B. G. Mende, K. Köhler, et al. 2013. "Lathe Neolithic Human Samples Used for TB Paleomicrobial Research." German Society of Anthropotlogy (GfA) September 2nd-6th 2013, EURAC Research—Bolzano/Bozen, Itatly. Program and abstracts, 35.

Povýšil, C. 1990. "Techniques and Principles of Histological Diagnosis in Osteopathies: Review and Report of Personal Experience." *Československá patologie* 26:179-189.

Povýšil, C. et al. 2017. *Patomorfologie chorob kostí a kloubů. Pathomorphology of Bone and Joint Diseases.* Prague: Galén.

Povýšil, C., I. Sotorník, and A. Válek. 1990. "Aluminium osteopathy." *Československá patologie* 26:65-71.

Price, T. D. 2000. "Lessons in the Transition to Agriculture." In *Europe's First Farmers*, edited by T. D. Price, 301-318. Cambridge: Cambridge University Press.

Price, T. D., J. H. Burton, and R. A. Bentley. 2002. "The Characterization of Biologically Available Strontium Isotope Ratios for the Study of Prehistoric Migration." *Archaeometry* 44:117-135.

Price, T. D., and G. M. Feinman. 2001. *Images of the Past.* 3rd ed. Mountain View, CA: Mayfield.

Price, T. D., J. Wahl, and R. A. Bentley. 2006. "Isotopic Evidence for Mobility and Group Organisation among Neolithic Farmers at Talheim, Germany, 5000 B.C." *European Journal of Archaeology* 9:259-284.

Prokop, M., C. Povýšil, and P. Novák. 1991. "A Program for Automated Histomorphometry of Bone Tissue." *Československá patologie* 27:41-47.

Raczky, P. 1974. "A lengyeli kultúra legkésőbbi szakaszának leletei a Dunántúlon." *Archaeologiai Értesítő* 101:185-210.

Raczky, P. 2002. "Evidence of Contacts between the Lengyel and Tisza-Herpály Cultures at the Late Neolithic Site of Polgár-Csőszhalom. Relationship between Central-European and Balkan Ritual Practice and Sacral Thought in the Upper Tisza Region." *Budapest Régiségei* 36:79-92.

Rajchl, R. 2002. "Archeoastronomická analýza orientace skeletů na pohřebišti v "Široké u lesa"." In *Dvě pohřebiště lidu s lineární keramikou ve Vedrovicích*, edited by V. Podborský, 275-291. Brno: Ústav archeologie a muzeologie FF MU.

Rakovský, I. 1985. "Morava na prahu eneolitu." Ph.D. diss. Brno.

Rakovský, I., and J. Čižmářová. 1988. "Sídliště s moravskou malovanou keramikou v Brně-Bystrci." *Archeologické rozhledy* 40:481-508.

Rascovan, N., K. G. Sjögren, K. Kristiansen, et al. 2019. "Emergence and Spread of Basal Lineages of Yersinia Pestis during the Neolithic Decline." *Cell* 176:295-305.

Regenye, J. 2002. "Chronological Situation of the Sopot Culture in Hungary." *A Veszprém Megyei Múzeumok Közleményei* 22:31-42.

Regöly-Mérei, G. 1960. "Palaeopathological vizsgálatok a Janus Pannonius Múzeum aeneolithkorból szarmazó emberi csontlelet anyagán." In *A Janus Pannonius Múzeum Évkönyve*, 75-83. Pécs: A Janus Pannonius Múzeum.

Regöly-Mérei, G. 1962. *Az ősemberi és későbbi emberi maradványok rendszeres kórbonctana.* Budapest: Medicina Kiadó.

Renfrew, C. 2018. "Introduction: Play as the Precursor of Ritual in Early Human Societies." In *Ritual, Play and Belief in Evolution and Early Human Societies*, edited by C. Renfrew, I. Morley, and M. Boyd 9-20. Cambridge: Cambridge University Press.

Resnick, D., and G. Niwayama. 1976. "Radiographic and Pathologic Features of Spinal Involvement in Diffuse Idiopathic Skeletal Hyperostosis (DISH)." *Radiology* 119:559-568.

Richards M. P, T. D. Price, and E. Koch. 2003. "Mesolithic and Neolithic Subsistence in Denmark: New Stable Isotope Data." *Current Anthropology* 44:288-295.

Řídký, J. 2011. *Rondely a struktura sídelních areálů v mladoneolitickém období.* Prague: FF UK.

Řídký, J., P. Květina, P. Limburský, M. Končelová, P. Burgert, R. Šumberová. 2018. *Big Men or Chiefs? Rondel Builders of Neolithic Europe.* Oxford: Oxbow Books.

Řídký, J., P. Květina, H. Stäuble, and I. Pavlů. 2015. "What Is Changing and When—Post Linear Pottery Culture Life in Central Europe." *Anthropologie* 53:333-39.

Rivera, F., and M. B. Mirazon Lahr. 2017. "New Evidence Suggesting a dissociated etiology for cribra orbitalia and porotic hyperostosis." *American Journal of Physical Anthropology* 164:76-96.

Roberts, C., and K. Manchester. 1995. *The Archaeology of Disease.* 2nd ed. Ithaca, NY: Cornell University Press.

Roberts, C., and K. Manchester. 2005. *The Archaeology of Disease.* 3rd ed. Ithaca, NY: Cornell University Press.

Roberts, C., and K. Manchester. 2007. *The Archaeology of Disease.* 3rd ed. Reprint. Ithaca, NY: Cornell University Press.

Rogers, J., and T. Waldron. 1987. "Consequences of Osteoarthritis in Early Neolithic Skeletons from Denmark." *Antiquity* 61:267-268.

Rogers, J., and T. Waldron. 2001. "DISH and the Monastic Way of Life." *International Journal of Osteoarchaeology* 11:357-365.

Rude, R. K., F. R. Singer, and H. E. Gruber. 2009. "Skeletal and Hormonal Effects of Magnesium Deficenci." *Journal of the American College of Nutrition* 28:131-141.

Ruttkay, E. 1970. "Das jungsteizeitliche Hornsteinbergwerk mit Bestattungen von der Antonshöhe bei Mauer (Wien 23)." *Mitteilungen der Anthropologischen Gesellschaft in Wien* 100:70-83.

Ruttkay, E. 1985. *Das Neolithikum in Niederösterreich.* Wien: Österreichische Arbeitsgemeinschaft für Ur- und Frühgeschichte.

Ruttkay, E., and M. Teschler-Nicola. 1985. "Zwei Lengyel-Gräber aus Niederöstereich." *Annalen des Naturhistorischen Museums in Wien* 87A:211-235.

Sadler, T. W. 2011. *Langmanova lékařská embryologie.* 10th ed. Prague: Grada.

Sadler, T. W. 2015. *Langman's Medical Embryology.* 13th ed. Philadelphia: Wolters Kluwer.

Salisbury, R. B. 2016. *Soilscapes in Archaeology. Settlement and Social Organization in the Neolithic of the Great Hungarian Plain.* Budapest: Archaeolingua.

Saluja, G., K. Fitzpatrick, M. Bruce, and J. Cross. 1986. "Schmorl's Nodes (Intravertebral Herniations of Intervertebral Disc Tissue) in Two Historic British Populations." *Journal of Anatomy* 145:87-96.

Sansone, V., D. Pagani, and M. Melato. 2013. "The Effects on Bone Cells of Metal Ions Released from Orthopedic Implants. A Review." *Clinical Cases in Mineral and Bone Metabolism* 10: 34-40.

Šantrůček, J., H. Šantrůčková, et al. 2018. *Stabilní izotopy biogenních prvků. Použití v biologii a ekologii.* Prague: Academia.

Sarastre, H. 1993. "Spondylolysis and spondylolisthesis." *Acta Orthopeadica Scandinavica* 251:84-96.

Schaefer, M., S. Black, and L. Scheuer. 2009. *Juvenile Osteology. A Laboratory and Field Manual.* Burlington: Elsevier.

Scheeres, M., C. Knipper, M. Hauschild, et al. 2014. "'Celtic Migrations': Fact or Fiction? Strontium and Oxygen Isotope Analysis of the Czech Cemeteries of Radovesice and Kutná Hora in Bohemia." *American Journal of Physical Anthropology* 155:496-512.

Schenk, Z., M. Kuča, M. Hložek, et al. 2007. "Pohřeb kultury s moravskou malovanou keramikou z polohy "Dolní újezd" na katastru Dluhonice, okr. Přerov." *Ročenka Archeologického centra Olomouc 2006*:38-56.

Schenk, Z., M. Kuča, P. Škrdla, and A. Roszková. 2008. "Spytihněv (okr. Zlín)." *Přehled výzkumů* 49:285-90.

Scheuer, L., and S. Black. 2004. *The Juvenile Skeleton.* London: Elsevier.

Schinz, H., W. Baensch, E. Uehlinger, and E. Friedl. 1952. "Ossifikationstabelle." In *Lehrbuch der Röntgen-Diagnostik.* 5th ed. Stuttgart: G. Thieme.

Schour, J., and M. Massler. 1941. "The Development of the Human Dentition." *Journal of American Dental Association* 28:1153-60.

Schranz, D., and G. Huszár, G. 1962. "Caries Findings on Prehistoric Human Dentitions from Hungary." *Zeitschrift für Morphologie und Anthropologie* 52:141-54.

Schrier, W. 2015. "Central and Eastern Europe." In *The Oxford Handbook of Neolithic Europe,* edited by C. Fowler, J. Harding, and D. Hofmann, 99-120. Oxford: Oxford University Press.

Schulting, R. J., and L. Fibiger, eds. 2012. *Sticks, Stones, and Broken Bones: Neolithic Violence in a European Perspective.* Oxford: Oxford University Press.

Schwartz, J. H. 1995. *Skeleton Keys: An Introduction to Human Skeletal Morphology, Development, and Analysis.* Oxford: Oxford Unversity Press.

Shboul, M., P. Roschger, R. Ganger, et al. 2018. "Bone Matrix Hypermineralisation Associated with Low Bone Turnover in a Case of Nasu-Hakola Disease." *Bone* 10:8-21.

Sherratt, A. "The Development of Neolithic and Copper Age Settlement in the Great Hungarian Plain. Part I: The Regional Setting." *Oxford Journal of Archaeology* 1:287-316.

Šimek, E. 1935. "Problémy moravské prehistorie." *Časopis Matice moravské* 59:1-66.

Simon, H. K. 2003. "A dunántúli neolitikum a kezdetektől a Lengyel-kultúra kialakulásáig." In *Magyar régészet az ezredfordulón,* edited by Z. Visy, 102. Budapest: NKÖM.

Simon, M. J., F. T. Beil, W. Rüther, et al. 2015. "High Fluoride and Low Calcium Levels in Drinking Water is Associated with Low Bone Mass, Reduced Bone Quality and Fragility Fractures in Sheep." *Osteoporosis International* 25:1891-93.

Sjøvold, T. 1990. "Estimation of Stature from Long Bones Utilizing the Line of Organic Correlation." *Human Evolution* 5:431-47.

Skeates, R. 1991. "Caves, Cult and Children in Neolithic Abruzzo, Central Italy." In *Sacred and Profane. Proceedings of a Conference on Archaeology, Ritual and Religion*, edited by P. Garwood et al., 122-34. Oxford: Oxford University Committee for Archaeology.

Sklenář, K. 2005. *Biografický slovník českých, moravských a slezských archeologů*. Prague: Libri.

Sklenář, K. 2013. "O rodu a rodině Jaroslava Palliardiho." *Studia Archaeologica Brunensia* 18: 79-83.

Smart, G. W., J. E. Taunton, and D. B. Clement. 1980. "Achilles Tendon Disorders in Runners." *Medicine and Scence in Sports and Exercise* 12:231-43.

Šmíd, M. 2012. *Kostrové a žárové pohřebiště kultury s lineární keramikou v Kralicích na Hané, střední Morava*. Brno: Ústav archeologické památkové péče Brno.

Smrčka, V. 2005. *Trace Elements in Bone Tissue*. Prague: Karolinum.

Smrčka, V., T. Berkovec, and V. Erban. 2019. "Children as Plants. Analyses of Skeletal Remains of Suspected Children Sacrifices of a Neolithic Settlement in Vedrovice, Czech Republic." *Anthropologie* 57:79-86.

Smrčka, V., F. Bůzek, V. Erban, et al. 2005. "Carbon, Nitrogen and Strontium Isotopes in the Set of Skeletons from the Neolithic Settlement at Vedrovice (Czech Republic)." *Anthropologie* 43:315-23.

Smrčka V., F. Bůzek, V. Erban, K. Neumannová, M. Dočkalová, and T. Berkovec. 2004. "Stabilní izotopy v kosterním souboru z neolitického sídliště ve Vedrovicích" In *Ve službách archeologie*. Vol. 5, *Sborník k sedmdesátinám RNDr. Emanuela Opravila, CSc.*, edited by V. Hašek, R. Nekuda, and M. Ruttkay, 274-276. Brno: Muzejní a vlastivědná společnost v Brně.

Smrčka, V., F. Bůzek, and J. Zocová. 2008. "C and N stable Isotopes in a Set of 17 Skeletons from the Vedrovice Cemetery." *Anthropologie* 46:227-31.

Smrčka, V., M. Dočkalová, F. Bůzek, V. Erban, M. Mihaljevič, and J. Zocová. 2008. "Rekonstrukce stravy a migrace populace z neolitických sídlišť na Moravě—na modelu Těšetic-Kyjovic / Reconstruction of Diet and Mobility in the Neolithic Settlements of Moravia—on the Model of Těšetice-Kyjovice." *Service to Archaeology* 2:219-230.

Smrčka, V., and I. Dylevský. 1999. *Flexory ruky*. Brno: Institut pro další vzdělávání pracovníků ve zdravotnictví.

Smrčka, V., V. Kuželka, and J. Melková. 2003. "Meningioma Probable Reason for Trephination." *International Journal of Osteoarchaeology* 13:325-30.

Smrčka, V., V. Kuželka, Z. Musilová, O. Gábor. 2018. "Bone Diseases at the Lengyel Culture Burial Site in Zengővárkony, Hungary." *Anthropologie* 56:53-62.

Smrčka, V., V. Kuželka, and C. Povýšil. 2009. *Atlas of Diseases in Dry Bones*. Prague: Academia.

Smrčka V., M. Mihaljevič, J. Zocová, A. Humpolová, and T. Berkovec. 2006. "Multielementární chemická analýza z kosterních pozůstatků lidí a zvířat neolitického sídliště ve Vedrovicích (Česká republika)." In *Ve službách archeologie*. Vol. 7, *Sborník věnovaný 85. narozeninám doc. PhDr. Karla Valocha, DrSc.*, edited by V. Hašek, R. Nekuda, and M. Ruttkay, 329-341. Brno: Muzejní a vlastivědná společnost v Brně.

Smrčka, V., and Z. Tvrdý. 2009. "Skeletal Evidence for Diseases in the Neolithic of Moravia." *Anthropologie* 47:295-303.

Sofaer Derevenski, J., ed. 2000. *Children and Material Culture*. London: Routledge.

Sofaer Derevenski, J. 2002. "Rings of Life: The Role of Early Metalworking in Mediating the Gendered Life Course." *World Archaeology* 31:389-406.

Spatz, H. 1998. "Krisen, Gewalt, Tod—zum Ende der ersten Ackerbauernkultur Mitteleuropas." In *Krieg oder Frieden? Herxheim vor 7000 Jahren. Katalog zur Sonderausstellung*, 10-19. Herxheim: Speyer-Landesamt für Denkmalpflege.

Spekker, O., G. Pálfi, G. Kozocsay, A. Pósa, Z. Bereczki, and E. Molnar. 2012. "New Cases of Probable Skeletal Tuberculosis from the Neolithic Period in Hungary—A Morphological Study." *Acta Biologica Szegediensis* 56:115-23.

Stabrava, P. 2008. "Opava (k. ú. Kylešovice, okr. Opava)." *Přehled výzkumů* 49:281-82.

Stabrava, P., and P. Kováčik. 2009. "Opava (k. ú. Kylešovice, okr. Opava)." *Přehled výzkumů* 50:255.

Stafford, T. W. Jr, K. Brendel, and R. C. Duhamel. 1988. "Radiocarbon, 13C and 15N Analysis of Fossil Bone: Removal of Humates with XAD-2 Resin." *Geochimica et Cosmochimica Acta* 52:2257-67.

Steinbock, R. T. 1976. *Paleopathological Diagnosis and Interpretation.* Springfield, IL: Charles C Thomas.

Stloukal, M., and H. Hanáková. 1978. "Die Länge der Längsknocken altslawischer Bevölkerungen unter besonderer Berücksichtigung von Wachstumsfragen." *Homo* 29:53-69.

Stloukal, M., and L. Vyhnánek. 1976. *Slované z velkomoravských Mikulčic.* Prague: Academia.

Strouhal, E. 1987. "La tuberculose vertébrale en Égypte et Nubie anciennes." *Bulletins et mémories de la Société d'Anthropologie de Paris* 14:261-71.

Strouhal, E. 1991. "Myeloma Multiplex versus Carcinomatous Metastases: Differential Diagnosis on Dry Bone." *International Journal of Osteoarchaeology* 1:219-24.

Strouhal, E., and J. Jungwirth. 1970. "Die menschlichen Skelette aus dem neolithischen Hornsteinbergwerk von Mauer bei Wien." *Mitteilungen der Anthropologischen Gesellschaft in Wien* 100:85-110.

Strouhal, E., and H. Kritscher. 1990. "Neolithic Case of a Multiplex Myeloma from Mauer (Vienna, Austria)." *Anthropologie* 28:79-87.

Strouhal, E., and A. Němečková. 2008. *Trpěli i dávní lidé nádory? Historie a palopatologie nádorů, zhláště zhoubných.* Prague: Karolinum.

Stuchlík, S. 1997. "Borotice (okr. Znojmo)." In *Přehled výzkumů 1993-1994,* 115. Brno: Archeologický ústav ČSAV.

Stuchlík, S. 2004. "Pes v neolitu." In *Otázky neolitu a eneolitu našich zemí,* edited by V. Janák and S. Stuchlík, 213-226. Opava: Ústav historie a muzeologie FPF Slezské univerzity v Opavě.

Swanson, A. B. 1976. "A Classification for Congenital Limb Malformations." *Journal of Hand Surgery* 1:8-22.

Szeverényi, V. 2013. "Pécs története a késő bronzkorig." In *Pécs története.* Vol. 1, *Az őskortól a püspökség alapításáig,* edited by J. Vonyó and Z. Visy, 37-68. Pécs: Pécs Története Alapítvány—Kronosz Kiadó.

Szilvássy, J. 1980. "Age Determination on the Sternal Articular Face of the Clavicula." *Journal of Human Evolution* 9:609-10.

Tauber, H. 1981. "13C Evidence for Dietary Habits of Prehistoric Man in Denmark." *Nature* 292:332-33.

Tihelka, K. 1956. "Sídliště lidu s moravskou malovanou keramikou na Cezavách u Blučiny." *Archeologické rozhledy* 8:773-74.

Točík, A. 1991. "Erforschungstand der Lengyel-Kultur in der Slowakei. Rückblick und Ausblick." In *Die Kupferzeit als historische Epoche,* edited by J. Lichardus, 301-17. Bonn: Habelt.

Todd, T. W. 1920. "Age Changes in the Pubis Bone I: The Male White Pubis." *American Journal of Physical Anthropology* 3:285-334.

Tóth, E. Á. 2006. "Derékfájdalommal járó gerincbetegségek." *LAM-tudomány* 16:453-59.

Tsutaya, T., T. Gakuhari, A. Asahara, et M. Yoneda. 2017. "Isotopic Comparison of Gelatin Extracted from Bone Powder with that from Bone Chunk and Development of a Framework for Comparison of Different Extraction Methods." *Journal of Archaeological Science*: Reports 11:99-105.

Turner, C. H., I. Owan, E. J. Brizendine, W. Zhang, M. E. Wilson, and A. J. Dunipace. 1996. "High Fluoride Intakes Causes Osteomalacia and Diminished Bone Strengh in Rats Renal Deficiency." *Bone* 19:595-601.

Tvrdý, Z. 2010. "Antropologický posudek kosterních nálezů z mladolengyelské těžní šachty v Krumlovském lese." In M. Oliva, *Pravěké hornictví v Krumlovském lese. Vznik a vývoj industriálně-sakrální krajiny na jižní Moravě,* 402-8. Brno: Moravské zemské muzeum.

Tvrdý, Z. 2016a. "Anthropology of the Neolithic Population from Nitra-Horné Krškany (Slovakia)." *Anthropologie* 54:231-84.

Tvrdý, Z. 2016b. "Lidské kosti s antropogenními zásahy z jeskyně Jestřábí skála v Moravském krasu." *Acta Musei Moraviae — Scientiae sociales* 101:3-13.

Ubelaker, D. H. 1978. *Human Skeletal Remains. Excavation, Analysis, Interpretation.* Chicago: Aldine.

Ubelaker, D. H. 1989. *Human Skeletal Remains. Excavation, Analysis, Interpretation.* Washington: Taraxacum.

Ubelaker, D. H., I. Pap, and S. Graver. 2006. "Morbidity and mortality in the Neolithic of Northeastern Hungary." *Anthropologie* 44:241-57.

USEPA 2007. "Toxicity and Exposure Assesment for Children's Health." Manganese TEACH Chemical Summary.

Uthus, E. O., and F. H. Nielsen. 1993. "Determination of the Possible Requirement and Reference Dose Levels for Arsenic in Humans." *Scandinavian Journal of Work, Environment and Health* 19 (Suppl. 1): 243-249.

Válek, D., J. Bíšková, and M. Kuča. 2016. "Výplň rondelového příkopu v Těšeticích-Kyjovicích na základě artefaktů a malakofauny z půdních vzorků." *Acta Musei Moraviae — Scientiae sociales* 101:137-55.

Válek, D., E. Kazdová, and J. J. Kovář. 2013a. "Cíle a průběh revizního výzkumu příkopu neolitického rondelu v Těšeticích-Kyjovicích." *Studia Archaeologica Brunensia* 18:159-69.

Válek, D., L. Lisá, N. Doláková, H. Uhlířová, and A. Bajer. 2013b. "Nové poznatky o genezi sedimentů a artefaktuální výpovědi výplně rondelového příkopu v Těšeticích-Kyjovicích (okr. Znojmo)." *Acta Musei Moraviae — Scientiae sociales* 98:215-38.

Valoch, K. 1997. "Jaroslav Mikulášek." *Acta Musei Moraviae — Scientiae Sociales* 82:283-84.

Vaškových, M. 2006. "Vývoj osídlení středního a severní části dolního Pomoraví v neolitu a na počátku eneolitu." Ph.D. diss. Brno.

Vaškových, M. 2010. "Bánov (okr. Uherské Hradiště)." *Přehled výzkumů* 51:305.

Vencl, S. 1985. "Žaludy jako potravina; k poznání významu sběru pro výživu v pravěku." *Archeologické rozhledy* 37:516-65.

Vencl, S. 1999. "Stone Age Warfare." In *Ancient Warfare: Archaeological Perspectives*, edited by J. Carman and A. Harding, 57-72. Stroud, UK: Sutton.

Verhagen, P., S. A. Crabtree, H. Peeters, and D. Raemaekers. 2021. "Reconstructing Human-Centered Interaction Networks of the Swifterbant Culture in the Dutch Wetlands: An Example from the ArchaeoEcology Project. *Applied Sciences*, https://doi.org/10.3390/app11114860.

Videiko, M. 2003. *Tripillia Culture.* 2nd ed. Kiev: Akademperiodika.

Vigorita, V. J. 1999. *Orthopaedic Pathology.* Philadelphia: Lippincott Williams and Wilkins.

Vildomec, F. 1928/1929. "O moravské neolithické keramice malované." *Obzor praehistorický* 7-8:1-43.

Vildomec, F. 1949. "O mých nálezech neolitických sošek." *Z dávných věků* 2:6-26.

Virág, Z. M. 2003. "Korai fémművesség a Kárpát-medencében." In *Magyar régészet az ezredfordulón*, edited by Z. Visy, 129-30. Budapest: Teleki László Alapítvány.

Visy, Z. 2003. *Magyar régészet az ezredfordulón.* Budapest: NKÖM.

Vladár, J. 1969. "Frühäneolitische Siedlung und Gräberfeld in Branč." *Štúdijné zvesti AÚ SAV* 17:497-512.

Vladár, J., and J. Lichardus. 1968. "Erforschung der frühäneolithischen Siedlungen in Branč." *Slovenská archeológia* 16:263-352.

Voerkelius, S., G. D. Lorenz, S. Rummel, et al. 2010. "Strontium Isotopic Signatures of Natural Mineral Waters, the Reference to a Simple Geological Map and Its Potential for Authentication of Food." *Food Chemistry* 118:933-40.

Vogel, M., M. Hahn, and G. Delling. 1995. "Trabecular Bone Structure in Patients with Primary Hyperparathyroidism." *Virchows Archiv* 426:127-34.

Vokolek, V., and M. Zápotocká. 1997. "Neolithische Gräber und Gräberfelder in Plotiště n. Labem und Předměřice n. Labem, Bezirk Hradec Králové." *Památky archeologické* 88:5-55.

Vyhnánek, L. 1976. "Kostní variety a patologické změny." In *Slované z velkomoravských Mikulčic*, edited by M. Stloukal and L. Vyhnánek, 91-165, Prague: Academia.

Wahl, J., and I. Trautmann. 2012. "The Neolithic Massacre at Talheim: A Pivotal Find in Conflict Archaeology." In *Sticks, Stones and Broken Bones: Neolithic Violence in a European Perspective*, edited by R. J. Schulting and L. Fibiger, 77–100. Oxford: Oxford University Press.

Währen, M. 1984. "Brote und Getreidebreinvon Twann aus dem 4. Jahrtausend vor Christus." *Archäologie der Schwediz* 7:2–6.

Walker, P., R. R. Bathurst, R. Richman, T. Gjerdrum, and V. A. Andrushko. 2009. "The Causes of Porotic Hyperostosis and cribra orbitalia: A Reappraisal of the Iron-Deficiency-Anemia Hypothesis." *American Journal of Physical Anthropology* 139:109–25.

Wankel, J. 1873. "Eine Opferstätte bei Raigern in Mähren." *Mittheilungen der Anthropologischen Gesellschaft in Wien* 3:75–94.

Wapler, U., E. Crubézy, and M. Schultz. 2004. "Is cribra orbitalia Synonymous with anemia? Analysis and Interpretation of Cranial Pathology in Sudan." *American Journal of Physical Anthropology* 123:333–39.

Warman, M. L., V. Cormier-Daire, C. Hall, et al. 2011. "Nosology and Classification of Genetic Skeletal Disorders—2010. Revision." *American Journal of Medical Genetics* 155A:943–68.

Watts, J., O. Sheehan, Q. D. Atkinson, J. Bulbulia, and R. D. Gray. 2016. "Ritual Sacrifice Promoted and Sustained the Evolution of Stratified Societies." *Nature* 532:228–31.

Weinreb, F. 1995. *Symbolika biblického jazyka*. Prague: Herrmann a synové.

Welcker, H. 1888. "Cribra Orbitalia, ein etiologisch. Diagnostisches Merkmal am Schädel Mehrerer Menschenrassen." *Archiv für Anthropologie* (Braunsweig) 17:1–18.

Whitehouse, H., P. François, P. E. Savage, et al. 2019. "Complex Societies Precede Moralizing Gods throughout World History." *Nature* 568:226–29.

Whittle, A. 1966. *Europe in the Neolithic. The Creation of New Worlds*. Cambridge: Cambridge University Press.

Whittle, A., R. A. Bentley, P. Bickle, et al. 2013. "Moravia and Western Slovakia." In *The First Farmers of Central Europe: Diversity in LBK Lifeways*, edited by P. Bickle and A. Whittle, 101–58. Oxford: Oxbow Books.

Windl, H. 2001. "Erdwerke der Linearbandkeramik in Asparn an der Zaya/Schletz, Niederösterreich." *Preistoria Alpina* 37:137–44.

Wolff, K., Z. Bernert, T. Balassa, T. Szeniczey, C. K. Kiss, and T. Hajdu. 2014. "Two Suture Craniosynostoses: A Presentation that Needs to be Noted." *Journal of Craniofacial Surgery* 25:714–15.

Wosinsky, M., 1885. "Funde von der urzeitlichen Siedlung von Lengyel." *Archaeologiai Közlemének* 14:1–89.

Wright, L. E. 1997. "Intertooth Patterns of Hypoplasia Expression: Implications for Childhood Health in the Classic Maya Collapse." *American Journal of Physical Anthropology* 102:233–47.

Zalai-Gaál, I. 1982. "A lengyeli kultúra a Dél-Dunántúlon (Die Lengyel-Kultur in Südtransdanubien)." *A Szekszárdi Béri Balogh Ádám Múzeum Évkönyve* 10–11:3–58.

Zalai-Gaál, I. 1984. "Mórágy—Tüzkődomb: Entwurf sozialarchäologischer Forschungen." In *Internationales Symposium über die Lengyel-Kultur*, 333–38. Nitra and Vienna.

Zalai-Gaál, I. 1988. "Közép-európai neolitikus temetők szociálarchaeológiai elemzése (Sozialarchäologische Untersuchungen des mitteleuropäischen Neolithikums aufgrund der Gräberfeldanalyse)." *A Szekszárdi Béri Balogh Ádám Múzeum Évkönyve* 14:3–178.

Zalai-Gaál, I. 1990a. "Neue Daten zur Erforsung der spätneolithischen Schanzweke in sündlichen Transdanubien (Újabb adatok a késöneolitikus körsáncok kutatásához a Déldunántúlon)." *Zalai Múzeum* 2:31–46.

Zalai-Gaál, I. 1990b. "A neolitikus körárokrendszrek kutatása a Dél-Dunántúlon." *Archaelogiai Értesítö* 117:3–24.

Zalai-Gaál, I. 1994. "Betrachtungen über die kultische Bedeutung des Hundes im mitteleuropäischen Neolithikum." *Acta Archaeologica Academiae Scientiarum Hungaricae* 46:33–57.

Zalai-Gaál, I. 2001. "Die Gräbergruppe B2 von Mórágy-Tűzkődomb und der ältere Abschnitt der Lengyel-Kultur." *Acta Archaeologica Academiae Scientiarum Hungaricae* 52:5–48.

Zalai-Gaál, I. 2002. *Die neolithische Gräbergruppe-B1 von Mórágy-Tűzkődomb*. Szekszárd: Wosinsky Mór Múzeum.

Zalai-Gaál, I. 2003. "Das Henkelgefäß aus Györe. Ein Beitrag zu den chronologischen und kulturellen Beziehungen der Lengyel-Kultur." In *Morgenrot der Kulturen. Frühe Etappen der Menschheitsgeschichte in Mittel- und Südosteuropa. Festschrift für Nándor Kalicz zum 75. Geburtstag*, edited by E. Jerem and P. Raczky, 285-309. Budapest: Archaeolingua.

Zalai-Gaál, I. 2010. *Die soziale Differenzierung im Spätneolithikum Südtransdanubiens: die Funde und Befunde aus den Altgrabungen der Lengyel-Kultur*. Budapest: Archaeolingua.

Zalai-Gaál, I., E. Gál, K. Köhler, A. Osztás, and K. Szilágyi. 2012. "Präliminarien zur Sozialarchäologie des lengyelzeitlichen Gräberfeldes von Alsónyék-Bátaszék, Südtransdanubien." *Praehistorische Zeitschrift* 87:58-82.

Zalai-Gaál, I., and A. Osztás. 2009. "Neue Aspekte zur Erforschung des Neolithikums in Ungarn. Ein Fragenkatalog zu Siedlung und Gräberfeld der Lengyel-Kultur von Alsónyék, Südtransdanubien." In: *Zeiten—Kulturen—Systeme. Gedenkschrift für Jan Lichardus*, edited by V. Becker, M. Thomas, and A. Wolf-Schuler, 111-39. Langenweißbach: Beier & Beran.

Zápotocká, M. 1981. "Bi-ritual Cemetery of the Stroked-Pottery Culture at Miskovice, Distr. of Kutná Hora." In *Nouvelles archéologiques dans La République socialiste tchèque. Xe Congrès international des Sciences préhistoriques et protohistoriques Mexico 1981*, edited by J. Hrala, 26-31. Prague: ČSAV.

Zápotocká, M. 2009. "Der Übergang von der Linear- zur Stichbandkeramik in Böhmen." In *Krisen—Kulturwandel—Kontinuitäten. Zum Ende der Bandkeramik in Mitteleuropa. Beiträge der Internationalen Tagung in Herxheim bei Landau (Pfalz) vom 14.-17. 06. 2007*, edited by A. Zeeb-Lanz, 303-315. Rahden, Westfalen: Marie Leidorf.

Zeeb-Lanz, A. 2009. "Gewaltszenarien oder Sinnkrise? Die Grubenanlage von Herxheim der und das Ende der Bandkeramik." In *Krisen- Kulturwandel-Kontinuitäten. Zum Ende der Bandkeramik in Mitteleuropa. Beträge der Internationalen Tagung in Herxheim bei Landau(Pfalz) vom 14.-17. 6. 2007*, edited by A. Zeeb-Lanz, 87-101. Rahden, Westfalen: Marie Leidorf.

Zeman, T. 2013. "Mohelnice (okr. Šumperk)." *Přehled výzkumů* 54:147-48.

Zias, J. 1998. "Tuberculosis and the Jew in the ancient Near East: the biocultural interaction." In *Digging for Pathogen Ancient Emerging Diseases—Their Evolutionary Anthropological and Archaeological Context*, edited by C. L. Greebnlatt, 277-297. Rehovot: Balaban Publisher.

Zoffmann, Z. 1965. "Data to the Burial Rites of the Lengyel Culture." *A Janus Pannonius Muzeum Evkonyve* 10:55-58.

Zoffmann, Z. 1968. "An Anthropological Study of the Neolithic Cemetery at Villánykővesd (Lengyel culture), Hungary." *A Janus Pannonius Múzeum Évkönyve* 13:25-38.

Zoffmann, Z. 1969-70. "Anthropological Analysis of the Cemetery at Zengővárkony and the Neolithic Lengyel Culture in SW Hungary." *A Jannus Pannonius Múzeum Évkönyve* 14-15:53-73.

Zoffmann, Z. 2004. "A Lengyeli kultúra Mórágy B. 1. temetkezési csoportjának embertani ismertetése." *A Wosinszky Mór Megyei Múzeum Évkönyve* 26:137-79.

Zoffmann, Z. 2007. "Anthropological Material from a Neolithic Common Grave Found at Esztergályhorváti (Lengyel Culture, Hungary)." *Folia Anthropologica* 6:53-60.

Zoffmann, Z. 2011. "Kárpát-medence területéről származó neolitikus, réz-, bronz-, és vaskori antropológiai sorozatok halandósági táblái (Adatközlés)." *Folia Anthropologica* 10:17-57.

Zoffmann, Z. 2015-16. "Anthropologic Remains from Feature 2 at the Site Borjád-Kenderföldek." In *Communicationes Archaeologicae Hungariae*, 70. Budapest. Magyar Nemzeti Múzeum.

Zoffmann, Z., and T. Hadu. 2013. "Anthropological Bibliography of the Prehistoric Periods of the Carpathian Basin." *Annales Historico-Naturales Musei Nationalis Hungarici* 105:321-56.

Zuscik, M., L. Ma, T. Buckley, J. E. Punzas, H. Drissi, E. M. Schwarz, and R. J. O'Keefe. 2007. "Lead Induces Chondrogenesis and Alters Transforming Growth Factor-Beta and Bone Morphogenetic Protein Signaling in Mesenchymal Cell Populations." *Environmental Health Perspectives* 115:1276-82.

Полосъмак, Н. В. 2001: Всадники Укока. Новосибирск.

LIST OF CONTRIBUTORS

František Bůzek
Czech Geological Survey
Geologická 6
15200 Prague 5
Czech Republic

Alžběta Čerevková
Moravian Museum
Archaeological Institute
Zelný trh 6
65937 Brno
Czech Republic

Eva Čermáková
Palacký university
Department of Sociology, Andragogy
and Cultural Anthropology
třída Svobody 8
77900 Olomouc
Czech Republic

David Dick
Charles University
First Faculty of Medicine
U nemocnice 4
12108 Prague 2
Czech Republic

Marta Dočkalová
Moravian Museum
Anthropos Institute
Zelný trh 6
65937 Brno
Czech Republic

Vojtěch Erban
Czech Geological Survey
Geologická 6
15200 Prague 5
Czech Republic

Martina Fojtová
Moravian Museum
Anthropos Institute
Zelný trh 6
65937 Brno
Czech Republic

Olivér Gábor
Janus Pannonius Muzeum
Káptalan u. 5.
7621 Pécs
Hungary

Csila Gáti
Janus Pannonius Muzeum
Káptalan u. 5.
7621 Pécs
Hungary

Zdeněk Hájek
Moravian Museum
Archaeological Institute
Zelný trh 6
65937 Brno
Czech Republic

Martin Hill
Charles University
First Faculty od Medicine
Národní třída 139/8
116 94 Prague 1
Czech Republic

Ivana Jarošová
Freelancer in Anthropology
Czech Republic

Sylva Kaupová
National Museum
Anthropological Department
Cirkusová 1740
19300 Prague-Horní Počernice
Czech Republic

Kitti Köhler
Hungarian Academy of Sciences
Research Centre for the Humanities
Tóth Kálmán u. 4
1097 Budapest
Hungary

Vítězslav Kuželka
National Museum
Anthropological Department
Cirkusová 1740
19300 Prague-Horní Počernice
Czech Republic

Martin Mihaljevič
Charles University
Faculty of Science
Albertov 6
12843 Prague 2
Czech Republic

Zdenka Musilová
Municipality of the Town Letovice
Masarykovo náměstí 19
67961 Letovice
Czech Republic

Ivo Němec
Military University Hospital Prague
U vojenské nemocnice 1200
16902 Prague 6
Czech Republic

Lenka Půtová
Charles University
First Faculty of Medicine
U nemocnice 4
12108 Prague 2
Czech Republic

Štefan Rástočný
Charles University
First Faculty of Medicine
U nemocnice 4
12108 Prague 2
Czech Republic

Václav Smrčka
Charles University
First Faculty of Medicine
U nemocnice 4
12108 Prague 2
Czech Republic

Jakub Trubač
Charles University
Faculty of Science
Albertov 6
12843 Prague 2
Czech Republic

Zdeněk Tvrdý
Moravian Museum
Anthropos Institute
Zelný trh 6
65937 Brno
Czech Republic

Ivan Zoc
Charles University
Faculty of Science
Albertov 6
12843 Prague 2
Czech Republic

Jarmila Zocová
Charles University
Faculty of Science
Albertov 6
12843 Prague 2
Czech Republic